T0213694

# Lecture Notes in Artificial Intelligence 9919

Subseries of Lecture Notes in Computer Science

More information about this series at http://www.springer.com/series/1244

Giorgio A. Ascoli · Michael Hawrylycz
Hesham Ali · Deepak Khazanchi
Yong Shi (Eds.)

# Brain Informatics and Health

International Conference, BIH 2016
Omaha, NE, USA, October 13–16, 2016
Proceedings

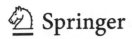 Springer

*Editors*

Giorgio A. Ascoli
George Mason University
Fairfax, VA
USA

Michael Hawrylycz
Department of Modeling,
  Analysis and Theory
Allen Institute for Brain Science
Seattle, WA
USA

Hesham Ali
University of Nebraska Omaha
Omaha, NE
USA

Deepak Khazanchi
Information Science and Technology
University of Nebraska Omaha
Omaha, NE
USA

Yong Shi
College of Information Sciences and
  Technology
University of Nebraska Omaha
Omaha, NE
USA

ISSN 0302-9743                ISSN 1611-3349   (electronic)
Lecture Notes in Artificial Intelligence
ISBN 978-3-319-47102-0        ISBN 978-3-319-47103-7   (eBook)
DOI 10.1007/978-3-319-47103-7

Library of Congress Control Number: 2016952873

LNCS Sublibrary: SL7 – Artificial Intelligence

Printed on acid-free paper

This Springer imprint is published by Springer Nature
The registered company is Springer International Publishing AG
The registered company address is: Gewerbestrasse 11, 6330 Cham, Switzerland

# Preface

This volume contains papers selected for presentation in the technical and invited special sessions of the 2016 International Conference on Brain Informatics and Health (BIH 2016), which was held at Hilton Omaha, Nebraska, USA, during October 13–16, 2016. The conference was co-organized by the University of Nebraska at Omaha College of Information Science and Technology, the Web Intelligence Consortium (WIC), and IEEE Computational Intelligence Society Task Force on Brain Informatics (IEEE-CIS TF-BI), and jointly held with The IEEE/WIC/ACM International Conference on Web Intelligence 2016 (WI 2016).

Brain research is rapidly advancing with the application of big data technology to neuroscience, as reflected in major international initiatives throughout the world. The paradigm of brain informatics (BI) is becoming mainstream and crosses the disciplines of neuroscience, cognitive science, computer science, signal processing, and neuroimaging technologies as well as data science. BI investigates essential functions of the brain, in a wide range of areas from perception to thinking, and encompassing areas such as multi-perception, attention, memory, language, computation, heuristic search, reasoning, planning, decision-making, problem-solving, learning, discovery, and creativity. The current goal of BI is to develop and demonstrate a systematic approach to achieving an integrated understanding of working principles of the brain from macroscopic to microscopic levels, by means of experimental, computational, and cognitive neuroscience studies, not least utilizing advanced Web intelligence-centric information technologies.

The series of BI Conferences had started with the First WICI International Workshop on Web Intelligence Meets Brain Informatics (WImBI 2006), held in Beijing, China, in 2006. The Second, the Third, and the 4th Conference on Brain Informatics (BI 2009, BI 2010, and BI 2011) were jointly held with the International Conferences on Active Media Technology (AMT 2009, AMT 2010, and AMT 2011), in Beijing, China; Toronto, Canada; and Lanzhou, China, respectively. The 5th Conference on Brain Informatics was held jointly with other international conferences (AMT 2012, WI 2012, IAT 2012, and ISMIS 2012) in Macau, China, in 2012. The 2013 International Conference on Brain and Health Informatics was held in Maebashi-City, Japan, and it was the first conference specifically dedicated to interdisciplinary research in brain and health informatics. The BIH 2014 and 2015 conferences were held in Warsaw, Poland, and London, UK, respectively. Following the success of past conferences in this series, BIH 2016 placed a strong emphasis on emerging trends of big data analysis and management technology for brain research, behavior learning, and real-world applications of brain science in human health and wellbeing, especially highlighting the theme "Connecting Network and Brain with Big Data."

BIH 2016 aimed to give a common thesis of Informatics for Human Brain, Behavior, and Health. The conference gathered researchers at the cutting edge of BI, bringing together investigators and practitioners from neuroscience, cognitive science, computer science, data science, and neuroimaging technologies with the purpose of exploring the fundamental roles, interactions, and practical impact of BI. This year, the BIH 2016 conference was especially dedicated to the celebration of the 60th anniversary of artificial intelligence (AI). While neuroscientists are making breakthrough progress in understanding brain function, AI researchers also have been striving to formalize the organization and function of the human brain, aiming at creating computer hardware and software with a capacity for intelligent behavior. The integration of technological advancements with fundamental academic research yielded a plethora of brain-inspired achievements. By leveraging AI, BI has produced new products, services, and frameworks empowered by the World Wide Web. Neuromorphic computer architectures, chips that mimic brain dynamics, show promise in the quest to extract context and meaning from big data through both analytical and heuristic means. There has never been a more exciting moment than now, in neuroscience, cognitive science, computer science, and AI.

BIH 2016 involved an inspiring cadre of world leaders in brain research, including keynote speakers Stephen Smith, Senior Investigator of the Allen Institute for Brain Science, and Ivan Soltesz, James R. Doty Professor of Neurosurgery and Neurosciences, at Stanford School of Medicine; and feature speakers Steven Schiff, Brush Chair Professor of Engineering in the Departments of Neurosurgery, Engineering Science and Mechanics, Physics, and BioE, at Pennsylvania State University; Kristen Harris, Professor of Neuroscience at University of Texas at Austin; Giulio Tononi, Professor of Psychiatry, Distinguished Professor in Consciousness Science, and the David P. White Chair in Sleep Medicine, at University of Wisconsin - Madison; Bob Jacobs, Professor of Psychology, at Colorado College; Partha Mitra, Professor at Cold Spring Harbor Laboratory; and Paola Pergami, Associate Professor in Pediatric Neurology, at George Washington University. BIH 2016 also included a panel discussion among the leaders of brain researchers in the world.

Here we would like to express our gratitude to all members of the Conference Committee for their instrumental and unwavering support. BIH 2016 had a very exciting program with a number of features, ranging from keynote talks to technical sessions, workshops/special sessions, and social programs. This would not have been possible without the generous dedication of the Program Committee members in reviewing the papers submitted to BIH 2016, the BIH 2016 workshop and special session chairs and organizers, and our keynote and feature speakers in giving outstanding talks at the conference. BIH 2016 could not have taken place without the great team effort of the local Organizing Committee and generous support from sponsors.

Special thanks go to the Steering Committee co-chairs, Ning Zhong and Hanchuan Peng, for their help in organizing and promoting BIH 2016. We also thank Juzhen Dong and Yang Yang for their assistance with the CyberChair submission system. We are grateful to Springer's *Lecture Notes in Computer Science* (LNCS/LNAI) team for their support. We thank Springer for their help in coordinating the publication of this special volume in an emerging and interdisciplinary research field.

October 2016

Giorgio A. Ascoli
Michael Hawrylycz
Hesham Ali
Deepak Khazanchi
Yong Shi

# Organization

## General Chairs

Hesham Ali — University of Nebraska at Omaha, USA
Deepak Khazanchi — University of Nebraska at Omaha, USA
Yong Shi — University of Nebraska at Omaha, USA
Chinese Academy of Sciences, China

## Program Committee Chairs

Giorgio A. Ascoli — George Mason University, USA
Michael Hawrylycz — Allen Institute for Brain Science, USA

## Workshop/Special Session Chairs

Bingni Wen Brunton — University of Washington, USA
Arvind Ramanathan — Oak Ridge National Laboratory, USA
Yi Zeng — Institute of Automation, Chinese Academy of Sciences, China

## Publicity Chairs

Kate Cooper — University of Nebraska at Omaha, USA
Weidong Cai — University of Sydney, Australia
Henning Müller — University of Applied Sciences and Arts Western Switzerland (HES-SO), Switzerland

## Steering Committee Co-chairs

Ning Zhong — Maebashi Institute of Technology, Japan
Hanchuan Peng — Allen Institute for Brain Science, USA

## WIC Co-chairs/Directors

Ning Zhong — Maebashi Institute of Technology, Japan
Jiming Liu — Hong Kong Baptist University, SAR China

## IEEE-CIS TF-BI Chair

Ning Zhong — Maebashi Institute of Technology, Japan

## Program Committee

| | |
|---|---|
| Samina Abidi | Dalhousie University, Canada |
| Ajith Abraham | Norwegian University of Science and Technology, Norway |
| Anil Anthony Bharath | Imperial College London, UK |
| Luiz Baccala | University of Sao Paulo, Brazil |
| Sanghamitra Bandyopadhyay | Indian Statistical Institute, India |
| Alan J. Barton | Carleton University, Canada |
| Jan G. Bazan | University of Rzeszow, Poland |
| Przemyslaw Biecek | University of Warsaw, Poland |
| Katarzyna Blinowska | University of Warsaw, Poland |
| Piotr Bogorodzki | Warsaw University of Technology, Poland |
| Nizar Bouguila | Concordia University, Canada |
| Zhigang Cao | Chinese Academy of Sciences, China |
| Mirko Cesarini | University of Milano-Bicocca, Italy |
| W. Art Chaovalitwongse | University of Washington, USA |
| Phoebe Chen | La Trobe University, Australia |
| Yiu-ming Cheung | Hong Kong Baptist University, SAR China |
| Jonathan Y. Clark | University of Surrey, UK |
| Frank Emmert-Streib | Tampere University of Technology, Finland |
| Massimo Ferri | University of Bologna, Italy |
| Huiguang He | Chinese Academy of Sciences, China |
| Wilko Heuten | OFFIS Institute for Technology, Germany |
| Daniel Howard | Howard Science Limited, UK |
| D. Frank Hsu | Fordham University, USA |
| Bin Hu | Lanzhou University, China |
| Xiaohua Hu | Drexel University, USA |
| Zhisheng Huang | Vrije University of Amsterdam, The Netherlands |
| Tianzi Jiang | Chinese Academy of Sciences, China |
| Ernesto Jimenez-Ruiz | University of Oxford, UK |
| Colin Johnson | The University of Kent, UK |
| Peter Konig | University of Osnabrück, Germany |
| Renaud Lambiotte | University of Namur, Belgium |
| Yan Li | The University of Southern Queensland, Australia |
| Sidong Liu | University of Sydney, Australia |
| Tony T. Luo | Institute for Infocomm Research, Singapore |
| Marcello Pelillo | University of Venice, Italy |
| Andrzej Przybyszewski | University of Massachusetts Medical School, USA |
| Koichi Sameshima | University of Sao Paulo, Brazil |
| Hideyuki Sawada | Kagawa University, Japan |
| Christina Schweikert | St. John's University, USA |
| Zhongzhi Shi | Chinese Academy of Sciences, China |
| Andrzej Skowron | Warsaw University, Poland |
| Neil Smalheiser | University of Illinois, USA |

# Contents

**Brain Big Data Analytics, Curation and Management**

**New Methodologies for Brain and Mental Health**

**Brain-Inspired Intelligence and Computing**

**Workshop on Brain and Artificial Intelligence (BAI 2016)**

# Cognitive and Computational Foundations of Brain Science

# Robust Neuron Counting Based on Fusion of Shape Map and Multi-cue Learning

Alexander Ekstrom[1], Randall W. Suvanto[1], Tao Yang[2], Bing Ye[2], and Jie Zhou[1(✉)]

[1] Department of Computer Science, Northern Illinois University, DeKalb, IL 60115, USA
{z1664374,z1779093}@students.niu.edu, jzhou@niu.edu
[2] Life Sciences Institute and Department of Cell and Developmental Biology, University of Michigan, Ann Arbor, MI 48109, USA
{taoyang,bingye}@umich.edu

**Abstract.** Automatic counting of neurons in fluorescently stained microscopic images is increasingly important for brain research when big imagery data sets are becoming a norm and will be more so in the future. In this paper, we present an automatic learning-based method for effective detection and counting of neurons with stained nuclei. A shape map that reflects the boosted edge and shape information is generated and a learning problem is formulated to detect the centers of stained nuclei. The method combines multiple cues of edge gradient, shape, and texture during shape map generation, feature extraction and final count determination. The proposed algorithm consistently delivers robust count ratios and precision rates on neurons in mouse and rat brain images that are shown to be better than alternative unsupervised and supervised counting methods.

**Keywords:** Neuron counting · Machine learning · Shape map · Microscopic neuronal image · Nuclei staining

## 1 Introduction

Along with the recent advancement of imaging and florescent staining, automatic counting of neurons using microscopic images is seeing increasingly important applications in neuroscience including developmental neuroscience, study of the neural functions, as well as the effects of neural diseases and their cures [1–3]. When the volume and the scale of the neural imagery data grow, as the inevitable trend at the big data era, automatic counting of cells and neurons is expected to be more essential in scientific discovery. To promote and evaluate the computational methods for automatic neuron counting, several competitions have been held, with a recent example being the Nucleus Counting Challenge at the 2015 Bioimage Informatics Conference.

However, obtaining a robust neuron count remains a very challenging task for several reasons. First of all, the staining of the neurons can be fuzzy due to the imaging technique. Second, intensity and patterns vary greatly among different types of staining labels. Even for the same type of nuclear label, there often exist intensity variations

© Springer International Publishing AG 2016
G.A. Ascoli et al. (Eds.): BIH 2016, LNAI 9919, pp. 3–13, 2016.
DOI: 10.1007/978-3-319-47103-7_1

among different nuclei or within the same nucleus, which make it difficult to tell them apart from background and artifacts. In addition to the complexity and variability of morphology and intensity of the stained objects, cells or nuclei are often clustered in the image, which further increases the level of difficulty for automatic counting. As a result, current automatic software for cell counting falls short on providing the robustness needed in neuroscience research. Figure 1 shows the images of several popular staining of nuclei. We can see non-uniform and fuzzy objects from multiple staining techniques.

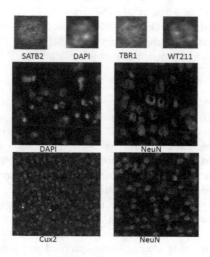

**Fig. 1.** Nuclei staining. Images are from BII 2015 nuclei counting challenge or Bing Ye lab. Some are ubiquitous stains of all nuclear DNA (e.g. DAPI) and some are only expressed in neurons (e.g. NeuN).

A majority of current automatic counting methods for neurons – and for cells in general – are based on the principle of image segmentation. The stained components of different neurons (often nuclei) are considered as the individual objects to be segmented from the image background and separated apart from each other. Counting is then performed after the segmentation. The specific method varies from local or global thresholding to region-based watershed to dynamic models [1, 2]. Counting methods relying on image processing/segmentation are unsupervised traditionally. A relatively recent category of methods, on the other hand, makes use of supervised machine learning. A cell counting method using machine learning starts by labeling some training samples. The counting is then performed using pattern recognition [3, 4].

While both methods have their uses, they also have shortcomings. The unsupervised category suffers from many traditional obstacles of image segmentation, which has been a knowingly difficult problem in image processing, especially with fuzzy and/or clustered objects in images. It also requires more parameter tuning to overcome over-segmentation or under-segmentation. In contrast, the learning-based approach for cell counting builds the model using known examples. It potentially requires fewer critical parameters. It also has the advantage of a more flexible problem formulation if full segmentation is not needed for counting. Yet pattern recognition algorithms are trained based on the features extracted from the training samples. The relevance of the features directly impacts the result of detection. For example, features extracted from the intensities of regions of interest may not make full use of the object properties such as shape and neighborhood gradient.

In this paper, we report an approach that aims to combine these two methods to achieve improved robustness for automatic counting of neurons using microscopic images with florescent staining. The core of the approach is a learning-based detection for the centers of stained nuclei. As a hybrid solution that combines traditional segmentation and machine learning, the proposed method is able to integrate multiple cues including neuron edges, shapes, intensity distribution and texture, and achieve a robust count for images with intensity variety and clustered objects. We will explain our method in Sect. 2, followed by experimental results and discussions.

## 2  Method

### 2.1  Rationale

For microscopic images with staining of neuron nuclei such as STAB2 or DAPI as shown in Fig. 1, the neurons are counted using the stained nuclei.

Traditional counting methods using segmentation approaches such as thresholding or watershed are insufficient for the problem of nuclei counting. Figure 2 shows some example results. We can see that simple thresholding such as Fig. 2B is apparently insufficient. Figure 2C and D show that, on one hand, bright noise is counted by watershed leading to false positives. On the other hand, clustered cells especially those close together will be counted as one cell. This leads to false negatives.

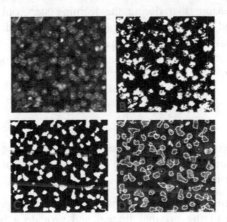

**Fig. 2.** Effects of common segmentation methods. (A) Raw image (B) ImageJ thresholding (C) and (D) Watershed and the resulting counting. False positives are circled in D for annotation.

Learning-based models have also been experimented. Trainable segmentations that classify every pixel to detect the nuclei have similar issues as other traditional segmentation-based methods for counting. An alternative formulation is to detect the center of stained nuclei, instead of all pixels of the nuclei. It, however, encounters issues when a nuclei stain such as DAPI leads to multiple bright spots in the same cell nucleus. Other stains tend to have the similar problem of uneven staining. This issue tends to lead towards over counting when a cell is counted multiple times as each bright spot is detected as a separate center. However, if the features exacted from the region of interest surrounding the center of nucleus reacts better to shape data, then we hypothesize that the combination of the two methods may lead to better results.

To this end, we decided that the unsupervised stage can be more aggressive to segment the objects and effectively reduce clustering when extracting the object shapes. As long as the machine learning phase can smartly reject the over-segmented parts, it will not lead to over count. Aggressive segmentation also reduces the counting problem to only be a matter of reducing the objects, rather than both reducing and attempting to split. We thus design several steps to achieve this in the proposed algorithm. We incorporate aggressive background subtraction to enhance contrast before edges are extracted and watershed is applied. A distance transform map replaces the original intensity information with distances from edges, which are essentially shape information and are named *shape-map* in the algorithm.

With the motivation to boost a machine learning-based counting method using multiple cues from the image, we propose to apply learning on the *shape-map* image. Compared with the original microscopic image, the shape-map image will be edge-boosted, pre-segmented, and distance-transformed with shape and boundary information better reflected. It will serve as the base for further feature extraction and learning. In addition, multiple cues of nuclei properties such as texture and geometry will be included in the features when a classifier is applied for the detection of nuclei centers. As a result, the proposed method, surrounding a machine learning backbone, provides a fusion of intensity, edge and shape information in the detection and counting of neurons. In addition, to ensure that during the learning step, only the relevant shape information is extracted from the region surrounding the center of nuclei, we also incorporated a flood-mask step to exclude nearby objects.

Summarizing the rationale above, we have the resulting proposed counting algorithm described in Sect. 2.2.

## 2.2   Algorithm Flow

The proposed method contains three phases: Generate the shape-map image, identify the centers of nuclei using machine learning based detection, and come up with a final neuron count after post processing.

**Shape-Map Image Generation.** The emphasis of the first stage is to boost the edge and shape information of the original image, and provide a base for the machine learning step.

First, if the image contains clustered objects or is very noisy, an initial background subtraction is performed using a rolling ball algorithm, which corrects or uneven illuminated background, since a cleared background improves the contrast of the edges. A relatively small radius for the rolling ball is used to make this fairly aggressive. The second step is finding edges using Sobel-Feldman filtering [5]. As stated above, this is done to convert the original image into a set of shape data. Several actions taken from this point will be altering and enhancing the shape information. Specifically, a histogram equalization is done followed by a despeckling to remove noise. The edge image is then binarized using local adaptive thresholding, followed by watershed to split the nearby objects. Two final steps are applying the distance transform and another histogram equalization which boosts the distance map image. The whole process results in the shape-map image.

Note that although thresholding and watershed steps are applied in the process of generating the shape-map, the purpose here is to create the image that highlights the edge and shape information. The shape map contains objects that may or may not be the neurons to be counted. However, this carefully designed process converted the original raw image to an image where shapes are emphasized. As the result, the following learning will be less sensitive to uneven intensities within a nucleus, as well as staining variation among different neurons. Figure 3 shows two examples of generated shape maps.

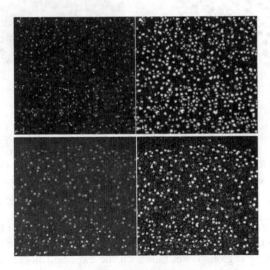

**Fig. 3.** The shape-map images. Left column: raw images. Right column: shape-maps. Top row: DAPI stained rat brain neurons. Bottom row: STAB2 stained mouse brain neurons

**Learning the Centers of Neuron Nuclei.** The shape-map images, as shown in Fig. 3, are transformed images that highlight the edge and shape information. A machine learning engine is then applied to the shape-map image for learning.

The pattern recognition formulation at this stage has several possibilities. One is to classify each pixel to see if it belongs to *any* part of nuclei as often employed in trainable segmentation. However, in our context, counting instead of segmentation is the main goal, and shape-map highlights the centers of shapes, so we formulate the problem as the identification of the *center* of the nuclei. It is a binary problem to tell if a pixel is a center of cell nuclei or not.

As needed by supervised learning, the first task is to label the positive and negative samples. Objects in the shape map image may correspond to actual cells or noise arising from edges of background artifacts. The task of labeling training samples is to tell apart two types of objects. We developed an ImageJ plugin for this purpose as shown in Fig. 4. For an improved usability, the tool provides an automatic mapping of the selected regions in the shape-map back to the raw image, so that the user can confidently decide positive or negative objects on the shape map. For cells that were split into many pieces during the generation of shape-map, the tool marks the largest subsection positive, and the rest as negative. This is to facilitate the classifier to pick out only one representative portion of each cell from the shape-map in the detection stage.

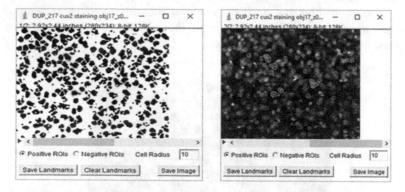

**Fig. 4.** Labeling positive and negative training samples on the shape-map image. The cyan-circled shapes are the positive objects correspond to cells in the raw image. The red ones are the negative ROIs. The user selects objects on the shape-map image (left panel), and corresponding regions on the raw image are automatically marked (right panel) to facilitate the labeling

About ten positive samples and ten negative samples are chosen for training. Features are extracted from the surrounding regions of each center pixel of the sample ROI. The size of the surrounding regions is set based on the expected nuclei size. Assume the radius of the expected nuclei is r, then the neighborhood size is $(2r + 1) * (2r + 1)$. This region centered around the pixel-in-question is used for feature extraction, with a modification: since the object shape is what is being dealt with now, it is important not to include nearby objects in the case of clusters. A flood masking is applied starting from the center and stopping at the object boundary, so that only data from one object in the region is used for feature extraction. This prevents nearby objects from confounding the details of the object of question. Multiple features are then extracted from the modified surrounding region. The following features are used:

- Wavelet-based texture features:

$$f(k,n) = \iint \emptyset_{k,n}(i,j) I(i,j) didj$$

where $\phi$ is the two dimensional discrete wavelet Haar base function [6]. k is set to 0,1 for two level transform. n is the index at the specific level, $n = 1 \ldots |i| * |j|$, where $|i|$ and $|j|$ are the width and height of the sub-image analyzed at the level. $I(i,j)$ is the intensity at the location of the subimage for the specific level. The total number of texture features equals to the size of the surrounding region.

- The Gaussian correlation coefficient with a Gaussian template

$$f = \iint I(x,y) * \theta(x,y) dxdy$$

where $\Theta$ (x, y) is intensity at location (x, y) of the 2D Gaussian approximation centered at the pixel of question, with $\sigma$ set to the expected radius of the nuclei r.

- Four image statistics are used. Geometry symmetry at x, y directions, as well as the mean and standard deviation of the region intensities.

The total number of features depends on the nuclei radius parameter r which decides the size of ROI centered by the pixel of question. For a radius of 3 and a surrounding region of 7 * 7, the number of features is 54. Learning is then performed by training a support vector machine with a linear kernel [7] to maintain speed efficiency without sacrificing reliability.

To detect of the centers of nuclei in an image, foreground pixels of the shape-map are fed to the learned classifier. If the prediction is positive for the pixel, it is a candidate to be a nuclei center. The pixels of positive candidates are then mean-shifted to the closest center of mass, and merged with others if multiple predictions are shifted to the same center of mass. The resulting number yields the tentative count of cells.

A post-processing is then performed to finalize the count. The post-processing stage links the results obtained from the shape-map image back to the original florescent stained image to perform double-checking. Mean shifting of the detected centers is re-attempted in the original image based on the florescent intensity to offset the effects of aggressive splitting. In addition, intensities surrounding the detected center in the original image are examined to avoid dim spots from being counted in order to alleviate false positives.

## 3   Results and Discussions

The following measures are used to quantitatively assess the proposed counting algorithm: Count Ratio, Precision and Recall. Manually counted results are used as a golden standard in calculation.

Count ratio is defined as the ratio of automatically counted neurons to the golden standard count. We define a detected cell as precise if the computationally detected nuclei center is within the boundary of a cell marked manually. The precision is then calculated as the ratio of precise cells to all detected cells. The recall rate is calculated as the ratio of true positive cells to total golden standard cells.

**Experimental Results.** We report our results on two types of stained neuronal images as shown in Fig. 3. One is STAB2 stained mouse brain neurons, the other is the DAPI stained rat brain neurons. Table 1 lists the count ratios. Table 2 lists the precisions and recalls obtained on these images. From Tables 1 and 2, we can see that the proposed neuron counting algorithm delivers a robust count ratio of 95 % or above on the STAB stained mouse brain images, and an average 90 % count ratio on the NeuN stained rat brain image. It also consistently delivers precision mostly around or above 95 %.

**Table 1.** Count ratios. Different rolling ball radii for background subtraction are tested. Image 1–6 are STAB2 stained. Image 7 is a DAPI-stained image from BII 2015 nuclei counting challenge. Radius for image 1–6 is set to 3 pixels. For image 7 the radius is set to 7 pixels.

| Image | 1 | | 2 | | 3 | | 4 | | 5 | | 6 | | 7 | |
|---|---|---|---|---|---|---|---|---|---|---|---|---|---|---|
| Standard | 312 | | 347 | | 324 | | 325 | | 319 | | 305 | | 801 | |
| Rolling ball | Count | Ratio | Count | Ratio | Count | Ratio | Count | Ratio | Count | Ratio | Count | Ratio | Count | Ratio |
| 10 | 301 | 0.96 | 337 | 0.97 | 317 | 0.98 | 297 | 0.91 | 284 | 0.89 | 284 | 0.93 | 756 | 0.94 |
| 20 | 326 | 1.04 | 332 | 0.96 | 300 | 0.93 | 299 | 0.92 | 306 | 0.96 | 293 | 0.96 | 753 | 0.94 |
| 30 | 319 | 1.02 | 341 | 0.98 | 325 | 1.00 | 311 | 0.96 | 311 | 0.97 | 319 | 1.05 | 672 | 0.84 |
| 40 | 313 | 1.00 | 336 | 0.97 | 325 | 1.00 | 323 | 0.99 | 312 | 0.98 | 261 | 0.86 | 704 | 0.88 |
| Average | 315 | 1.01 | 337 | 0.97 | 317 | 0.98 | 308 | 0.95 | 303 | 0.95 | 289 | 0.95 | 721 | 0.90 |

**Table 2.** The precisions and recalls of the STAB2-stained images using different expected nuclei radius.

| Image | Rolling ball size | Radius | 3 | 5 | 7 | 10 | Avg. |
|---|---|---|---|---|---|---|---|
| 1 | 10 | Precision | 0.95 | 0.96 | 0.96 | 0.98 | 0.96 |
| | | Recall | 0.91 | 0.90 | 0.88 | 0.90 | 0.90 |
| 2 | 20 | Precision | 0.93 | 0.95 | 0.95 | 0.95 | 0.95 |
| | | Recall | 0.89 | 0.87 | 0.84 | 0.82 | 0.86 |
| 3 | 30 | Precision | 0.92 | 0.95 | 0.95 | 0.98 | 0.95 |
| | | Recall | 0.92 | 0.89 | 0.87 | 0.85 | 0.88 |
| 4 | 40 | Precision | 0.94 | 0.96 | 0.96 | 0.93 | 0.95 |
| | | Recall | 0.94 | 0.87 | 0.84 | 0.78 | 0.86 |
| 5 | 20 | Precision | 0.90 | 0.94 | 0.95 | 0.96 | 0.94 |
| | | Recall | 0.86 | 0.84 | 0.81 | 0.79 | 0.83 |
| 6 | 30 | Precision | 0.91 | 0.93 | 0.95 | 0.97 | 0.94 |
| | | Recall | 0.95 | 0.86 | 0.86 | 0.83 | 0.88 |
| Avg. | | Precision | 0.93 | 0.95 | 0.95 | 0.96 | 0.95 |
| | | Recall | 0.90 | 0.87 | 0.85 | 0.82 | 0.86 |

The shape-image generation and the labeling tool were implemented in Java as an ImageJ plugin. The learning and counting were implemented in C++ as a Vaa3D plugin [8]. On a typical laptop (2.3 GHz i5 processor with 4 GB of RAM), the algorithm counts 700 cells in about 3 s.

**Algorithm Comparison.** Figure 5 shows the detected cells on a STAB-stained image using the proposed method, as well as two alternatives. One alternative method is the unsupervised watershed in ImageJ and the other is the same machine learning based formulation but applied directly to the raw image without shape map.

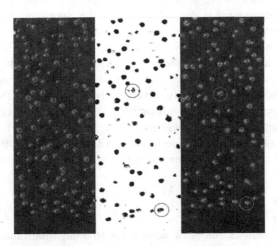

**Fig. 5.** Counting results and algorithm comparison on various images. The left panel: the proposed method. The middle panel: watershed-based counting. The right panel: machine learning based counting without shape map. The red circles indicate examples of over count.

From Fig. 5, we can see that the two alternative methods suffer from several issues. The watershed algorithm splits several cells into multiple components, resulting in over-count. For example, on test image 1, when the expected radius is set to 5, 18 % more cells were counted by the watershed approach. Meanwhile it also misses some dim objects. Figure 5 shows that the machine learning algorithm by itself tends to overcount as well, due to detecting multiple positive centers when the staining is uneven. The precisions of the alternative algorithms are also lower. We calculated the learning-based algorithm's precision for radius of 3, 5, 7 and 10 on the same testing images as in Table 2. The average of the precision range from 85 % to 89 % for the STAB-stained images, which are significantly lower than the proposed method that achieved an average of 95 % precision on the same images. The similar phenomenon was observed on the NeuN stained rat brain image. Detailed statistics of alternative methods are omitted due to space limit

Several parameters are used in the algorithm. Most importantly the rolling ball size for clearing the background, and the expected nuclei radius used in feature extraction, mean-shifting, and the calculation of precision. As shown by Table 1, the rolling ball size seems to be a relatively insensitive although some variations are observed. The nuclei radius parameter impacts the results in multiple ways and should be determined carefully based on the expected size of the stained nuclei: With a small expected radius, more cells could be counted, partially related to a smaller region during mean-shifting.

Meanwhile, the measure of precision is stricter with a smaller nuclei boundary. As a result, a smaller radius sees relatively higher recall but a lower precision rate. On the other hand, if the expected radius is set to be larger, the cell counts are lower which reduces the recall as the result.

In addition to the need of choosing the proper nuclei radius, the proposed method also expects that the objects are of somewhat uniform size. While the stained neuron nuclei satisfy this requirement in general, the use of the algorithm to count other types of objects can be less effective if their sizes are dramatically different. The proposed algorithm can be extended to 3D. Some cells are uncounted in the testing images because the confocal imaging focused on a different z-layer with respect to their optimal z-position. It caused some ambiguity during manual labeling. We will experiment using the extended algorithm to count the neurons in the three dimensional image, which is expected to alleviate this problem and further improve the recall rates. However, implementing the same image processing techniques in a three dimensional image will prove to be challenging due to the fact that many of the image processing algorithms used do not support volumetric data.

# 4    Conclusions

In this paper, we present an automatic neuron counting algorithm that reliably detects and counts stained neuron nuclei in microscopic images. In addition to providing the advantage of a learning-based approach, the hybrid method also makes use of edge gradient, shape and texture information during decision making, which resulted in improved count ratios and precision rates for neuron counting. The proposed method is expected to provide useful assistance in current and future neuroscience research.

**Acknowledgements.** We thank Dr. Dragan Maric for providing the image for Bioimage Informatics Conference 2015 Nucleus Counting Challenge. The work was partially supported by NIH NIMH R15 MH099569 (Zhou) and R21 NS094091 from NIH and a Seed Grant from the Brain Research Foundation (Ye).

# References

1. Lin, G., Adiga, U., Olson, K., Guzowski, J.F., Barnes, C.A., Roysam, B.: A hybrid 3D watershed algorithm incorporating gradient cues and object models for automatic segmentation of nuclei in confocal image stacks. Cytom. A **56**, 23–36 (2003)
2. Oberlaendera, M., Dercksenb, V.J., Eggera, R., Genselb, M., Sakmanna, B., Hegeb, H.-C.: Automated three-dimensional detection and counting of neuron somata. J. Neurosci. Methods **180**, 147–160 (2009)
3. Zhou, J., Peng, H.: Counting cells in 3D confocal images based on discriminative models. In: ACM Conference on Bioinformatics, Computational Biology and Biomedicine (ACM BCB) (2011)
4. Sanders, J., Singh, A., Sterne, G., Ye, B., Zhou, J.: Learning-guided automatic three dimensional synapse quantification for drosophila neurons. BMC Bioinform. **16**, 1–13 (2015)

5. Sobel, I., Feldman, G.: A 3×3 isotropic gradient operator for image processing. In: The Stanford Artificial Intelligence Project (SAIL) (1968)
6. Mallat, S.: A Wavelet Tour of Signal Processing. Academic, San Diego (1999)
7. Chang, C.-C., Lin, C.-J.: LIBSVM: a library for support vector machines. ACM Trans. Intell. Syst. Technol. **2**, 1–27 (2011)
8. Peng, H., Ruan, Z., Long, F., Simpson, J.H., Myers, E.W.: V3D enables real-time 3D visualization and quantitative analysis of large-scale biological image data sets. Nat. Biotechnol. **28**, 348–353 (2010)

# Identification of Relevant Inter-channel EEG Connectivity Patterns: A Kernel-Based Supervised Approach

Juana Valeria Hurtado-Rincón[1]([✉]), Juan David Martínez-Vargas[1],
Sebastian Rojas-Jaramillo[1], Eduardo Giraldo[2],
and German Castellanos-Dominguez[1]

[1] Signal Processing and Recognition Group, Universidad Nacional de Colombia,
Manizales, Colombia
{jvhurtador,jmartinezv,cgcastellanosd}@unal.edu.co
[2] Universidad Tecnológica de Pereira, Pereira, Colombia
egiraldos@utp.edu.co

**Abstract.** Extraction of brain patterns from electroencephalography signals to discriminate brain states has been an important research field to the develop of non-invasive applications like brain-computer-interface systems or diagnosis of neurodegenerative diseases. However, most of the state-of-the-art methodologies use observations derived from each electrode independently, without considering the possible dependencies between channels. To improve understanding of brain functionality, connectivity analysis have been developed. Nevertheless in those works, where connectivity measures are included, the total number of connections is high dimensional, and the relevance of connectivity values is not considered. To cope with this issue, we propose a kernel-based inter-channel connectivity relevance analysis (termed ConnRA), for such a purpose, linear dependencies between channel signals are extracted using coherence measures over specific sub-frequency bands, and a similarity criterion is implemented to rank the contribution of each channel-to-channel connection for a specific task. Experimental validation carried out on a database of brain-computer interfaces, demonstrate very promising results, making the proposed methodology a suitable alternative to support many neurophysiological applications.

## 1 Introduction

Description of separable patterns of brain activity has been a research field of interest to support the diagnosis of neurophysiological disease and to inferring

J.V. Hurtado-Rincón—This research is supported by *Programa Jóvenes Investigadores e Innovadores convocatoria 645-2014 Manizales* funded by Colciencias and Universidad Nacional de Colombia, it is also supported by COLCIENCIAS project *Evaluación asistida de potenciales evocados cognitivos como marcador del transtorno por déficit de atención e hiperactividad (TDAH)* and Programa Nacional de Formacion de Investigadores "Generacion del Bicentenario", 2011. The authors also thank to "Maestría en Ingeniería Eléctrica" and research project "6-14-1" at "Universidad Tecnológica de Pereira" for the financial support.

© Springer International Publishing AG 2016
G.A. Ascoli et al. (Eds.): BIH 2016, LNAI 9919, pp. 14–23, 2016.
DOI: 10.1007/978-3-319-47103-7_2

about a person thoughts for the development of brain-computer-interface (BCI) systems. For this purpose, the monitoring of brain activity is commonly performed by the non-invasive measurement of the electrical activity projected over the brain scalp surface, (electroencephalogram – EEG). Because of high temporal resolution and low cost, EEG signals have been widely used in many neurophysiological applications related to brain-computer interfaces (BCI) [1], automated diagnosis of neurological diseases like epilepsy [2], neuromarketing [3], among others.

In practice, most of the approaches for brain activity discrimination are based on time-frequency representations of individual channels. Nevertheless, the dynamic behavior of neural activity can also be assumed as a combination of interactions among different brain areas [4]. Therefore, the patterns of brain connections should be included with the aim of analyzing all possible communicated networks between EEG signals measured from electrodes located in various areas of the scalp.

So far, connectivity methods have been applied on EEG signals, in order to estimate functional connectivity between scalp electrodes [5–9], however, reproduction of these interactions across spatial scales, by using EEG inter-channel connectivity measures, leads to high-dimensional spaces that may include redundant or worthless information for a specific task, not mentioning further computational cost issues. Hence, it is necessary to extract a set of the most relevant connectivity patterns that better encodes the main connection information to enhance discrimination performances for neurophysiological applications.

In this work, we propose to use the Magnitude Square Coherence as a measure of both linear dependencies (in amplitude and phase) to compute the degree of similarity between all possible pairs of EEG-channel signals, so that the interactions between the whole scalp areas can be detected. Also, we introduce a methodology to extract the most relevant EEG channel-to-channel connections for a specific task using prior information within a kernel-based analysis. This method may facilitate the physiological interpretation and improve the brain activity discrimination performance.

## 2  Methods

### 2.1  Magnitude Square Coherence

*Magnitude Square Coherence.* (MSC) is a large-scale measure of the underlying dynamic neural interactions, where higher coherence values indicate greater functional interplay between the two underlying neural networks [10]. Consequently, given a set of $N$ EEG recordings $\{Z_i \in \mathbb{R}^{C \times T}, i \in [1, N]\}$, where the $i$-th EEG is measured at $C$ electrodes and $T \in \mathbb{N}$ time samples, the pair-wise MSC between two channels $c$ and $c'$ can be computed as [11]:

$$\gamma_{z_i^c, z_i^{c'}}(f) = \frac{|S_{z_i^c z_i^{c'}}(f)|^2}{S_{z_i^c z_i^c}(f) S_{z_i^{c'} z_i^{c'}}(f)}, \ \gamma_{z_i^c, z_i^{c'}}(f) \in \mathbb{R}^+ \tag{1}$$

where $z_i^c \in \mathbb{R}^T$ is the $c$-th channel of $i$-th recording, $S_{z_i^c z_i^{c'}}(f) \in \mathbb{R}^+$ is the cross-spectral density between channels $c$ and $c'$ at the frequency bin $f$, and $S_{z_i^c z_i^c}(f) \in \mathbb{R}^+$ and $S_{z_i^{c'} z_i^c}(f) \in \mathbb{R}^+$ are the auto-spectral density of $z_i^c$ and $z_i^{c'}$, respectively.

Moreover, to quantify the dependencies, the averaged MSC, $\overline{\gamma}_{z_i^c, z_i^{c'}} \in \mathbb{R}^+$, is computed over a predefined frequency rank $f \in [f_1, f_2]$. Therefore, the feature representation matrix $X \in \mathbb{R}^{N \times Q}$ is built by computing the connections between all the possible pair of channels, being $Q$ the number of concatenated connections for the $i$-th trial.

## 2.2 Kernel-Based Relevance Analysis of EEG Channel-to-Channel Connections

With the aim of finding the most relevant channel-to-channel connections for a given task (i.e. Motor Imagery discrimination), we compute all relationships over pairs of feature vectors of $X$, namely $(x_i, x_j) \in \mathbb{R}^Q$, through the introduced similarity kernel $K \in \mathbb{R}^{N \times N}$ with elements defined like $k_{ij} = \kappa(\mathrm{d}_A(x_i, x_j)), \forall i, j \in [1, N]$, where the distance $\mathrm{d}_A : \mathbb{R}^Q \times \mathbb{R}^Q \mapsto \mathbb{R}$ is an operator related to the positive definite kernel function $\kappa(\cdot)$. Here, the Mahalanobis distance is used that defined in a $Q$-dimensional space with inverse covariance matrix $AA^\top$ computed as below:

$$\mathrm{d}_A^2(x_i, x_j) = (x_i, x_j)AA^\top(x_i, x_j)^\top, \tag{2}$$

where matrix $A \in \mathbb{R}^{Q \times M}$ holds the linear projection $y_i = x_i A$, with $y_i \in \mathbb{R}^M$, $M \leq Q$.

The matrix $A$ is computed by adding the available prior knowledge about the task of interest, in our case, the motor imagery paradigm with imagination of left or right motor action. The prior information is enclosed into the matrix $B \in \mathbb{R}^{N \times N}$ with elements $b_{ij} = \delta(l_i - l_j) \in [0, 1]$, being $\delta(\cdot)$ – the delta function. Besides, the relationship between $K$ and $B$ is computed by the following kernel target centered alignment function [12]:

$$\rho(K, B; A) = \frac{\langle HKH, HBH \rangle_F}{\|HKH\|_F \|HBH\|_F}, \rho \in [0, 1] \tag{3}$$

where $H = I - N11^\top$ is a centering matrix, $I \in \mathbb{R}^{N \times N}$ is the identity matrix, $1 \in \mathbb{R}^N$ is an all-ones vector, $K \in \mathbb{R}^{N \times N}$ is the computed similarity kernel for a given matrix $A$, and notations $\langle \cdot, \cdot \rangle_F$ and $\|\cdot, \cdot\|_F$ stand for the Frobenius inner product and norm, respectively.

Consequently, the prior knowledge about the EEG trials can be used to highlight relevant features by learning the matrix $A$ that parameterizes a Mahalanobis distance between pairwise samples. Therefore, the function that implements the Centered Kernel Alignment can be formulated to compute the projection matrix $A$ as follows:

$$A^* = \arg\max_A \rho(K, B; A), \tag{4}$$

From the obtained matrix $\boldsymbol{A}^*$, a relevant feature matrix $\boldsymbol{Y} \in \mathbb{R}^{n \times M}$ is estimated encoding a linear combination of EEG discriminative features according to the prior knowledge considered in $\boldsymbol{B}$.

At the end, the relevance for each input feature can be estimated by analyzing its contribution to building the projection matrix $\boldsymbol{A}^*$, resulting in the following feature relevance vector $\varrho \in \mathbb{R}^Q$:

$$\varrho_q = \sum_{m=1}^{M} |a_{qm}|; \forall q \in Q, a_{qm} \in \boldsymbol{A} \tag{5}$$

The main assumption behind the introduced relevance index is that the largest values of $\varrho_q$ should point out to better input attributes since they exhibit higher overall dependencies to the estimated embedding. The $M$ value is fixed as the number of dimensions needed to preserve some percentage of the input data variability [13]. So, the calculated relevance vector $\varrho$ is used to rank the inter-channel connections.

# 3   Experimental Set-Up

## 3.1   Tested Dataset and Preprocessing

In order to assess the proposed methodology as a tool to support BCI systems, experimental testing is carried out over a two-class Motor Imagery (MI) Database[1]. The EEG signals are provided by *Berlin Brain-Computer Interface group for a BCI* and include the 59-channel recording acquired for seven subjects who were instructed to perform the imaginary movement of the left or right hand indicated by a pointing arrow on a screen. All the recordings are band-pass filtered between 0.05 and 200 Hz and then submitted to a 10-order low-pass Chebyshev II filter with a stop-band ripple of 50 $dB$ down and stop-band edge frequency of 49 Hz. All EEG signals are further digitized at 1000 Hz and down-sampled to supply the sampling frequency at 100 Hz. The whole session is performed without feedback, and 100 repetitions are recorded for each of two MI classes per person for a total of 200 trials per subject. The section of interest is 4 $s$ during when the subject is instructed to perform the MI task. These periods, lasting 4 $s$, are interleaved with a blank screen and a fixation cross in the screen center.

The design procedure for the preprocessing stage is as follows: first, a 5-order band-pass Butterworth filter is implemented with bandwidth ranging from 30 till 30 Hz. Later, a data-driven supervised decomposition of the EEG multi-channel data is carried out based on the Common Spatial Patterns (CSP) algorithm. In this step, a spacial filter matrix is calculated projecting the original EEG signals to space where the differences in variance between the two labels of the MI task are maximized [14]. Finally, an empirical mode decomposition (EMD) is used, to extract adaptively components carrying MI information that better fits for the frequency band selection needed in the CSP method [15].

---

[1] http://bbci.de/competition/iv/desc_1.html. BCI competition IV 2008, Dataset 1.

## 3.2   Inter-channel Connectivity Extraction

In general, the EEG rhythms carrying out motor imagery interest include, mainly, the sub-bands Alpha $(\alpha, f \in [8, 13])$ Hz and Beta $(\beta, f \in [14, 30])$ Hz [16]. Consequently, the underlying dynamic interactions are computed across those frequency bandwidths by filtering each preprocessed EEG trial $\boldsymbol{Z}_i$ using a 5-order band-pass Butterworth filter. Moreover, to obtain a holistic view of the information transfer using this linear metric, MSC is also calculated for the entire range $(f \in [8, 30])$ Hz. As a result, MSC is computed over all EEG trials for each frequency range.

Consequently, all row channel vectors are considered in pairs over which coherence measurement is calculated as explained in Sect. 2.1, building the channel-to-channel connection matrix for each trial $\boldsymbol{\Upsilon}_i \in \mathbb{R}^{C \times C}$ with elements $v_i^{c,c'} \in \mathbb{R}[0, 1]$ defined as follows: $v_i^{c,c'} = \overline{\gamma}(\boldsymbol{z}_i^c, \boldsymbol{z}_i^{c'})$, $\forall c, c' \in [1, C]$ with $v_i^{c,c'} \in \mathbb{R}^+$.

Given that the coherence is a measure that assumes linear relationships, the square matrix $\boldsymbol{\Upsilon}$ becomes symmetric with ones on the main diagonal and zeros elsewhere. Accordingly, only the values of the upper diagonal of $\boldsymbol{\Upsilon}$ are contemplated to create a feature representation matrix $\boldsymbol{X}$ with the minimum possible redundant information. As a result, each row vector of $\boldsymbol{X}$ comprises $Q = 3 \times C(C-1)/2$ features, corresponding to the $C(C-1)/2$ possible connections over the three studied frequency ranks of interest.

## 3.3   Classifier Training and Validation

The proposed approach is used as a tool to select the most relevant channel-to-channel connections, providing a better understanding of the relations of brain electrical signals projected over the scalp in a specific task as MI paradigm. Hence, the approach generates by feature transformation, new composites of the input feature set to improve overall brain activity discrimination performance. Consequently, the accuracy of the approach for an MI task is carried out.

Prior to classification, the feature relevance analysis is performed as stated in Sect. 2.2. As a result, the estimated relevance vector $\boldsymbol{\rho}$ is employed to rank the original features. Further, the $k$-Nearest-Neighbor ($k$-nn) classifier is trained. The number of nearest neighbor is fixed automatically for each subject according to the training set accuracy. Finally, the accuracy curve performed for the MI classification is computed through the 10-folds cross-validation scheme, adding one by one the features ranked by the relevance vector. Also, the average of each feature relevance for all the cross-validation iterations is computed, aiming to obtain a representative relevance vector of the complete features set.

## 4   Results and Discussion

As described before, we consider the relevance analysis as a channel-to-channel connections selection tool. Thus, Fig. 1a shows the coherence matrix for subject labeled as #6 obtained in the three considered frequency sub-bands: Alpha,

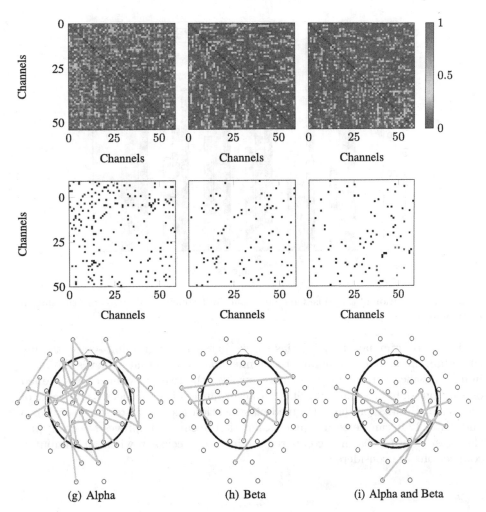

**Fig. 1.** Estimated values of the connectivity measure and the most relevant connections for subject # 6 for the subfrequency bands: Alpha, Beta, and the interval that holds both frequency ranges.

Beta, and the interval that holds both frequency ranges. Each matrix position designates the connection weight between channels $c$ and $c'$. Further, Fig. 1b shows with black points the inter-channel connections that are selected as the most relevant for the discrimination between left-right motor imagery classes.

For the sake of visual representation, Fig. 1c displays only the 50 most relevant connections, drawn as linked lines between electrode locations. As seen in Fig. 1b and 2, the majority of relevant connections for the discrimination of the contemplated MI tasks is extracted from $\alpha$ sub-band. This behavior holds for the majority of subjects of this study (in five of seven). Also, different patterns for each frequency band are noticed in Fig. 1c.

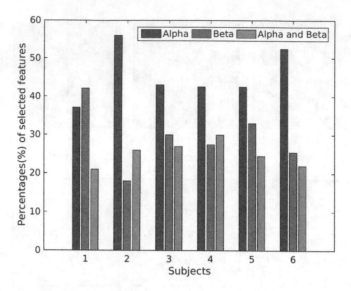

**Fig. 2.** Contribution of the considered sub-bands of frequency to the MI discrimination performance.

In the discrimination of MI classes, we just select a training set containing the minimum amount of channel-to-channel connections that achieves the maximum classification accuracy. For this purpose, the relevant connections are fed one by one into the $k$-nn classifier in accordance with the decreasing rank of relevance. Results for the performed classification accuracy are shown in Fig. 3 and Table 1. It can be seen that classification accuracy improves selecting just the most relevant features compared against the accuracy when all computed connections are considered.

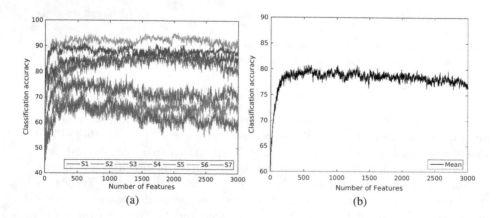

**Fig. 3.** Learning curves for classification accuracy.

Besides, we analyze the suggested Kernel-based relevance analysis of inter-channel connectivity selection concerning the classification accuracy achieved for the contemplated MI task, where the proposed methodology reaches an averaged accuracy $84.64 \pm 0.544$ as shown for all subjects in Table 1. With the aim of comparing our methodology, we add the accuracy estimated by the approach submitted in [14] where spatio-temporal features are selected and a non-linear regression for predicting the time-series of class labels is applied. The work in [17] that employs spatial preprocessed features and an SVM classifier is also compared. Note that either examined training approach does not take in account spatial dependencies between brain electrical signals, underperforming the proposed *ConnRA* method.

**Table 1.** Classification accuracy [%]. Figures remarked in bold are the best performed for each subject. Notation # is the subject label. (–) Results not provided

| # | He [14] | Zhang [17] | ConnRA |
|------|---------|------------|--------|
| #1 | 67.7±2.20 | 77.2±0.03 | **91.0±6.00** |
| #2 | 70.7±1.20 | 70.8±0.02 | **80.5±9.27** |
| #3 | **83.9±1.30** | - | 73.0±7.54 |
| #4 | **93.0±1.20** | - | 73.0±9.48 |
| #5 | **93.2±1.20** | - | 88.0±5.38 |
| #6 | - | 76.8±0.03 | **95.5±5.00** |
| #7 | - | 80.0±0.03 | **91.5±5.83** |
| *Mean* | 81.7±12.1 | 76.2±3.87 | **84.6±6.92** |

## 5   Discussion and Concluding Remarks

In this work, we discuss a novel methodology for selecting the most relevant EEG channel-to-channel interactions to enhance the automatic identification of brain connectivity patterns. For such a purpose, a similarity criterion to rank the contribution of inter-channel connectivity values for classifying two tasks of brain activity in an MI paradigm is proposed. So, experimental results are carried out on real EEG Data in motor imagery paradigm, i.e., a real BCI application.

The values calculated for connectivity over the sub-frequency band Alpha are more relevant for the discrimination of the considered MI task; this fact can be seen in Fig. 1. Furthermore, the classification accuracy of the proposed methodology outperforms the accuracy presented in works where dependencies between the EEG signals are not considered explicitly. This behavior can also be noticed in Fig. 3 showing that the highest accuracy rates are obtained for a low amount of features (connections). In turn, the accuracy rate considerably decreases when the entire set of connections considered (See also Table 1). Consequently, we can conclude that the selected features are the most relevant ones to discriminate between MI tasks. Moreover, the proposed approach is a suitable alternative to support straightforward BCI systems.

The proposed methodology is tested through the 10-folds cross-validation scheme, but due to the phenomenon is not universal for all subjects as a future work new data can be used and hypothesis tests can be implemeted.

The feature extraction in [14] is made by measuring signal dynamics both in time and frequency over each channel. Hence, this dynamics could also create a favorable representation for the label discrimination given specific subjects and conditions, and this might explain the outcomes of this method for some subjects in the considered dataset. Therefore, as a future work, we propose to implement both feature extraction: to represent the individual channel dynamics and to find channel-to-channel relations, to lately use the feature selection stage based on the similarity criterion applied in this work to rank the contribution of each set of features. Also, it is suitable to compare different methods of connectivity selection, including supervised and unsupervised schemes.

Given that the electrical brain activity measured over the scalp is affected by volume conduction factors and do not faithfully represent the information in the brain source space, neurophysiological interpretation in EEG channels spaces is difficult and no accurate [18]. Therefore, as a future work a EEG source imaging stage can be included to implement the proposed methodology over the estimated brain source signals.

Recently, connectivity analysis has been used as a biological marker to the support of the diagnosis of Attention deficit hyperactivity disorder, using evoked response potentials [19, 20]. Consequently, also as a future work we propose to use the proposed methodology to find the most relevant inter-channel connections in the support of diagnosis of this disorder.

# References

1. Nicolas-Alonso, L.F., Gomez-Gil, J.: Brain computer interface: a review. In: Hassanien, A.B., Azar, A.T. (eds.) Brain-Computer Interfaces, vol. 74, pp. 3–30. Springer, Heidelberg (2012)
2. Faust, O., Acharya, U.R., Adeli, H., Adeli, A.: Wavelet-based EEG processing for computer-aided seizure detection and epilepsy diagnosis. Seizure **26**, 56–64 (2015)
3. Maglione, A.G., Vecchiato, G., Babiloni, F.: On the use of cognitive neuroscience in industrial applications by using neuroelectromagnetic recordings. In: Liljenström, H. (ed.) Advances in Cognitive Neurodynamics (IV), pp. 31–37. Springer, Heidelberg (2013)
4. Ingber, L., Nunez, P.L.: Neocortical dynamics at multiple scales: EEG standing waves, statistical mechanics, and physical analogs. Math. Biosci. **229**(2), 160–173 (2011)
5. Tononi, G., Sporns, O., Edelman, G.M.: A measure for brain complexity: relating functional segregation and integration in the nervous system. Proc. Nat. Acad. Sci. **91**(11), 5033–5037 (1994)

6. Stam, C.J., Van Dijk, B.W.: Synchronization likelihood: an unbiased measure of generalized synchronization in multivariate data sets. Phys. D: Nonlinear Phenom. **163**(3), 236–251 (2002)
7. Lithari, C., Klados, M.A., Bamidis, P.D.: Graph analysis on functional connectivity networks during an emotional paradigm. In: Bamidis, P.D., Pallikarakis, N. (eds.) XII Mediterranean Conference on Medical and Biological Engineering and Computing 2010, vol. 29, pp. 115–118. Springer, Heidelberg (2010)
8. Kim, S.-P., Chung, Y.G., Kim, M.-K.: Inter-channel connectivity of motor imagery EEG signals for a noninvasive bci application. In: International Workshop on Pattern Recognition in NeuroImaging. IEEE (2011)
9. Chen, M., Han, J., Guo, L., Wang, J., Patras I.: Identifying valence and arousal levels via connectivity between EEG channels. In: 2015 International Conference on Affective Computing and Intelligent Interaction (ACII), pp. 63–69. IEEE (2015)
10. Gupta, R., Falk, T.H., et al.: Relevance vector classifier decision fusion and EEG graph-theoretic features for automatic affective state characterization. Neurocomputing **174**, 875–884 (2016)
11. Srinivasan, R., Winter, W.R., Ding, J., Nunez, P.L.: EEG and MEG coherence: measures of functional connectivity at distinct spatial scales of neocortical dynamics. J. Neurosci. Methods **166**(1), 41–52 (2007)
12. Brockmeier, A.J., Choi, J.S., Kriminger, E.G., Francis, J.T., Principe, J.C.: Neural decoding with kernel-based metric learning. Neural Comput. **26**(6), 1080–1107 (2014)
13. Velasquez-Martinez, F., Alvarez-Meza, A.M., Castellanos-Dominguez, G.: Connectivity analysis of motor imagery paradigm using short-time features and kernel similarities. In: Vicente, J.M.F., Álvarez-Sánchez, J.R., Paz López, F., Toledo-Moreo, F.J., Adeli, H. (eds.) Artificial Computation in Biology and Medicine. LNCS, vol. 9107, pp. 439–448. Springer, Heidelberg (2015)
14. He, W., Wei, P., Wang, L., Zou Y.: A novel emd-based common spatial pattern for motor imagery brain-computer interface. In: IEEE EMBC (2012)
15. Álvarez-Meza, A.M., Velásquez-Martínez, L.F., Castellanos-Dominguez, G.: Time-series discrimination using feature relevance analysis in motor imagery classification. Neurocomputing **151**, 122–129 (2015)
16. Rodríguez, G., García, P.J.: Automatic and adaptive classification of electroencephalographic signals for brain computer interfaces. Med. Syst. **36**(1), 51–63 (2012)
17. Zhang, H., Guan, C., Ang, K.K., Wang, C.: BCI competition iv-data set i: learning discriminative patterns for self-paced EEG-based motor imagery detection. Front. Neurosci. **6**, 7 (2012)
18. Haufe, S., Nikulin, V.V., Müller, K.-R., Nolte, G.: A critical assessment of connectivity measures for eeg data: a simulation study. Neuroimage **64**, 120–133 (2013)
19. Murias, M., Swanson, J.M, Srinivasan, R.: Functional connectivity of frontal cortex in healthy and ADHD children reflected in EEG coherence. Cereb. Cortex **17**(8), 1788–1799 (2007)
20. Rodrak, S., Wongsawat, Y.: EEG brain mapping and brain connectivity index for subtypes classification of attention deficit hyperactivity disorder children during the eye-opened period. In: 2013 35th Annual International Conference of the IEEE Engineering in Medicine and Biology Society (EMBC), pp. 7400–7403. IEEE (2013)

# Computational Role of Astrocytes in Bayesian Inference and Probability Distribution Encoding

Martin Dimkovski[(⊠)] and Aijun An

York University, Toronto, ON, Canada
martin@cse.yorku.ca

**Abstract.** The past few years have seen new research methods confirming more confidently that glia have a key information processing role in the brain, specifically in relation to learning capability. However, many details Tof glia's role remain unknown, including a gap between cellular and behavioural level findings. Based on $Ca^{2+}$ wave mechanics in astrocytes, we derive a theoretical capability of astrocytes to encode cognitive representations as probability distributions over synapses. The process is analogous to MCMC Bayesian inference that samples a neural network configuration from a prior in the astrocyte and then uses its performance to update to a posterior distribution. The proposed model explains recent behavioural results where obstructing astrocytes leads to deficiencies in learning new knowledge without affecting ability to recall existing knowledge. The model is also a novel Bayesian brain theory which uniquely addresses the cellular and synaptic levels.

**Keywords:** Glia · Astrocytes · Bayesian brain · Neural networks

## 1 Introduction

An article published this year in Nature Neuroscience [1] describes a recent 3rd wave in the debate about information processing by astrocytes, the principal type of glia in the cortex. The 1st wave, which had began more than two decades ago, started reporting relationships between neurotransmitters in synapses and $Ca^{2+}$ flows inside astrocytes. The 2nd wave followed with critical studies in response, mostly showing discrepancies in terms of the $Ca^{2+}$ dynamics in the cell soma. The 3rd wave is a result of new methods for tracking $Ca^{2+}$ activity, which have clarified some discrepancies as a consequence of compartmentalization of the $Ca^{2+}$ dynamics: at least eight times as many $Ca^{2+}$ transients were found in the fine cellular branching near synapses compared to transients in the soma. Other discrepancies were also clarified in terms of how astrocytes affect synapses.

In addition to the astrocyte role at cellular levels, recent results also show behavioural effects from tampering with the signalling in astrocytes. Results across a series of tests consistently show effects on learning and formation of new memory, while having no effect on recall of existing memory [2–5]. The proposed model is particularly capable of explaining these findings.

© Springer International Publishing AG 2016
G.A. Ascoli et al. (Eds.): BIH 2016, LNAI 9919, pp. 24–33, 2016.
DOI: 10.1007/978-3-319-47103-7_3

Marr's tri-level hypothesis on information processing systems [6] suggests the need for analysis on three levels: a physical implementation level, an algorithmic or representation level above it, and a level for computational objectives on top. Current findings and models of the computational role of astrocytes relate to the physical level (synaptic effects) and computational level (behavioural effects). To the best of our knowledge, there is no model currently that addresses the algorithms and information representations that link the physical and computational levels.

In Sect. 2 we present an overview of the argument for astrocytes having some information processing role in the brain. In Sect. 3 we present arguments for this role being specifically related to learning capability. In Sect. 4 we derive a theoretical capability of the $Ca^{2+}$ wave mechanics in astrocytes to encode a probability distribution over synapses in its domain, and to facilitate a process analogous to Markov Chain Monte Carlo (MCMC) Bayesian inference by which the distribution is updated by the performance of the associated neural network. In Sect. 5 we discuss the new Bayesian brain theory that is implied by this astrocyte model, and which uniquely extends to the cellular and synaptic levels. Section 6 ends with a conclusion.

## 2    Having a Role in Information Processing

Shigetomi et al. [7] describe how the new methods of the 3rd wave, especially Genetically Encoded Calcium Indicators (GECIs) and two-photon fluorescence imaging, have produced in-vivo results suggesting that astrocytes display behaviorally relevant $Ca^{2+}$ signaling. The authors also state that "it is now well established that astrocytes serve diverse and important roles for the brain ... includ[ing]... ion homeostasis, neurotransmitter clearance, synapse formation/removal, and synaptic modulation..." Similar arguments about the shift due to the new methods are made in [8], and about glia signalling in [9,10].

Perea et al. [11] define three aspects required for an information processing role and elaborate how astrocytes satisfy all of them: they receive incoming information, integrate and code information in a way that is not a side-effect of neural processing, and transmit the results to other cells.

To begin with, glia create the neurons in all stages of life. During prenatal neurogenesis, radial glia create the scaffolding over which neurons are positioned into physical arrangements [12]. Radial glia are also the progenitor cells for cortical neurons and astrocytes during this period. In adulthood, radial glia transform into astrocyto-like neural stem cells that provide adult neurogenesis [13]. In addition to creating the neurons, glia also induce the creation of synapses and their removal [13,14]. Adult astrocytes can remodel the neuropil in the hippocampus in a matter of minutes [15].

Astrocytes partition the neuropil into functional islands called *micro-domains* with an overlap under than 5 % [16], where they engulf millions of synapses and neurons have a tendency to be under a unique micro-domain [17].

Astrocytes are not just passive neural network builders because they form a feedback loop with the *tripartite synapses* [18,19] under their micro-domains.

Synaptic activity causes activation of second messengers inside the astrocyte, of which the best-known are $Ca^{2+}$ flows. These flows undergo their own temporal and spatial dynamics, including accumulating into $Ca^{2+}$ waves across the astrocyte which can reach remote and otherwise unrelated synapses. In the return direction, $Ca^{2+}$ flows affect a synapse in various ways. A now non-controversial effect is by changing the activity of transporters in the astrocyte membrane that affect GABA, glutamate, or $Na^+$ already in the synapse. Another way is due to the astrocyte volume and shape changes around the synapses it engulfs. In addition, some findings suggest astrocytes exocytose gliotransmitters such as glutamate, ATP, D-serine, and GABA, though the jury is still out on this point. Aside from $Ca^{2+}$, other second messengers such as $cAMP$ are also suspected [1].

The information flow inside an astrocyte has considerably different spatial and temporal characteristics. While neurons communicate in a point-to-point manner with a specific peer, astrocyte communication is of a broadcast nature. In addition, neural communication is on a scale of milliseconds, where as intracellular astrocyte communication is on a scale of seconds and minutes [20].

## 3 Affecting Learning Without Affecting Recall

Lee et al. [3] found that by selectively disabling astrocyte communication and without affecting neurons, mice spent less time exploring new objects (NOR test) compared to healthy mice. The tampering with the astrocytes did not change the mice behaviour with familiar objects, and the modified mice did not have deficits in attention, sensory functions, or exploratory drive. The mice were tested in both the Y-maze task and the NOR test, and although both involve exploratory behaviour only the NOR test showed impairment. This implies that the defect is not in exploratory drive but specifically in the ability to detect and encode a new object.

Jahn et al. [21] review several studies where genetic control is used to show how preventing glia from listening to neural activity affects higher cognitive functions such as learning and working memory. Miranda et al. [4] found that obstructing astrocyte communication does not affect recall of existing memory but causes defects in forming new memories.

Han et al. [2] engrafted human glia progenitor cells in neonatal mice, which later developed in hominid astrocytes, which are considerably larger and more complex, covering even 2 millions synapses compared to the 20,000–120,000 synapses of a murine astrocyte. In addition, hominid astrocytes communicate faster. Mice with hominid glia showed improved learning and activity-dependent plasticity, assessed by Barnes maze navigation, object-location memory, and both contextual and tone fear conditioning.

Besides astrocytes, other types of glia such as oligodendrocytes and microglia have also been found to have a key role in learning [22]. McKenzie et al. [23] show how if the ability to make new oligodendrocytes is turned off in mice, they become unable to master running on a complex wheel while not losing any ability to recall any previously learned skill. The experiments confirm that the effect is not because of a neural or physical impairment due to the genetic control setup for the allele for myelin regulatory factor (MyRF), since if the mice were trained on the complex wheel before MyRF deactivation, they could recall this skill after the deactivation, even though they couldnt learn it anymore. This research was also highlighted in Nature Reviews Neuroscience [24].

Markham and Greenough [25] speculated based on histological studies that "astrocytic changes might be necessary to induce, but not to maintain, adaptive changes in the brains 'wiring diagram' in response to experience."

## 4   $Ca^{2+}$ Waves and Bayesian Inference

Most previous computational models of astrocytes do not present astrocytes as processing or encoding information separate from neurons, but attribute them with a secondary synapse potentiation and depression role [26–28]. A couple of studies [29,30] however describe an information encoding capability of $Ca^{2+}$ waves in terms of bifurcations, amplitude and frequency modulation, and oscillatory properties. These studies are based on simulating differential equations for minute physical properties of a cell, and due to this complexity they have a couple of cells and few synapses in their models. Also, they use low-level computational concepts that don't extend into Marr's algorithmic and computational levels. None of the previous models are probabilistic.

There are intuitive examples in physics which link wave mechanics to information encoding. Eddi et al. [31] show one such example with a bouncing droplet coupled to a vibrating fluid surface. If the vibrating amplitude approaches the Faraday instability threshold the droplet couples to a "pilot" wave and starts moving with it. With every bounce, the droplet causes ripples, which interfere with ripples from previous activity and create a path memory. At the point of next contact, the path memory in turn "reads out" the droplets next movement. The authors point out the interpretation in terms of information encoding: "The dual nature ... is contained in the path memory dynamics: the wave nature lies in the coding while the particle nature lies in the reading." Such memory function based on wave mechanics with a coupled point-centred process has been also found in the study of crack propagation in a physical medium [32]. Goldman et al. note how the crack tip point can be dominated by memory encoded in superimposed elastic waves caused in the past, reflected from boundaries and inhomogeneous zones.

A parallel can be drawn with astrocytes, where a tripartite synapse can be described as a coupled point-centered process to the $Ca^{2+}$ wave dynamics inside the astrocyte. In such a perspective, the $Ca^{2+}$ waves can be seen as coding information based on perturbations from connected synapses, while the $Ca^{2+}$ wave effect on the synapse can be seen as a read-out of the collectively coded information at the point location of each synapse. The longer time frame and cumulative nature of $Ca^{2+}$ waves allows for many synapse interaction to accumulate in the memory they encode, similar to previous scenarios in other physical systems.

Seeking a modeling approach which is more scalable than using differential equations for the $Ca^{2+}$ waves, we turn to a probabilistic interpretation of wave dynamics. A well-studied example of that nature is the Copenhagen interpretation of quantum mechanics, where Schroedingers wave equation is interpreted probabilistically, by relating it to the concept of a probability current, derived from fluid mechanics. In fluid mechanics the concept of *current* **j** is described by the continuity equation:

$$\frac{\partial \rho}{\partial t} = -\nabla \cdot \mathbf{j}, \tag{1}$$

which is characteristic when there is some physical quantity $Q$ which moves continuously and is conserved [33]. Known types of $Q$ include dissolved ions, which is the case of $Ca^{2+}$ ions inside the astrocyte. $\rho$ is the density of $Q$, i.e. the quantity in a unit volume, $t$ is the time of change, **j** is the current (sometime called *flux*) which is a vector field which tells how much $Q$ passes through a unit area in the cross-section perpendicular to **j** in a unit time, and $\nabla$ is the divergence of **j**. In summary, **j** describes how density changes in a unit volume.

The probability of finding a $Ca^{2+}$ ion in a specific location is proportional to its density $\rho$ in that location. In addition, probability is also conserved because its integral is always 1. Therefore, a *probability current* can be defined in the same form as Eq. (1), since divergence is a linear operator, as follows:

$$\frac{\partial P}{\partial t} = \frac{\alpha(\partial \rho)}{\partial t} = -\alpha(\nabla \cdot \mathbf{j}_\rho) = -\nabla \cdot \mathbf{j}_P, \tag{2}$$

where $\alpha$ is the proportionality constant, and $\mathbf{j}_P$ is the probability current.

Given the probability current we can get the probability by integrating across a cross-section and time [33]. Therefore, the probability $P_A$ that a $Ca^{2+}$ ion inside the astrocyte affects a specific surface on the astrocyte membrane $\Delta S$ (where a particular synapse might be) during $\Delta t$ is:

$$P_A = \int_{\Delta t} \left[ \int_{\Delta S} \mathbf{j}_P \cdot dS \right] dt. \tag{3}$$

Equation (3) above explains how changes in density of $Ca^{2+}$ ions, caused by activity of all the tripartite synapses, can translate into a probability density function $P_A$ that applies to the whole micro-domain. $P_A$ represents wave memory encoded by the astrocyte due to historical activity in its associated neural network. If we describe a tripartite synapse located within $\Delta S$ as the point process enacting the information reading of wave memory $P_A$, then it follows that synapse changes are analogous to sampling from $P_A$. Therefore, if the neural network in the astrocyte micro-domain is parametrized by a set of synapses $\mathbf{s} = \{s_1, s_2, \dots\}$, and the data propagated in this neural network is **D**, then $P(\mathbf{s}|\mathbf{D}) \equiv P_A$. In other words, the propagation of data **D** through the network builds up $P_A$ over time, which then in return re-parametrizes the neural network as $P(\mathbf{s}|\mathbf{D})$.

To be able to use Eq. (3) in that form we need to be able to get the probability current $\mathbf{j}_P$ of the $Ca^{2+}$ waves. Theoretically, this can be accomplished with any mathematical model for $\partial Ca^{2+}/\partial t$ since $Ca^{2+}$ is proportional to its density $\rho$, and using a derivation similar to Eq. (2) and another proportionality constant $\beta$ we can get:

$$\frac{\partial Ca^{2+}}{\partial t} = -\beta(\nabla \cdot \mathbf{j}_P).\qquad(4)$$

However, using inverse divergence to get $j_P$ from Eq. (4) is not trivial. Therefore, we use other aspects of the $\partial Ca^{2+}/\partial t$ dynamics to frame a more practical approach. In particular, Wade et al. [30] computationally model $\partial Ca^{2+}/\partial t$ in astrocytes and suggest how individual puffs of $Ca^{2+}$ remain mostly self-contained, while their intra-cellular propagation effect is caused by cascade activation of puffs in neighbouring areas. With this, in place of $P(\mathbf{s}|\mathbf{D})$ above, we imply a conditional probability distribution $P(s_i|s_{-i},\mathbf{D})$ of a single synapse given the state of all other synapses and the processed data.

The order in which synapses are updated is determined by how the $Ca^{2+}$ wave interacts with the astrocyte membrane on the inside. The update order can be described as stochastic, since at worst it is pseudorandom due to the chaotic interaction patterns of the wave and the membrane, or it could be random due to randomness in the biological processes that underpin it. For simplicity, we can assume a single synapse updating at one time, by considering an arbitrary level of precision in measuring the update periods. This view can be extended to blocks of synapses updating simultaneously.

The effect of the astrocyte on its tripartite synapses can now be described as continually updating them one by one in a stochastic order, by sampling the parametrization of each synapse $s_i$ from $P(s_i|s_{-i},\mathbf{D})$ during each update. Each update conditions on the current state of all other synapses, and the states of all synapses are therefore continually interpolated across the astrocyte. This update process is mathematically equivalent to Gibbs sampling [34], which is an MCMC Bayesian inference method which guarantees that the sampled synapse will all together asymptotically converge to the joint distribution $P(\mathbf{s}|\mathbf{D})$. The equivalence with Bayesian inference implies the Bayes theorem relationship:

$$P(\mathbf{s}|\mathbf{D}) \propto P(\mathbf{s})P(\mathbf{D}|\mathbf{s}),\qquad(5)$$

where *prior* probability distribution $P(\mathbf{s})$ is updated to a *posterior* distribution $P(\mathbf{s}|\mathbf{D})$ after the *likelihood* of new data $P(\mathbf{D}|\mathbf{s})$ is accounted for. The astrocyte encodes $P(\mathbf{s})$ before data is accounted for, and encodes $P(\mathbf{s}|\mathbf{D})$ afterwards. The likelihood value $P(\mathbf{D}|\mathbf{s})$ is produced by propagating the data $\mathbf{D}$ through the neural network which at that moment is parameterized by $\mathbf{s}$. The interpretation of the likelihood is based on the function of that neural network. For example, if the micro-domain belongs to a neural circuit which recognizes a particular cognitive symbol (eg. a visual receptive field), then the likelihood will measure the relevance of that symbol to the current data $\mathbf{D}$.

A biologically plausible model must describe how continually streaming data from the environment are incrementally processed, i.e. it must not require the explicit storage of all the data seen. The wave memory provides this since it integrates previous data into the $Ca^{2+}$ current $\mathbf{j}$. This means that at time $t-1$, $\mathbf{j}^{(t-1)}$ represents the effect of all $\mathbf{D}^{(t-1)} = \{D_1, D_2, \ldots, D_{t-1}\}$, and can be thought of a surrogate sufficient statistics for them. The difference between $P_A^{(t)}$ and $P_A^{(t-1)}$ should be describable using only $D_t$, i.e. only $D_t$ is used for the likelihood. This gives us a conditional probability distribution of the form $P(s_i|s_{-i}, D_t, \xi^{(t-1)})$ instead of $P(s_i|s_{-i}, \mathbf{D})$, and the Bayesian inference relationship becomes:

$$P(s_i|s_{-i}, D_t, \xi^{(t-1)}) \propto P(s_i|s_{-i}, \xi^{(t-1)})P(D_t|\mathbf{s}). \qquad (6)$$

An implementation of Eq. (6) is not straightforward because the standard MCMC algorithms are not incremental. Even though Gibbs sampling can be modified for incremental use [35] by integrating sufficient statistics $\xi^{(t-1)}$ from previous data $\mathbf{D}^{(t-1)}$ into $P(s_i|s_{-i}, D_t, \xi^{(t-1)})$, we have found it better to use Metropolis-Hastings sampling. Gibbs sampling is a special case of the more general Metropolis-Hastings algorithm [34]. Metropolis-Hastings is also not incremental, but it has a more flexible incremental extension [36] which recursively uses the previous posterior as a new prior through kernel density estimations, and requires only the last data $D_t$ from the input data stream.

The key points of the proposed model can be summarized as follows:

1. Based on likelihood derived from propagating new data through a neural network, the astrocyte learns an empirical prior distribution over synapses in its micro-domain for the functional interpretation of that likelihood/neural network.
2. The synapses of a neural network are continually sampled from the prior distribution and thus continually fluctuate. This implies a level of constant noise in the neural network. There may be a link between the near-Poisson nature of experimentally known neural noise [37] and the Poisson model of waves breaking thresholds at particular points in their domains [38].
3. Each new data that propagates through the neural network results in a new posterior distribution through Bayesian inference, which then becomes a new prior for upcoming data.
4. If the $Ca^{2+}$ mechanism is blocked, the neural network would continue to be able to use prior knowledge, however it will not be able to do the Bayesian inference and update the distribution after new data. Therefore this model fits the experimental findings described in Sect. 3.

## 5   Bayesian Brain

The Bayesian brain hypothesis [39] proposes that the brain somehow internally encodes probability distributions for prior beliefs which are updated to posterior beliefs after processing sensory information. Tenenbaum et al. [40] describe how many aspects of higher-level cognition can be explained through Bayesian inference, and make the argument how the brain must have some way of encoding prior distributions. The challenge for Bayesian brain theories has been in explaining how all this is implemented on the physical level in neural circuits and across all the synapses.

Some authors have presented Bayesian brain models [37, 41–43] where the axon output of a separate neuron is used to encode a separate point from the probability distribution or a separate statistical moment. In the latter case the distribution must take on density shape limitations. In all these models the representation for the probability distribution does not span all the synapses of the neural network, which is why the different authors state the same challenge of not being able to learn the synapse parameters for base representations directly from data.

By considering the proposed role of astrocytes a new Bayesian brain theory becomes possible, which addresses the above challenges: probability distributions of unconstrained density shapes can be encoded by ion wave mechanics, and an explicit Bayesian inference process is inherently bound between the distributions and all the synapses across many neurons in a micro-domain.

# 6   Conclusion

Existing information processing theories of glia are lacking perspectives for Marr's algorithmic level. Existing Bayesian brain theories are lacking perspectives for Marr's physical level. The proposed model establishes complementing relationships between these two sets of theories, allowing them to span all three levels.

Perhaps most interesting is that the model uniquely fits recent experimental results where obstructing astrocytes leads to deficiencies in learning new knowledge without affecting ability to recall existing knowledge. In future work we would like to find a way to quantify the actual $Ca^{2+}$ activity observed in astrocytes against the supposed Bayesian processes of the model.

# References

1. Bazargani, N., Attwell, D.: Astrocyte calcium signaling: the third wave. Nat. Neurosci. **19**, 182–189 (2016)
2. Han, X., Chen, M., Wang, F., Windrem, M., Wang, S., Shanz, S., Xu, Q., Oberheim, N.A., Bekar, L., Betstadt, S., Silva, A.J., Takano, T., Goldman, S.A., Nedergaard, M.: Forebrain engraftment by human glial progenitor cells enhances synaptic plasticity and learning in adult mice. Cell Stem Cell **12**, 342–353 (2013)
3. Lee, H.S., Ghotti, A., Pinto-Duarte, A., Wang, X., Dziewczapolski, G., Galimi, F., Huitron-Resendiz, S., Pia-Crespo, J.C., Roberts, A.J., Verma, I.M, Sejnowski, T.J., Heinemann, S.F.: Astrocytes contribute to gamma oscillations and recognition memory. Proc. Natl. Acad. Sci. **111**, E3343–E3352 (2014)
4. Miranda, M.I., Gonzlez-Cedillo, F.J., Daz-Muoz, M.: Intracellular calcium chelation and pharmacological SERCA inhibition of Ca2+ pump in the insular cortex differentially affect taste aversive memory formation and retrieval. Neurobiol. Learn. Mem. **96**, 192–198 (2011)

5. Han, J., Kesner, P., Metna-Laurent, M., Duan, T., Xu, L., Georges, F., Koehl, M., Abrous, D.N., Mendizabal-Zubiaga, J., Grandes, P.: Acute cannabinoids impair working memory through astroglial CB 1 receptor modulation of hippocampal LTD. Cell **148**, 1039–1050 (2012)

6. Marr, D.: Vision: A Computational Investigation into the Human Representation and Processing of Visual Information. Freeman and Company, San Francisco (1982)

7. Shigetomi, E., Patel, S., Khakh, B.S.: Probing the complexities of astrocyte calcium signaling. Trends Cell Biol. **26**, 300–312 (2016)

8. Haydon, P.G., Nedergaard, M.: How do astrocytes participate in neural plasticity? Cold Spring Harb. Perspect. Biol. **7**, a020438 (2015)

9. Oliveira, J.F., Sardinha, V.M., Guerra-Gomes, S., Araque, A., Sousa, N.: Do stars govern our actions? Astrocyte involvement in rodent behavior. Trends Neurosci. **38**, 535–549 (2015)

10. Clarke, L.E., Barres, B.A.: Emerging roles of astrocytes in neural circuit development. Nat. Rev. Neurosci. **14**, 311–321 (2013)

11. Perea, G., Sur, M., Araque, A.: Neuron-glia networks: integral gear of brain function. Front. Cell. Neurosci. **8**, 378 (2014)

12. Ma, D.K., Ming, G., Song, H.: Glial influences on neural stem cell development: cellular niches for adult neurogenesis. Curr. Opin. Neurobiol. **15**, 514–520 (2005)

13. Corty, M.M., Freeman, M.R.: Cell biology in neuroscience: architects in neural circuit design: glia control neuron numbers and connectivity. J. Cell Biol. **203**, 395–405 (2013)

14. Allen, N.J., Bennett, M.L., Foo, L.C., Wang, G.X., Chakraborty, C., Smith, S.J., Barres, B.A.: Astrocyte glypicans 4 and 6 promote formation of excitatory synapses via GluA1 AMPA receptors. Nature **486**, 410–414 (2012)

15. Haber, M., Murai, K.K.: Reshaping neuron glial communication at hippocampal synapses. Neuron Glia Biol. **2**, 59 (2005)

16. Nedergaard, M., Ransom, B., Goldman, S.A.: New roles for astrocytes: redefining the functional architecture of the brain. Trends Neurosci. **26**, 523–530 (2003)

17. Nakae, K., Ikegaya, Y., Ishikawa, T., Oba, S., Urakubo, H., Koyama, M., Ishii, S.: A statistical method of identifying interactions in neuron glia systems based on functional multicell Ca2+ imaging. PLoS Comput. Biol. **10**, e1003949 (2014)

18. Volterra, A., Magistretti, P.J., Haydon, P.G. (eds.): The Tripartite Synapse: Glia in Synaptic Transmission. Oxford University Press, New York (2002)

19. Araque, A., Parpura, V., Sanzgiri, R.P., Haydon, P.G.: Tripartite synapses: glia, the unacknowledged partner. Trends Neurosci. **22**, 208–215 (1999)

20. Araque, A., Carmignoto, G., Haydon, P.G.: Dynamic signaling between astrocytes and neurons. Ann. Rev. Physiol. **63**, 795–813 (2001)

21. Jahn, H.M., Scheller, A., Kirchhoff, F.: Genetic control of astrocyte function in neural circuits. Front. Cell. Neurosci. **9**, 310 (2015)

22. Fields, R.D., Araque, A., Johansen-Berg, H., Lim, S.S., Lynch, G., Nave, K.A., Nedergaard, M., Perez, R., Sejnowski, T., Wake, H.: Glial biology in learning and cognition. Neuroscientist **20**, 426–431 (2014)

23. McKenzie, I.A., Ohayon, D., Li, H., Paes de Faria, J., Emery, B., Tohyama, K., Richardson, W.D.: Motor skill learning requires active central myelination. Science **346**, 318–322 (2014)

24. Bray, N.: GLIA: oligodendrocytes rev up motor learning. Nat. Rev. Neurosci. **15**, 766–767 (2014)

25. Markham, J.A., Greenough, W.T.: Experience-driven brain plasticity: beyond the synapse. Neuron Glia Biol. **1**, 351 (2005)

26. Porto-Pazos, A.B., Veiguela, N., Mesejo, P., Navarrete, M., Alvarellos, A., Ibez, O., Pazos, A., Araque, A.: Artificial astrocytes improve neural network performance. PLoS ONE **6**, e19109 (2011)
27. Ikuta, C., Uwate, Y., Nishio, Y.: Performance and features of multi-layer perceptron with impulse glial network. In: The 2011 International Joint Conference on Neural Networks (IJCNN), pp. 2536–2541. IEEE Press, New York (2011)
28. Reid, D., Barrett-Baxendale, M.: Glial reservoir computing. In: Second UKSIM European Symposium on Computer Modeling and Simulation, EMS 2008, pp. 81–86. IEEE (2008)
29. De Pitt, M., Goldberg, M., Volman, V., Berry, H., Ben-Jacob, E.: Glutamate regulation of calcium and IP3 oscillating and pulsating dynamics in astrocytes. J. Biol. Phys. **35**, 383–411 (2009)
30. Wade, J.J., McDaid, L.J., Harkin, J., Crunelli, V., Kelso, J.A.S.: Bidirectional coupling between astrocytes and neurons mediates learning and dynamic coordination in the brain: a multiple modeling approach. PLoS ONE **6**, e29445 (2011)
31. Eddi, A., Sultan, E., Moukhtar, J., Fort, E., Rossi, M., Couder, Y.: Information stored in Faraday waves: the origin of a path memory. J. Fluid Mech. **674**, 433–463 (2011)
32. Goldman, T., Livne, A., Fineberg, J.: Acquisition of inertia by a moving crack. Phys. Rev. Lett. **104**, 114301 (2010)
33. Kroemer, H.: Quantum Mechanics: For Engineering, Materials Science, and Applied Physics. Prentice Hall, Englewood Cliffs (1994)
34. Gelman, A., Carlin, J.B., Stern, H.S., Rubin, D.B.: Bayesian Data Analysis, vol. 2. Chapman & Hall/CRC, Boca Raton (2014)
35. Guhaniyogi, R., Qamar, S., Dunson, D.B.: Bayesian conditional density filtering (2014). arXiv preprint: arXiv:1401.3632
36. Dimkovski, M., An, A.: A Bayesian model for canonical circuits in the neocortex for parallelized and incremental learning of symbol representations. Neurocomputing **149**, 1270–1279 (2015)
37. Knill, D.C., Pouget, A.: The Bayesian brain: the role of uncertainty in neural coding and computation. Trends Neurosci. **27**, 712–719 (2004)
38. Sharkov, E.A.: Breaking Ocean Waves: Geometry, Structure and Remote Sensing. Springer Science & Business Media, Heidelberg (2007)
39. Friston, K.: The free-energy principle: a unified brain theory? Nat. Rev. Neurosci. **11**, 127–138 (2010)
40. Tenenbaum, J.B., Kemp, C., Griffiths, T.L., Goodman, N.D.: How to grow a mind: statistics, structure, and abstraction. Science **331**, 1279–1285 (2011)
41. Deneve, S.: Bayesian inference in spiking neurons. In: Advances in Neural Information Processing Systems, vol. 17, pp. 353–360 (2005)
42. Rao, R.P.: Hierarchical Bayesian inference in networks of spiking neurons. In: Advances in Neural Information Processing Systems, pp. 1113–1120 (2004)
43. George, D., Hawkins, J.: Towards a mathematical theory of cortical micro-circuits. PLoS Comput. Biol. **5**, e1000532 (2009)

# An Automatic Neuron Tracing Method Based on Mean Shift and Minimum Spanning Tree

Zhijiang Wan[1,2(✉)], Yishan He[2], Ming Hao[2], Jian Yang[2,3,4],
and Ning Zhong[1,2,3,4,5]

[1] Department of Life Science and Informatics,
Maebashi Institute of Technology, Maebashi, Japan
wandndn@gmail.com
[2] International WIC Institute, Beijing University of Technology, Beijing, China
[3] Beijing Key Laboratory of MRI and Brain Informatics, Beijing, China
[4] Beijing International Collaboration Base on Brain Informatics and Wisdom
Services, Beijing, China
[5] Beijing Advanced Innovation Center for Future Internet Technology,
Beijing, China

**Abstract.** Digital reconstruction of 3D neuron structures is an important step toward reverse engineering the wiring and functions of a brain. Toward this end, the BigNeuron project bench testing was launched to gather a worldwide community to establish a Big Data resource and a set of the state-of-the-art of single neuron reconstruction algorithms for neuroscience community. As one of the communities, we contribute a Mean shift and Minimum Spanning Tree (M-MST) algorithm to trace single neuron morphology. In our experiment, we have successfully reconstructed 120 Drosophila neurons by using the M-MST algorithm and achieved relatively good difference scores compared with other four algorithms by using APP2 as a reference object.

## 1 Introduction

Understanding how the brain works from the angle of cognition and structure is undoubtedly one of the greatest challenges for modern science [1]. On the one hand, in order to develop algorithmic methods enlightened by cognition and speed up the development of computer technology, it is significant to learn the mechanism of thinking, induction and reasoning at human behavioral and brain region levels. On the other hand, acquiring knowledge of the morphological structure of brain nervous system at the molecular and cellular levels is also of particular importance. For understanding the morphological structure of brain nervous system deeply, the BigNeuron project [2] was launched to specially deal with the image processing problems exists in the deluge of complicated molecular and cellular microscopic images. The method of extracting the neuronal morphology from the image data can be called as neuron reconstruction or neuron tracing.

For neuron reconstruction methods, varieties of image processing theories based neuron tracing techniques have been proposed, such as fuzzy set [3], level set [4, 5], active contour model [6, 7], graph theory [8], and clustering [9, 10]. The BigNeuron

G.A. Ascoli et al. (Eds.): BIH 2016, LNAI 9919, pp. 34–41, 2016.
DOI: 10.1007/978-3-319-47103-7_4

project aims at gathering a worldwide community to define and advance the state-of-the-art of single neuron reconstruction by bench-testing as many varieties of automated neuron reconstruction methods as possible against as many neuron datasets as epossible following standardized data protocols. For example, the APP2 algorithm based on level set theory is the fastest tracing algorithm among the existing methods, the Micro-Optical Sectioning Tomography ray-shooting tracing (MOST) achieves a good result in terabytes 3D datasets of the whole mouse brain [11]. SIMPLE is a DT-based tracing approach and produces better reconstruction in dragonfly thoracic ganglia neuron images compared to several methods [12]. Additionally, other neuron reconstruction methods based on graph theory such as neuron tracing minimum spanning tree (N-MST for short), which is also a neuron tracing algorithm developed by one of the BigNeuron groups, also got reasonable reconstructions for several image datasets.

In this paper, we mainly focus on introducing our contribution to the BigNeuron project. Specifically, a neuron reconstruction method based on mean shift and minimum spanning tree (M-MST) algorithm is proposed to reconstruct the neuron images. The procedures of the M-MST algorithm are outlined and illustrated in Fig. 1. Firstly, input an original single neuron image (Fig. 1(a)) and use a certain voxel interval as step length to move the voxel to its local mean until convergence by mean shift algorithm. The voxel which is already located the peak in the density of local area is regarded as the node in the skeleton of neuron and is defined as marks which indicate a classification mark for other voxels. Notably, the marks and other voxels are collectively known as nodes in the following text. The Fig. 1(b) shows the marks extracted by mean shift algorithm in green. Secondly, because of the voxels in the neuron image will have radius property which is greater or equal then 1.0, the marks or other voxels might be covered within the area of other nodes. That situation is deemed as the repeat expression of neuron topology or over reconstruction. In response, we prune the marks or other voxels overlapped or covered by others by a node pruning method. The nodes after pruning (Fig. 1(c)) will be considered as the seeds and input into the MST to build the tree structure of neuron image. Thirdly, connect each pair of nodes and form an undirected graph. The weight of each edge in the graph can be regarded as the Euclidean distance of the corresponding two nodes. Based on the weights calculated, use the MST to find the minimum spanning tree in the graph and consider the tree as the final neuron reconstruction (Fig. 1(d)).

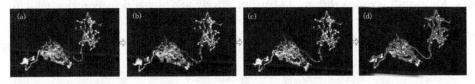

**Fig. 1.** The procedures of the M-MST algorithm. (a) An original neuron image. (b) The nodes in green color extracted by mean shift algorithm were located the peak in the density of local area and called as marks. (c) The red nodes mean the remaining nodes after pruning. (d) The final reconstruction result in red color is overlaid on the top of original neuron image. (Color figure online)

The paper is organized as follows. Firstly, the key steps of the M-MST algorithm were discussed. Secondly, the implementation and the availability of the algorithm were described. Thirdly, the experimental results between the M-MST and other algorithms on real neuron image data were presented, finally gave a brief discussion for the pros and cons and future work of the M-MST.

## 2 Method

### 2.1 Voxel Clustering Using Mean Shift Algorithm

For each voxel, we calculated the ratio of the number of background and foreground voxels surrounding it to determine whether it is a noise. Here, we set the threshold as 10 and define the voxel whose value is less then it as background and otherwise is foreground. The ratio of the number of background and foreground is set to be 0.3. In order to get an initial topological structure, mean shift algorithm is adopted to obtain a more detailed description of the neuronal tree since it always searches the direction of maximum increase in the density gradient. Those areas should be located in the center of the axon, soma or dendrite of neuron. In other words, mean shift starts at each voxel to iteratively estimate the local density gradient until locate the peak which can be interpreted as the convergence point that should be located in the centerlines of neuron skeleton. This is the mainly reason for selecting mean shift to finish the skeletonization step and hence get the preliminary neuronal topology.

The implementation of mean shift in this paper is interpreted as the following steps:

(1) For each voxel P in a 3D neuron image, assume a sphere region which centered at P and has a radius r, provide the weight W for every voxels located in the sphere area by

$$W = \exp(-\mathrm{sqrt}(2 * \mathrm{IS} + \mathrm{D})), \tag{1}$$

$$\mathrm{IS} = (\mathrm{I_{cur}} - \mathrm{I_{cen}})^2 \big/ I^2, \tag{2}$$

where D and IS mean the distance and the intensity similarity between the center node and the current node respectively, I equals 255.

(2) Mean shift involves shifting a kernel iteratively to a higher density region until to the centroid. We shift the current node using the Gaussian formula which is described as follow:

$$K(O_{cen} - O_{cur}) = \frac{1}{2\pi\delta^2} \exp(-C * \frac{|O_{cen} - O_{cur}|^2}{2\delta^2}), \tag{3}$$

where C is a scaling coefficient which is set to 0.1 and $\delta$ is standard deviation which is set to 1. $O_{cen}$ and $O_{cur}$ are the order number of center node and current node in the image.

(3) The order number $O_{new}$ of the new sphere center in region S is calculated by

$$O_{new} = \frac{\sum_s K(O_{cen} - O_{cur}) * W(O_{cur}) * O_{cur}}{\sum_s K(O_{cen} - O_{cur}) * W(O_{cur})}, \tag{4}$$

where $W(O_{cur})$ means the weight value of the current node in the region S.

## 2.2   Neuron Reconstruction Adopting MST Algorithm

After pruning the overlapped or covered nodes in the node set, we use the remaining nodes to reconstruct a tree structure in SWC format adopting the MST algorithm. Three steps are used to implement the MST and described as follow:

Firstly, we build an undirected graph by connecting each pair of nodes.

Secondly, the weight for each edge in the graph is the spatial distance between the corresponding two nodes. The calculation method of weight for the edge between each pair of nodes descripted as follow:

$$W = Dis(p_i, p_j), \tag{5}$$

where $p_i$ means the $i^{th}$ node ordered in the remaining node set, Dis() is the function to calculate the Euclidean distance between $p_i$ and $p_j$, W is the weight of the edge.

Thirdly, the weight for the edge of each pair of node can be formed as a diagonal matrix, which can be acted as the input of MST algorithm.

## 3   Experimental Results and Evaluation

In comparison with other three reconstruction algorithms, we selected APP2 as the reference object since the APP2 tracing algorithm is the fastest tracing algorithm among the existing methods and is reliable in generating tree shape morphology for neuron reconstructions to our best knowledge. We also calculated four difference scores of reconstruction produced by the other four reconstruction methods: M-MST, MOST, SIMPLE, N-MST. The four difference scores are called entire structure average, different structure average, percentage of different structure and max distance of neurons' nodes respectively. Correspondingly, the difference scores measure the overall average spatial divergence between two reconstructions, the spatial distance between different structures in two reconstruction, and the percentage of the neuron structure that noticeably varies in independent reconstruction, as well as the maximum distance to the nearest reconstruction elements compared with the reference algorithm. To make a fair comparison, the reported results of competing methods correspond to the default parameters used by respective plugins.

The histogram and boxplot are adopted to analyze and compare the performance between the four algorithms. Figure 2 shows the histogram of the four average difference-scores of four algorithms reconstruction compared with the APP2 reconstructions. Figure 3 shows the box plots of the four difference-scores for four

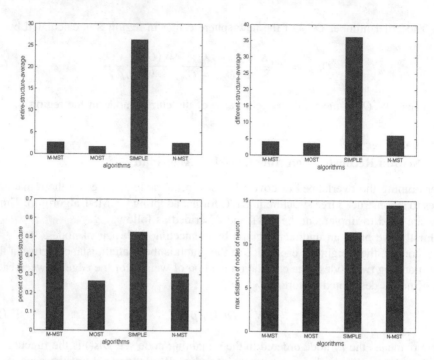

**Fig. 2.** The four average difference-scores of four algorithms reconstruction compared with the APP2 reconstructions of 120 Drosophila neuron images.

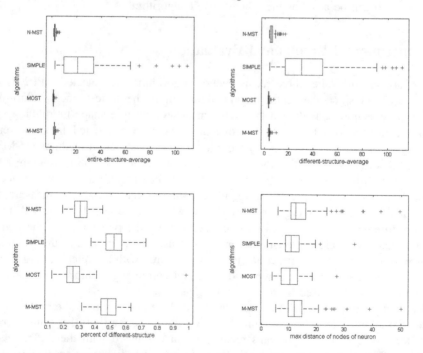

**Fig. 3.** Box plots of the four difference-scores for four algorithms of 120 neuron reconstructions obtained.

algorithms of 120 neuron reconstructions obtained by comparing with the APP2 reconstructions. As we can see, MOST achieves the best difference scores distribution for 120 reconstructions and the M-MST gets the relative good results. Comparing with N-MST, the entire structure average, the different structure average and the maximum distance of neurons' node of M_MST is higher which indicate the local reconstructions of M_MST is closer to the APP2 reconstruction. This result can be explained that benefiting from using mean shift algorithms to extract centroid of neuronal segments and form skeleton. The result of percentage of different structure of the M-MST is lower than N-MST probably due to the mean shift algorithm always keeps the nodes surround the local convergence point and do not generate the sufficient nodes to represent the whole topology. The same conclusions mentioned above can be got from the score distribution showed in Fig. 3. To sum up, compared with other three algorithms, although M_MST did not achieve the lowest difference scores, it still achieved relative good reconstructions referenced with APP2 reconstructions.

## 4  Discussion

In summary, the M-MST mainly adopts mean shift and the MST algorithm to reconstruct the neuron image. The reasons for using mean shift can be concluded in two aspects:

(1)  The mean shift is a clustering algorithm which possesses local convergence and can move and cluster each voxel to the nearest marks. We can segment the neuron image more elaborate based on every classification node set.

(2)  The marks which cannot move or shift one step by mean shift can be regarded as the centroid points of neuron segments. By observed, we find the most of centroid points located at the centerline of neuron which can also be considered as skeleton. Based on this, we can easily build a preliminary neuronal morphology by connect those points in SWC format.

As we know, the intensity variation of the neuron image has an influence on the reconstruction effect. For example, the APP2 algorithm got a less precise reconstruction if there are many image parts with low intensity. We call the image part with low intensity between two neuronal segments as the gap. However, due to the MST algorithm only considers the spatial information between each pair of nodes, the gap problem in the neuron image would never affect the reconstruction of the M-MST. The two nodes belonged to the minimum spanning tree will be built a paternity even if there is a gap between them. Additionally, the MST algorithm is initiative and easy to implement. Based on the node set extracted by mean shift algorithm, we can always build an undirected graph and extract a minimum spanning tree as the neuron reconstruction.

Comparing with the other three algorithms, although the M-MST got a relative good neuron reconstruction result, there are several limitations can be analyzed:

(1)  Although mean shift algorithm can always move each voxel to its local mean until automatically get the convergence points which can be regarded as the voxels in

the skeleton, it always keeps the nodes surround the local convergence point and do not generate the sufficient nodes to represent the whole topology.

(2) As mentioned above, the BigNeuron project aims at gathering the state-of-the-art of single neuron reconstruction by bench-testing as many varieties of automated neuron reconstruction methods as possible against as many neuron datasets as possible following standardized data protocols. In our experiment, we only bench test the M-MST against one kind of neuron image. The performance of reconstructing the other variety of images (especially the neuron image with low signal-noise ratio) will be further tested.

(3) Another limitation of the M-MST is the relatively high computational complexity. So far, the algorithm procedures with high computational complexity are proportional to the image size. For the former procedure, we can improve the performance of computer and adopt parallel computation framework to increase the image processing speed.

## 5 Conclusion

In this paper, we introduced an automatic neuron tracing method based on the M-MST algorithm. For the mean shift algorithm, it can move and cluster every foreground voxel to the nearest marks which are regarded as the centroid points of neuron segments. For the minimum spanning tree algorithm, not only it is initiative and easy to implement, but also it can build a paternity for the pair of nodes even if there is an image part with low intensity between them. Comparing with the other three algorithms, the M-MST got a relative good neuron reconstruction result.

**Acknowledgements.** This work was funded by National Basic Research Program of China (2014CB744600), International Science & Technology Cooperation Program of China (2013DFA32180), National Natural Science Foundation of China (61420106005, 61272345), and JSPS Grants-in-Aid for Scientific Research of Japan (26350994), and supported by Beijing Municipal Commission of Education, and Beijing Xuanwu Hospital.

## References

1. Meijering, E.: Neuron tracing in perspective. Cytom. A **77**, 693–704 (2010)
2. Peng, H., Meijering, E., Ascoli, G.A.: From DIADEM to BigNeuron. Neuroinformatics **13**, 259–260 (2015)
3. Pal, S.K.: Fuzzy sets in image processing and recognition. In: IEEE International Conference on Fuzzy Systems, San Diego, CA, pp. 119–126 (1992)
4. Malladi, R., Sethian, J.A.: Level set and fast marching methods in image processing and computer vision. In: International Conference on Image Processing, Lausanne, pp. 489–492 (1996)
5. Xiao, H., Peng, H.: APP2: automatic tracing of 3D neuron morphology based on hierarchical pruning of a gray-weighted image distance-tree. Bioinformatics **29**, 1448–1454 (2013)

6. Wang, Y., Narayanaswamy, A., Tsai, C.-L., Roysam, B.: A broadly applicable 3-D neuron tracing method based on open-curve snake. Neuroinformatics **9**, 193–217 (2011)
7. Cai, H., Xu, X., Lu, J.: Repulsive force based snake model to segment and track neuronal axon in 3D microscopy image stacks. NeuroImage **32**, 1608–1620 (2006)
8. Peng, H., Ruan, Z., Atasoy, D., Sternson, S.: Automatic reconstruction of 3D neuron structures using a graph-augmented deformable model. Bioinformatics **26**, 38–46 (2010)
9. Cai, H., Xu, X., Lu, J.: Using nonlinear diffusion and mean shift to detect and connect cross-selections of axons in 3D optical microscopy images. Med. Image Anal. **12**, 666–675 (2008)
10. Oliver, A., Munoz, X., Batlle, J., Pacheco, L., Freixenet, J.: Improving clustering algorithms for image segmentation using contour and region information. In: IEEE International Conference on Automation, Quality and Testing, Robotics, Cluj-Napoca, pp. 315–320 (2006)
11. Wu, J., He, Y., Yang, Z., Guo, C., Luo, Q., Zhou, W., Chen, S., Li, A., Xiong, B., Jiang, T., Gong, H.: 3D BrainCV: simultaneous visualization and analysis of cells and capillaries in a whole mouse brain with one-micron voxel resolution. NeuroImage **87**, 199–208 (2014)
12. Yang, J., et al.: A distance-field based automatic neuron tracing method. BMC Bioinform. **14**, 93 (2013)

# Graph Theoretic Compressive Sensing Approach for Classification of Global Neurophysiological States from Electroencephalography (EEG) Signals

Mohammad Samie Tootooni[1], Miaolin Fan[3],
Rajesh Sharma Sivasubramony[1], Chun-An Chou[3],
Vladimir Miskovic[2], and Prahalada K. Rao[4(✉)]

[1] Systems Science and Industrial Engineering Department,
State University of New York, Binghamton, NY, USA
[2] Psychology Department,
State University of New York, Binghamton, NY, USA
[3] Mechanical and Industrial Engineering Department,
Northeastern University, Boston, MA, USA
[4] Mechanical and Materials Engineering Department,
University of Nebraska-Lincoln, Lincoln, NE, USA
Rao@unl.edu

**Abstract.** We present a data fusion framework integrating graph theoretic and compressive sensing (CS) techniques to detect global neurophysiological states using high-resolution electroencephalography (EEG) recordings. Acute stress induction (and control procedures) were used to elicit distinct states of neurophysiological arousal. We recorded EEG signals (128 channels) from 50 participants under two different states: hand immersion in room temperature water (control condition) or in chilled ($\sim 3$ °C) water (stress condition). Thereafter, spectral graph theoretic Laplacian eigenvalues were extracted from these high-resolution EEG signals. Subsequently, the CS technique was applied for the classification of acute stress using the Laplacian eigenvalues as features. The proposed method was compared to a support vector machine (SVM) approach using conventional statistical features as inputs. Our results revealed that the proposed graph theoretic compressive sensing approach yielded better classification performance ($\sim 90$ % F-score) compared to SVM with statistical features ($\sim 50$ % F-Score). This finding indicates that the spectral graph theoretic compressive sensing approach presented in this work is capable of classifying global neurophysiological arousal with higher fidelity than conventional signal processing techniques.

**Keywords:** Graph theory · Compressive sensing · Laplacian eigenvalues · Electroencephalography · Stress · Classification

## 1 Introduction

Electroencephalography (EEG) is a neurophysiological method for non-invasively monitoring the large-scale electrical activity of the human brain. The objective of our work was to classify the global neurophysiological state of human subjects from

© Springer International Publishing AG 2016
G.A. Ascoli et al. (Eds.): BIH 2016, LNAI 9919, pp. 42–51, 2016.
DOI: 10.1007/978-3-319-47103-7_5

multichannel EEG signals using a novel spectral graph theoretic compressive sensing approach.

Specifically, we wished to use the raw, time domain EEG signals in order to discriminate brain electrical signals collected during either an acute stress induction period or an appropriate, non-stressful comparison condition. Detecting stress using non-invasive physiological sensing can serve as a critical indicator of the onset of fatigue in mission-critical human activity, such as hazardous cargo trucking, air traffic control and railroad operation, to name a few examples. Thus, being able to detect stress from recordings of ongoing brain activity would have clear real-world applications.

In this context, the real-time monitoring of high-resolution EEG signals with compressive sensing (CS) has attracted considerable attention in recent years. CS is an $\ell_1$-norm regularization-based signal compression and reconstruction approach that provides a sparse representation of the information in the original signal or image. Previous studies have shown the practical value of CS in EEG monitoring or brain computer interface systems for addressing problems, such as signal reconstruction and power consumption [1–3]. CS yields a more efficient representation, particularly with multi-channel EEG systems, of the original signal with a relatively smaller number of projected components for information reconstruction compared to signal reconstruction techniques. This feature of CS allows for a lower sampling rate than the Nyquist rate without losing information in the original signals.

In previous literature, CS was applied as a signal reconstruction technique to multi-channel EEG signals based on various dictionaries, e.g. Gabor frame [1] or Slepian basis function [2]. Classification algorithms, i.e. Block sparse Bayesian learning, were performed on the reconstructed signals and showed that the CS-based compression was power-saving and effective compared to conventional transformation approaches, such as wavelets [4]. A review of CS applications to bioelectric signal processing is presented in [5].

The complexity of bio-sensor data arises from nonstationarity in the time domain [6], nonlinearity and quasi-periodicity in state-space [7], and intermittency [8]. Furthermore, the low signal to noise ratio (S/N), autocorrelation within and cross-correlation between sensor data, and the interactions across multiple neurological conditions [9] are other factors that impede the use of conventional statistical features for analysis of bio-sensor [10, 11].

Graph theory is an approach whereby multi-dimensional signals can be fused. The Laplacian eigenvalues of a signal represented in graph space is used as input features for classification. We applied CS using these features as representations of high-resolution, continuous EEG signals to classify the signal patterns recorded during acute stress versus those recorded during an appropriate control condition. Figure 1 depicts a five second segment of the EEG time series (from a single electrode) recorded from two human subjects serving in different experimental conditions.

The rest of this paper is organized as follows; Sect. 2 explains the graph representation of EEG signal and the Laplacian eigen-spectra extraction. It also describes the acute stress experiments. Section 3 presents the results and compares it with both graph-based SVM and conventional methods using statistical features. Finally, Sect. 4 summarizes the conclusions and suggests avenues for future research.

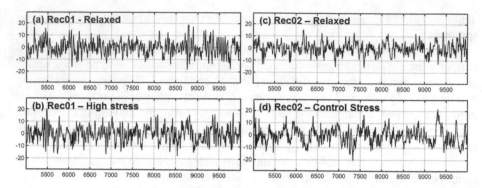

**Fig. 1.** Five second EEG fragment (single electrode) is depicted (a) when the first subject is relaxed; and (b) for the same subject during acute stress induction. Similarly, (c) and (d) depict EEG signals recorded from a different experimental subject, while relaxing, and during a control condition (hand immersion in room temperature water), respectively.

## 2  Methodology

In this section, we present our proposed approach which has two phases. First, the multi-channel EEG sensors will be fused using spectral graph theory and Laplacian eigenvalues will be extracted from the fused signals. In the second phase, the neuro-physiological states will be classified using CS with the Laplacian eigenvalues as inputs. The proposed methodology is schematically depicted in Fig. 2.

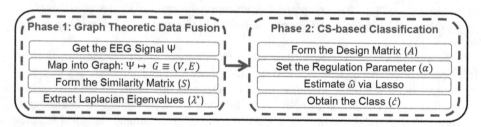

**Fig. 2.** The proposed graph theoretic compressive sensing classification approach

### 2.1  Phase 1 – Data Fusion with Graph Representation of EEG Signals

Let us consider matrix $\Psi \in \mathbb{R}^{q \times d}$ as a recorded EEG signal in which $q$ is the length of the signal and $d$ is number of EEG channels (in our practical case, $d = 128$ sensors and $q = 500$ data points ($\sim 1$ s). See Sects. 2.3 and 2.4).

$$
\Psi = \begin{bmatrix} \psi_1^1 & \cdots & \psi_1^d \\ \vdots & \ddots & \vdots \\ \psi_q^1 & \cdots & \psi_q^d \end{bmatrix}
$$

In this signal *window*, each row represents voltage fluctuation recorded by all $d$ sensors at a time instant. It is assumed that all sensors have equal recording rate (sampling rate). Choosing $q$ (window length) is a heuristic choice; it should not be either too large, since it increases the computational time, or too short, else the window is not representative of the whole signal.

A kernel function ($\Omega$) is chosen to capture the distance between each pair of rows $\psi_i, \psi_j \in \mathbb{R}^{1 \times d}$ of the matrix $\Psi$. In this paper, Gaussian kernel function is utilized to get the pairwise comparison matrix $\Upsilon$ (Eqs. (1) and (2)); where $\sigma^2$ is the total variance of the pairwise Euclidean distance matrix. A threshold function ($\Theta$) is then applied on $\Upsilon$ (Eq. (3)). This threshold is set as the average of all element of matrix $\Upsilon$. Rao *et al.* have discussed on setting the threshold value ($r$) [12]. A similarity matrix ($S$) is then acquired (Eq. (4)) to represent the corresponding unweighted and undirected network graph for matrix $\Psi$.

$$w_{ij} = \Omega(\psi_i, \psi_j) = e^{-\left(\frac{\|\psi_i - \psi_j\|^2}{\sigma^2}\right)} \; \forall\, i,j \in (1 \cdots q) \tag{1}$$

$$\Upsilon^{q \times q} = [w_{ij}] \tag{2}$$

$$\Theta(w_{ij}) = w_{ij} = \begin{cases} 1, & w_{ij} \le r \\ 0. & w_{ij} > r \end{cases} \tag{3}$$

$$S^{q \times q} = [w_{ij}] \tag{4}$$

The degree vector ($deg_i$) is formed then by row-wise summation of $w_{ij}$ as shown in Eq. (5) and by Eq. (6), it transforms into a diagonal matrix called *Degree Matrix* ($D$). Finally Eqs. (7) and (8) denote the formation of Laplacian matrix ($L$) and the normalized Laplacian matrix ($\mathcal{L}$), respectively.

$$deg_i = \sum_{j=1}^{j=q} w_{ij} \, \forall\, i,j \in (1 \cdots q) \tag{5}$$

$$D^{q \times q} = [d_{ij}] = \begin{cases} deg_i. & i = j \\ 0. & i \neq j \end{cases} \tag{6}$$

$$L^{q \times q} = D - S \tag{7}$$

$$\mathcal{L}^{q \times q} = D^{-\frac{1}{2}} \times L \times D^{-\frac{1}{2}} \tag{8}$$

$$\mathcal{L}v = \lambda^* v \tag{9}$$

In Eq. (9), $v \in \mathbb{R}^{q \times q}$ are the Laplacian eigenvectors; the Laplacian eigenvalues are indicated as $\lambda^* \in \mathbb{R}^{q \times q}$.

## 2.2    Phase 2 – Laplacian Eigen Compressive Sensing Classification

The aim of this phase is to classify the neurophysiological state of the subject using compressive sensing (CS) based on Laplacian eigenvalues $\lambda^*$ from phase 1 (Eq. (9)) as input features. We note that CS is a supervised learning technique, in other words, we will define *a priori* classes from offline sensor signals.

In this context, consider $A\omega = y$ to be an underdetermined system of equation with $N$ unknowns and $m$ equations. Matrix $A$ is referred as the training matrix which consists of Laplacian eigenvalues obtained from known-state EEG signal for each class. Where class refers to the neurophysiological state of the subject; in this case either relaxed vs. stressed. For instance, for a $C$-class classification problem, this matrix is designed as $A = [A_1, A_2, \ldots, A_C]$.

Zhan *et al.* [13] showed the first and last few eigenvalues have the highest variability among all Laplacian eigenvalues by analyzing their *relative deviation*. Accordingly in our paper, the first [Starting from the second eigenvalue since the first Laplacian eigenvalue is always zero $(\lambda_1 = 0)$] $m/2$ and the last $m/2$ of eigenvalues are chosen. We denote $\Lambda \in \mathbb{R}^{m \times 1}$ as the chosen eigenvalue vector for each window.

A *sample* vector $\bar{\Lambda} \in \mathbb{R}^{m \times 1}$ is then defined as average of $k$ randomly chosen eigenvalue vectors $(\Lambda)$ from each class. Although this averaging reduces the number of available samples for each class, it helps to increase the reliability of the training matrix $(A)$. Suppose we use $n$ sample vector to train the classification algorithm in each class. Therefore, a sample vectors is denoted by $\bar{\Lambda}_{j,c}$ where $c \in \{1, \ldots, C\}$ and $j \in \{1, \ldots, n\}$ are the class and sample indices, respectively. Ergo, the training matrix $(A \in \mathbb{R}^{m \times N})$ is designed as Eq. (10) where $N = n * C$.

$$A = \left[ \left[ \bar{\Lambda}_{1,1} \quad \ldots \quad \bar{\Lambda}_{n,1} \right] \left[ \bar{\Lambda}_{1,2} \quad \ldots \quad \bar{\Lambda}_{n,2} \right] \ldots \left[ \bar{\Lambda}_{1,C} \quad \ldots \quad \bar{\Lambda}_{n,C} \right] \right] \tag{10}$$

Also, measurement vector $Y \in \mathbb{R}^{m \times 1}$ represents the testing (new arrived information) set. This set is basically the average Laplacian eigenvalue vector $(\bar{\Lambda})$ extracted from the incoming EEG signal. Our aim is to find out unknown vector $\omega \in \mathbb{R}^{N \times 1}$ using compressive sensing to solve the linear system of equations mentioned $A\omega = y$ and eventually, to determine the class label of the incoming signal. Thereafter, an $\ell_0$-minimization problem should be formulated as Eq. (11). Equation (12) replaces it with its corresponding $\ell_1$-minimization problem [14]. To approximate a sparse solution, LASSO (Least Absolute Shrinkage and Selection Operator) algorithm is applied as shown in Eq. (13); where $\alpha$ is the regulation parameter for the LASSO algorithm. These concepts are clarified in detail in [15–18].

$$minimize \, \|\omega\|_0 \quad subject \, to \, A\omega = y \tag{11}$$

$$minimize \, \|\omega\|_1 \quad subject \, to \, A\omega = y \tag{12}$$

$$\hat{\omega} = \underset{\omega}{argmin} \, \alpha\|\omega\|_1 + \|Y - A\omega\|_2 \tag{13}$$

$$\acute{c} = \underset{c}{\operatorname{argmin}} A\delta_c(\hat{\omega}) - Y \tag{14}$$

vector $\hat{\omega} = [\hat{\omega}_1, \hat{\omega}_2, \ldots, \hat{\omega}_C]^T$ is obtained from Eq. (13) and eventually, Eq. (14) determines the class index of the new-arriving data where $\delta_c(\hat{\omega}) = [0^T, \ldots, \hat{\omega}_c^T, \ldots, 0^T]^T$.

## 2.3  Data Acquisition and Processing

We used a 128-channel EEG sensor network by Electrical Geodesics, Inc. (EGI), (HydroCel Geodesic Sensor Net) to collect the resting-state EEG data with subjects keeping their eyes open in two experiments with a sampling rate of 1 kHz and Net Station 4.5.6 software. In the first experiment (dataset 1), the resting-state EEG was recorded respectively from a *stress* condition of two male subjects who were instructed to place their hand into ice water (0–3 °C) and a pre-stimulus phase (*relaxed* condition). The length of EEG recording for each state was 2 min. In the second experiment (Dataset 2), we extended the study to 49 participants who were randomly assigned to either an acute stress or a comparison condition, where the ice water was replaced by lukewarm water. However, the subjects were not informed beforehand about which treatment they were assigned. Some participants in acute stress conditions do not have full length (2 min) recordings since they were unable to maintain their hand in the cold water. Furthermore, 1-min EEG recordings from *relaxed* condition was also collected.

The EEG recordings were down-sampled to 500 Hz for reducing the computational cost in the data analysis. After removing the facial sensors, a spatial principal component analysis (sPCA) was applied for the artifact correction, with 98 % of total variance explained. Furthermore, a reduced-rank independent component analysis (ICA) was performed to extract the same number of components as in sPCA. Finally, a binary classification on recorded EEG signals is performed to detect whether the participant is under stress in a within-participant manner.

## 2.4  Classification and Verification

When applying the Laplacian CS classification algorithm to the two datasets, the window size is chosen to be 1 s ($q = 500$), the number of features are $m = 20$, and the sample size is set to be $k = 5$ for the first dataset and $k = 3$ for the second dataset[1]. Among all the samples, we randomly allocate 60 % to training set which forms the design matrix ($A$). 30 % is randomly specified to validation set, which is used to find obtain the LASSO regularization parameter. An enumerative heuristic approach is applied to find a value which minimizes the overall classification error of the validation set. Finally, we use the remaining 10 % to evaluate the classification performance. Beside the proposed algorithm, to verify the capability of compressive sensing

---

[1] Due to lower length of available recorded signal for *Relaxed* class.

approach, the Laplacian eigen-spectra extracted from EEG signals are used in a Support Vector Machine with linear kernel function (LSVM).

To further verify the applicability of graph theoretic Laplacian eigenvalues in classification of EEG signals, we applied the CS and the SVM with the conventional statistical features, including 6 main chosen features: mean, median, standard deviation, kurtosis, skewness, and interquartile range of each signal *window*. However, having several channels in recorded EEG signals result in a large number of features (in our practical case $d = 128$, which results in $128 * 6 = 768$ features for each window) which intensely increases the computational time. Therefore, to make it comparable to other algorithms, we applied the ICA method on the acquired statistical features and chose the first $m$ independent components.

Moreover, to avoid bias due to random partition of training and test sets in classification, each Laplacian-based algorithm is run 20 times; and each statistical feature-based algorithm is run 10 times.

# 3   Results

In this section, we present the results of applying the proposed binary classification algorithm. To assess classification performance, we use a confusion matrix with F-score as the evaluation criterion to compare classification performances of selected algorithms $(F - score = 2 * (Precision.Recall)/(Precision + Recall))$ [19]. It should be noted that if either one of *precision* and *recall* does not exist, consequently, the F-score cannot be calculated which is shown as *NaN*.

## 3.1   Dataset 1

Table 1 shows the result confusion matrix for all discussed classification approaches. As shown in the table, the proposed graph theoretic CS approach has significantly higher F-score than graph theoretic SVM. Besides that, both Graph theoretic based approaches dominate the approaches based on conventional statistics. This result

**Table 1.** Confusion matrices for classification of the EEG signals. All numbers are reported as percentage. The two classes are *Relaxed* (Rel.) and *Stressed* (Str.) conditions.

| Confusion matrix | | Classifier | Laplacian eigenvalues | | | Conventional statistics | | |
|---|---|---|---|---|---|---|---|---|
| | | | Predicted | | Recall | Predicted | | Recall |
| | | | Rel. | Str. | | Rel. | Str. | |
| Actual | Rel. | CS (Proposed) | 85.0 | 15.0 | **85.0** | 73.3 | 26.7 | **73.3** |
| | Str. | | 5.0 | 95.0 | **95.0** | 70.0 | 30.0 | **30.0** |
| Precision | | | **94.4** | **86.4** | ***F* = 90.20** | 51.2 | 52.9 | ***F* = 51.86** |
| Actual | Rel. | SVM | 90.0 | 10.0 | **90.0** | 80.0 | 20.0 | **80.0** |
| | Str. | | 33.3 | 66.7 | **66.7** | 80.0 | 20.0 | **20.0** |
| Precision | | | **73.0** | **87.0** | ***F* = 79.14** | 50.0 | 50.0 | ***F* = 50.00** |

indicates that the proposed graph theoretic compressive sensing approach has higher fidelity compare to other conventional methods.

## 3.2   Dataset 2

In this dataset, there were many runs that F-score was not acquirable (the precision did not exist). Therefore, we introduced a metric, *Number of Success*, as number of the Runs that the F-score is estimable for each subject. This metric provides an appropriate criterion for evaluating the algorithms' performance. Indeed before comparing the average F-score, the *Success Rate* should be considered to compare the feasibility of the classification algorithms (*Success Rate* = (*Number of Success*)/(*Number of Runs*)).

Entirely 49 subjects participated in the second experiment, 17 of which did not have enough recorded signal to be considered in the analysis. Therefore, in this dataset there are 20 participants treated with warm water and 12 participants underwent cold water immersion. Figure 3 shows the performance (F-score and *Number of Successes*) of the graph theoretic features (Fig. 3(a) and (b)) as well as the statistical features (Fig. 3(c) and (d)). In this figure, the line charts represent the *number of success* and the bars show the average of available F-scores for each classification technique. As Fig. 3 (c) and (d) show, SVM with statistical features (SVM-ST) were unable to classify the state of the incoming signal almost in all runs; and the CS classifier with statistical (CS-ST) features had poor classification result as well as low success rate compare with CS based on graph theoretic features (CS-GT). This shows that using graph theoretic features for signal classification purposes is preferred over conventional statistics. We refer to the complex structure of EEG data, discussed in the Sect. 1, as one reason to make the statistical feature-based algorithms unable to capture the dynamics.

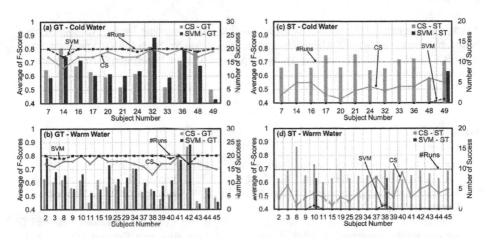

**Fig. 3.** Performance of the classifiers to detect stress for different participant. Bars show the average F-score in primary vertical axes; and lines represent the number of success in the secondary vertical axes. CS and SVM stand for Compressive Sensing and Support Vector Machine classifiers, respectively. Also GT and ST are representors of features: Graph Theoretic and Statistical features, correspondingly.

Also, Fig. 3(a) and (b) show the performance of the two graph theoretic classifiers for each participant, separately. The CS has a relatively lower F-score in warm water classification (Fig. 3(b)) compared to the cold water classification (acute stress, Fig. 3 (a)). This means that the proposed CS-GT was able to distinguish the acute stress easier than the control stress from the *relaxed* condition. Although the SVM has higher success rate in both groups of participants, the GT-CS has comparable F-score and success rate for detection of acute stress states (Fig. 3(a)). However, the SVM is highly sensitive to the size of the training and testing sets, and its performance is dependent on choosing the right kernel function and tuning parameters [20, 21]. In contrast, there is only LASSO regularization parameter to be set in the proposed CS-GT algorithm. It can thus be used to classify the neurophysiological signals in real-time with low computational load. Nonetheless, both CS and SVM with graph theoretic quantifiers outperformed the statistical features based approaches.

## 4  Conclusion

In this paper we applied a graph-based data fusion compressive sensing approach for high-dimensional signal classification. Two continuous EEG datasets we collected in an acute stress experiment to test the proposed graph-based compressive sensing (CS) approach. The validation procedure has two stages; first with graph-based SVM, and then, with other conventional-based methods. It was found that graph-based classifiers features were able to demarcate distinct states of neurophysiological arousal with higher fidelity compared to conventional statistical methods. The authors suggest two avenues for future research; using graph-theoretic features in other multi-class classification algorithms, and applying these features for prediction of high-stress conditions.

**Acknowledgements.** This research is made possible due to funding by the National Science Foundation under the Service, Manufacturing, and Operation Research (SMOR) program (grant number CMMI – 1538059), and the Transdisciplinary Area of Excellence (TAE) exploratory research grant by Binghamton University.

## References

1. Aviyente, S.: Compressed sensing framework for EEG compression (2007)
2. Senay, S., Chaparro, L.F., Sun, M., Sclabassi, R.J.: Compressive sensing and random filtering of EEG signals using Slepian basis. In: 16th European 2008 Signal Processing Conference, pp. 1–5. IEEE (2008)
3. Abdulghani, A.M., Casson, A.J., Rodriguez-Villegas, E.: Compressive sensing scalp EEG signals: implementations and practical performance. Med. Biol. Eng. Comput. **50**(11), 1137–1145 (2012)
4. Liu, B., Zhang, Z., Xu, G., Fan, H., Fu, Q.: Energy efficient telemonitoring of physiological signals via compressed sensing: a fast algorithm and power consumption evaluation. Biomed. Sig. Process. Control **11**, 80–88 (2014)

5. Craven, D., McGinley, B., Kilmartin, L., Glavin, M., Jones, E.: Compressed sensing for bioelectric signals: a review. IEEE J. Biomed. Health Inform. **19**(2), 529–540 (2015)
6. Kaplan, A.Y., Fingelkurts, A.A., Fingelkurts, A.A., Borisov, S.V., Darkhovsky, B.S.: Nonstationary nature of the brain activity as revealed by EEG/MEG: methodological, practical and conceptual challenges. Sig. Process. **85**(11), 2190–2212 (2005)
7. Pereda, E., Quiroga, R.Q., Bhattacharya, J.: Nonlinear multivariate analysis of neurophysiological signals. Progress Neurobiol. **77**(1), 1–37 (2005)
8. Siegel, M., Donner, T.H., Engel, A.K.: Spectral fingerprints of large-scale neuronal interactions. Nat. Rev. Neurosci. **13**(2), 121–134 (2012)
9. Hall, D.L., Llinas, J.: An introduction to multisensor data fusion. Proc. IEEE **85**(1), 6–23 (1997)
10. Stam, C.J.: Nonlinear dynamical analysis of EEG and MEG: review of an emerging field. Clin. Neurophysiol. **116**(10), 2266–2301 (2005)
11. Stam, C.J., Breakspear, M., van Walsum, A.M.V.C., van Dijk, B.W.: Nonlinear synchronization in EEG and whole-head MEG recordings of healthy subjects. Hum. Brain Mapp. **19**(2), 63–78 (2003)
12. Rao, P.K., Kong, Z., Duty, C.E., Smith, R.J., Kunc, V., Love, L.J.: Assessment of dimensional integrity and spatial defect localization in additive manufacturing using spectral graph theory. J. Manuf. Sci. Eng. **138**(5), 051007 (2016)
13. Zhan, C., Chen, G., Yeung, L.F.: On the distributions of Laplacian eigenvalues versus node degrees in complex networks. Phys. A: Stat. Mech. Appl. **389**(8), 1779–1788 (2010)
14. Chen, S.S., Donoho, D.L., Saunders, M.A.: Atomic decomposition by basis pursuit. SIAM Rev. **43**(1), 129–159 (2001)
15. Boche, H., Calderbank, R., Kutyniok, G., Vybíral, J.: Compressed Sensing and its Applications. Springer, Berlin (2015)
16. Foucart, S., Rauhut, H.: A mathematical introduction to compressive sensing, vol. 1, 3. Springer, Berlin (2013)
17. Qaisar, S., Bilal, R.M., Iqbal, W., Naureen, M., Lee, S.: Compressive sensing: from theory to applications, a survey. J. Commun. Netw. **15**(5), 443–456 (2013)
18. Bastani, K., Rao, P.K., Kong, Z.: An online sparse estimation-based classification approach for real-time monitoring in advanced manufacturing processes from heterogeneous sensor data. IIE Trans. **48**(7), 579–598 (2016)
19. Van Rijsbergen, C.: Information retrieval. Department of Computer Science, University of Glasgow (1979). citeseer.ist.psu.edu/vanrijsbergen79information.html
20. Suykens, J.A.: Advances in Learning Theory: Methods, Models, and Applications, vol. 190. IOS Press, Amsterdam (2003)
21. Burges, C.J.: A tutorial on support vector machines for pattern recognition. Data Min. Knowl. Disc. **2**(2), 121–167 (1998)

# Fast Marching Spanning Tree: An Automatic Neuron Reconstruction Method

Ming Hao[1,2,3](✉), Jian Yang[1,2,3,4](✉), Xiaoyang Liu[1,2,3,4], Zhijiang Wan[4,5], and Ning Zhong[1,2,3,4,5]

[1] International WIC Institute, Beijing University of Technology, Beijing, China
15201586114@emails.bjut.edu.cn, jianyang@bjut.edu.cn
[2] Beijing Key Laboratory of MRI and Brain Informatics, Beijing, China
[3] Beijing International Collaboration Base on Brain Informatics and Wisdom Services, Beijing, China
[4] Beijing Advanced Innovation Center for Future Internet Technology, Beijing, China
[5] Department of Life Science and Informatics, Maebashi Institute of Technology, Maebashi, Japan

**Abstract.** Neuron reconstruction is an important technique in computational neuroscience. There are many neuron reconstruction algorithms, but few can generate robust result, especially when a 3D microscopic image has low single-to-noise ratio. In this paper we propose a neuron reconstruction algorithm called fast marching spanning tree (FMST), which is based on minimum spanning tree method (MST) and can improve the performance of MST. The contributions of the proposed method are as follows. Firstly, the Euclidean distance weights of edges in MST is improved to be more reasonable. Secondly, the strategy of pruning nodes is updated. Thirdly, separate branches can be merged for broken neurons. FMST and several other reconstruction methods were implemented on the 120 confocal images of single neurons in the Drosophila brain downloaded from the flycircuit database. The performance of FMST is better than some existing methods for some neurons. So it is a potentially practicable neuron construction algorithm. But its performance on some neurons is not good enough and the proposed method still needs to be improved further.

**Keywords:** Neuron reconstruction · Neuron morphology · Minimum spanning tree

## 1 Introduction

With the development of modern scientific technology, understanding of brains becomes possible and attaches never seen before importance. For this purpose, the US BRAIN and the European Human Brain Project were launched to promote marshalling a vast amount of data and tools. One of the fundamental problem among these projects is that neuronal morphologies must be seamlessly reconstructed and aggregated on scales up to the whole rodent brain. Meanwhile

© Springer International Publishing AG 2016
G.A. Ascoli et al. (Eds.): BIH 2016, LNAI 9919, pp. 52–60, 2016.
DOI: 10.1007/978-3-319-47103-7_6

3D reconstruction of complex neuron morphology from light microscopic images is an important technique for computational neuroscience [1]. An important competition DIADEM (http://diademchallenge.org/) made neuron reconstruction becoming more popular. For better understanding the detailed morphology of neurons, 3D images of neurons are often acquired in high resolution, resulting in large volume datasets, which have posed substantial challenges in efficient and accurate reconstruction of complicated neuron Morphology [2].

Actually, in the past few decades, scientists have proposed many methods to solve the neuron reconstruction problem. The manual reconstruction of a neuron's morphology has been in practice for one century now since the time of Ramóy Cajal. Today, the technique has evolved such that researchers can quantitatively trace neuron morphologies in 3D with the help of computers [3]. A lot of automatic neuron tracing methods have been developed. In these algorithms, different methods have different strategies and models. App (All-path pruning) is a pruning over-complete neuron-trees method [4]. It firstly constructs an initial over-reconstruction by tracing the geodesic shortest path from the seed location to all possible destination voxels/pixels location in an image. Then it simplifies the entire reconstruction without compromising its connectedness by pruning the redundant structural elements. App2 is a new version of the APP algorithm [1]. The most important idea hidden in it is to prune an initial reconstruction tree of a neuron's morphology using a long-segment-first hierarchical procedure instead of the original termini-first-search process in APP. SimpleTracing is a DT-based method. It uses DF-Tracing to executes a coupled distance-field (DF) algorithm on the extracted foreground neurite signal and reconstructs the neuron morphology automatically [5]. Micro-Optical Sectioning Tomography (Most) ray-shooting tracing is a method based on the simulation of blood flow from initial seeds to compute centerlines and their corresponding radii [6]. All the initial seeds in Most are localized in the centroids of connected regions among evenly spaced 2D binaries images, and Most implements a voxel scooping algorithm to trace the blood vessels. There are many other 3D reconstruction algorithms for automated neuron tracing, such as Open-Curve Snake [7], graph-augmented deformable model [8], ray casting [9], tube-fitting model [10], and so on.

Last year, a project named BigNeuron was launched to bench-test existing algorithms on big dataset [11,12]. The project aims to both standardizing the methods to generate high quality and consistent data, and mobilizing the reconstruction community to generate interest in solving these complex and interesting algorithmic problems (http://alleninstitute.org/bigneuron/). It also enables anyone who wants to contribute a new reconstruction algorithm to compare it with existing ones, and to test it on the large set of image slices provided. The technical platform of BigNeuron is built upon the Vaa3D software (http://vaa3d. org) [13,14], an open-source visualization and analysis software suite created and maintained by Janelia Research Campus of Howard Hughes Medical Institute and the Allen Institute for Brain Science [15]. The BigNeuron has run a series of hackathons (http://alleninstitute.org/bigneuron/hackathons-workshops/) to help developers work with image reconstruction methods to make their algorithms available on the Vaa3D platform. Currently, BigNeuron incorporates around 30 reconstruction algorithms that can be applied to a set of 30,000+ multi-dimensional image stacks. This has so far resulted in more than one million reconstructed neurons from different species. For mouse and other mammal brains, there are hundreds of increasingly high-quality reconstructions [15].

The Bigneuron collected a neuron tracing algorithm called minimum spanning tree method (MST) as a plugin of Vaa3D. MST generates an initial reconstruction that covers all the potential signals of a neuron in a 3D image by minimum spanning tree method. Then it uses an optimal pruning procedure to remove the majority of spurs in the over-reconstruction to produce a final succinct representation of the neuron, which has a maximum coverage of all neuron signals. Concretely, MST method consists of four steps: getting foreground pixels through a threshold value, generating an initial reconstruction by minimum spanning tree method, using GD-tracing to get details of the neuron reconstruction, and pruning segments undetected by GD-tracing. In MST, one node is more likely to connect to nearer nodes but not farer nodes. But a reconstruction generated by MST may have some breakpoints due to pixels with poor quality. Sometimes, MST even can not get the whole skeleton of a neuron.

Fast marching (FM) algorithm is an essentially region-growing scheme, and is a key technique to extract the skeleton of neuron topology in many neuron tracing methods [16]. For example, in APP2, both grey-weighted distance transformation (GWDT) and the initial neuron reconstruction are implemented in the FM framework. By the way, FM method is so essentially that it makes the tracing method become much faster. FM helps APP2 to be one of the fastest method so far.

In this paper, we propose an automatic neuron reconstruction algorithm called fast marching spanning tree (FMST), which based on MST method. FMST follows the basic framework of MST, however, it enhances the key components of the original method. Our new method consists of four components: generating an over-reconstruction of a neuron, pruning redundant nodes, getting a reconstruction by minimum spanning tree, and recreate a tree. Compared with MST, the improvement of FMST includes the following two aspects. One is the changing of the coverage while pruning nodes. This is based on the fact that there is unnecessary to add so many points to the reconstruction and only the skeleton of a neuron is needed. Another is the merging of small trees reconstructed by MST. For more than one trees generated by MST, FMST recreates them as a tree by the minimum spanning tree method. By this means, small trees are connected, and the reconstruction of neuron has no breakpoints.

The paper is organized as follows. Section 2 discusses the important steps of FMST algorithm. Section 3 presents the experimental results on 120 Drosophila neurons dataset and comparisons between FMST and other algorithms. Finally, Sect. 4 gives a brief concluding and some release discussion.

# 2  Methods

## 2.1  Generating an Over-Reconstruction of a Neuron

We only focus on the reconstruction of a single neuron's morphology from a 3D image. To construct an over-reconstruction of a neuron, all foreground pixels must be identified firstly. We find all pixels with intensity larger than 30, calculate the mean intensity value of these pixels, and take pixels with intensity larger than the mean value as foreground pixels. A foreground pixel is connected to all its foreground neighbors, i.e., those neighbors who are foreground pixels. Following this rule, a graph G is constructed on all foreground pixels.

## 2.2  Implementing Fast Marching Method

The fast marching (FM) algorithm is essentially a region growing scheme and plays an important role in FMST. Both the calculation of the nodes' radii and weights of edges are implemented in FM framework. Denote the target node be *know*, its neighbors are set as *neighbor*, and others are set as *far*. FM consists of two steps. Firstly, calculate the $T$ value between all nodes in the *neighbor* set and the *know* set. Then, find the node $P$ in the *neighbor* set with minimum $T$ value to the *know* set, and extract it to *know* set. For the neighbor point $Q$ of $P$, if $Q$ in the *far* set, we extract it to *neighbor* set.

In FMST, the FM method is used to calculate nodes' radii and the weights of edges.

(1) Calculating nodes' radii. We get an initial over reconstruction, but there are too many points in the graph $G$ (all foreground pixels). It is not realistic to tracing neuron by minimum spanning tree method immediately. Since we only need important points that can generate the skeletons of the neuron, it is necessary to prune nodes that are not important. We prune nodes based on their radii. One common technique to calculate radius of node is expanding outward from the center and count the ratio of the foreground pixels and the background pixels, and we can get the radius when the ratio is below a certain threshold. But this method is infeasible in FMST because of too many nodes. We use FM method to calculate the radii of nodes. We set the background pixels as *know*, the edge of foreground pixels as *neighbor*, other foreground pixels as *far*. So moving surface is contracted gradually from the boundary to the interior in the neuron. We define the value of $T$ as:

$$T_{new} = T_{old} + 1, \tag{1}$$

$T_{new}$ is the value of the point in *far*, and $T_{old}$ is the value of the point in *neighbor* set. According to this strategy, the radii of all nodes can be obtained.

(2) Calculating the weights of edges. Our goal is to find the shortest pathway in a neuron image with little background pixels. Two factors impacting the pathway are its length and the number of background pixels on it. Let

$$W = a * Length - b * BackCount, \tag{2}$$

where *Length* and *BackCount* mean the length of a path and number of background pixels on the path, $a$ and $b$ are two positive coefficients. Actually, there are many pathways between any two nodes, and our goal is to look for the one with maximum weight $W$, that is to say, the path *maxEdge* satisfies

$$maxEdge = argmax(W). \tag{3}$$

The calculation of the weights of edges is implented in the FM framework. Let $x$ and $y$ be two foreground pixels, we set $x$ as *neighbor*, and set other nodes as *far*. Then FM propagates from the point $x$ with $T$ value. We repeat this iteration until $y$ is set as *know*, and the $T$ value of $y$ is the weight of the edge. By this mean, we can get the weights of all edges.

### 2.3  Pruning Nodes

The graph $G$ consists of all foreground pixels, so it has too many nodes. It is necessary to delete some nodes covered by other nodes (with bigger radius). We just want to find the skeleton of a neuron, and get a series of smooth connections of the sphere that can express the original three dimensional structure of the neuron. In order to get complete neuronal morphology with as few as possible nodes, we prune the redundant nodes and get a sufficient simplified neuronal topological structure. The node pruning method has two steps.

(1) The target node (with radius) is covered by another single node. We calculate the coverage of the target node and one of its neighbors with radii which are calculated by the FM method. The threshold value of coverage is set as 0. So if the target node is covered by a neighbor node or by contrast, we delete the small one. Then we change the connection relationships between these nodes and set the small node's child nodes as the big node's child nodes.

(2) The target node is covered by a set of nodes. The node coverage is very miscellaneous and different order of pruning node leads to different results. Our strategy is sorting the radii and deleting the node with smallest radius first. After pruning a node, its child nodes are reconnected each other. Of course, this approach has a shortcoming, i.e., it leads to an increase of edges after pruning nodes.

### 2.4  Generating Minimum Spanning Trees and Recreate a Tree

Minimum spanning tree method generates a tree from the perspective of edge. By connecting a target node with its all possible neighbors, we find out a pathway between each pair of nodes, but the graph model is not necessarily a connected graph. So we apply minimum spanning tree method in each connected domain in the graph model and may get some trees, rather than only one tree. One tree of a neuron can be constructed by minimum spanning tree method based on these small trees. We take every small tree as a node, and calculate the weights of these *nodes*. We set the weight between two trees as the minimum Euclidean distance:

$$W = argmin(E(a, b)), \qquad (4)$$

where $W$ means the weight of two trees, $a$, $b$ are nodes belong to the two trees, and $E(a, b)$ is the Euclidean distance between $a$ and $b$. Then all the local domains can be connected and a reconstruction with no breakpoints is obtained.

## 3   Experimental Results

We implement FMST as a plugin of Vaa3D which is the common platform to implement algorithms for the BigNeuron project (bigneuron.org) bench testing. Experiments on 120 Drosophila neurons dataset to compare the performance of FMST and MST, then we compare FMST with several previous automated methods in the public domain Vaa3D.

In our experiment, we successfully reconstructed complete neuron morphology of 120 Drosophila neurons, each of which has $1024 * 1024 * 120$ voxels. And we selected three groups of results to illustrate the effect of MST and FMST.

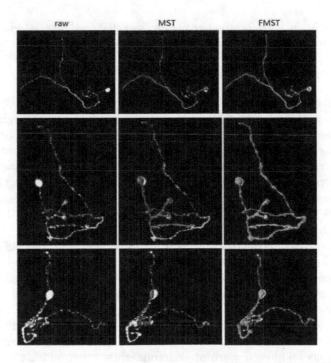

**Fig. 1.** The comparison of reconstruction results by MST and FMST for three Drosophila neuron images. The red parts are results of MST and the green parts are results of FMST, and reconstructions are overlaid on the top of original images for better visualization (Color figure online)

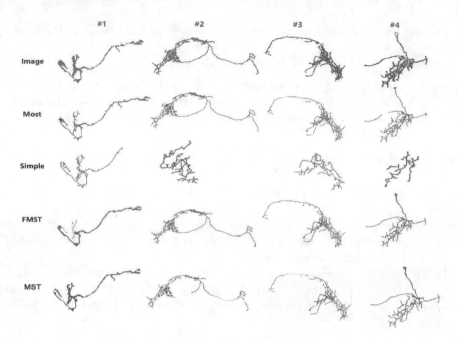

**Fig. 2.** Visualization of reconstructed neuron morphologies of 4 selected examples traced by different methods, the first line is the initial image, and the rest lines are the results of Most, Simple, FMST, MST, respectively

Figure 1 displays the reconstructions by MST and FMST, it can be seen that there may be a large fracture when the raw image has low noise-signal ratio, and this make the reconstruction more difficult. If a neuron has breakpoints, MST method can't trace it successfully, and often loss some important skeletons. FMST can overcome this difficulty and get a pretty good result. Compared with MST, reconstructions by FMST are more reasonable. The reason is that FMST reduces the weights of fracture paths instead of directly deleting them, but MST just considers the spatial distances between neuron segments and it is difficult to get whole reconstruction if the neuron has breakpoints.

We also compared reconstructions of Most, Simple, FMST and MST. Figure 2 displays raw images and reconstruction results of these four methods. It can be seen that reconstructions by Most method often have breakpoints, and the results consist of many small trees. For the Simple method, its results often lose some skeletons while the neuron is complex or the image quality is poor. Compared with these two methods, FMST can successfully overcome these difficulties and get the reconstructions with no breakpoints. For MST, its reconstructions also have breakpoints and lose important skeletons while a neuron has segments with low pixel.

# 4    Conclusion

In this paper, we present a method FMST for neuron tracing which is based on FM and minimum spanning tree. We compared our method to MST, and found that effect has been improved significantly. We also compared our method to several other methods on 120 Drosophila neurons dataset, and FMST performed better in some cases. FMST adopts FM algorithm to compute both nodes' radii and weights of edges, and this can speed up their execution. Another important improvement is that after the step of minimum spanning tree, FMST takes small trees as *nodes* and recreate a tree, which can fill the gaps between neuron segments.

There are some limitations of FMST. For example, if the image quality is too poor or the image with too much noise, FMST can't reconstruct well. The signal-to-noise ratio of the image is too low or the image is too big might also cause the failure of the reconstruction. On the one hand, if an image has low signal-to-noise ratio, noise might influence the selection of foreground pixels, which would leads to get some error nodes that don't belong to the skeleton. Sometimes because of the influence of the noise, we may prune nodes on the skeleton and lose important parts of the neuron. On the other hand, if the size of the image is too big, too many nodes will result in very long executing time including the time of deleting nodes, calculating radius and connecting edges. Anyway, FMST is an effective neuron tracing method and needs to be improved further.

**Acknowledgments.** This work is partially supported by the National Basic Research Program of China (No. 2014CB744600), National Natural Science Foundation of China (No. 61420106005), Beijing Natural Science Foundation (No. 4164080), and Beijing Outstanding Talent Training Foundation (No. 2014 000020124G039). The authors thank the BigNeuron project and Dr. Hanchuan Peng for providing the testing image data used in this article and many discussions.

# References

1. Xiao, H., Peng, H.: APP2: automatic tracing of 3D neuron morphology based on hierarchical pruning of a gray-weighted image distance-tree. Bioinformatics **29**, 1448–1454 (2013)
2. Zhou, Z., Sorensen, S., Peng, H.: Neuron crawler: an automatic tracing algorithm for very large neuron images. In: Procedings of IEEE 2015 International Symposium on Biomedical Imaging: From Nano to Macro, pp. 870–874 (2015)
3. Chen, H., Xiao, H., Liu, T., Peng, H.: SmartTracing: self-learning-based neuron reconstruction. Brain Inform. **2**, 135–144 (2015)
4. Peng, H., Long, F., Myers, G.: Automatic 3D neuron tracing using all-path pruning. Bioinformatics **27**, i239–i247 (2011)
5. Yang, J., Gonzalez-Bellido, P.T., Peng, H.: A distance-field based automatic neuron tracing method. BMC Bioinform. **14**, 93 (2013)
6. Wu, J., He, Y., Yang, Z., Guo, C., Luo, Q., Zhou, W., Chen, S., Li, A., Xiong, B., Jiang, T., Gong, H.: 3D BrainCV: simultaneous visualization and analysis of cells

and capillaries in a whole mouse brain with one-micron voxel resolution. Neuroimage **87**, 199–208 (2014)

7. Wang, Y., Narayanaswamy, A., Tsai, C.-L., Roysam, B.: A broadly applicable 3-D neuron tracing method based on open-curve snake. Neuroinformatics **9**, 193–217 (2011)

8. Peng, H., Ruan, Z., Atasoy, D., Sternson, S.: Automatic reconstruction of 3D neuron structures using a graph-augmented deformable model. Bioinformatics. **26**, i38–i46 (2010)

9. Ming, X., Li, A., Wu, J., Yan, C., Ding, W., Gong, H., Zeng, S., Liu, Q.: Rapid reconstruction of 3D neuronal morphology from light microscopy images with augmented rayburst sampling. PloS ONE **8**, e84557 (2013)

10. Feng, L., Zhao, T., Kim, J.: NeuTube 10: a new design for efficient neuron reconstruction software based on the SWC format. eNeuro **2**, 0049-0014 (2015)

11. Peng, H., Meijering, E., Ascoli, G.A.: From DIADEM to BigNeuron. Neuroinformatics **13**, 259–260 (2015)

12. Peng, H., Hawrylycz, M., Roskams, J., Hill, S., Spruston, N., Meijering, E., Ascoli, G.A.: BigNeuron: large-scale 3D neuron reconstruction from optical microscopy images. Neuron **87**, 252–256 (2015). doi:10.1016/j.neuron.2015.06.036

13. Peng, H., Ruan, Z., Long, F., Simpson, J.H., Myers, E.W.: V3D enables real-time 3D visualization and quantitative analysis of large-scale biological image data sets. Nat. Biotechnol. **28**, 348–353 (2010)

14. Peng, H., Bria, A., Zhou, Z., Iannello, G., Long, F.: Extensible visualization and analysis for multidimensional images using Vaa3D. Nat. Protoc. **9**, 193–208 (2014)

15. Shillcock, J., Hawrylycz, M., Hill, S., Peng, H.: Reconstructing the brain: from image stacks to neuron synthesis. Brain Inform. 1–5 (2016). doi:10.1007/s40708-016-0041-7

16. Sethian, J.: Level set methods and fast marching methods: evolving interfaces in computational geometry, fluid mechanics, computer vision, and materials science. In: Cambridge Monographs on Applied and Computational Mathematics, vol. 3, Cambridge University Press, Cambridge (1999)

# On Simple Models of Associative Memory: Network Density Is Not Required for Provably Complex Behavior

Predrag T. Tošić[(✉)]

School of Electrical Engineering and Computer Science,
Washington State University, Pullman, WA, USA
ptosic@eecs.wsu.edu

**Abstract.** It has been argued that complex behavior in many biological systems, including but not limited to human and animal brains, is to a great extent a consequence of high interconnectedness among the individual elements, such as neurons in brains. As a very crude approximation, brain can be viewed as an *associative memory* that is implemented as a large network of heavily interconnected neurons. *Hopfield Networks* are a popular model of associative memory. From a dynamical systems perspective, it has been posited that the complexity of possible behaviors of a Hopfield network is largely due to the aforementioned high level of interconnectedness. We show, however, that many aspects of provably complex – and, in particular, unpredictable within realistic computational resources – behavior can also be obtained in very sparsely connected Hopfield networks and related classes of *Boolean Network Automata*. In fact, it turns out that the most fundamental problems about the memory capacity of a Hopfield network are computationally intractable, even for restricted types of networks that are *uniformly sparse*, with only a handful neighbors per node. One implication of our results is that some of the most fundamental aspects of biological (and other) networks' dynamics do not require high density, in order to exhibit provably complex, computationally intractable behavior.

## 1 Introduction and Motivation: Brains as Dynamic Networks

From computational and dynamical systems standpoints, animal brains (and in particular, our own, human brains) are incredibly complex computational devices made of a large number of fairly simple basic elements (neurons) that are intricately interconnected with each other. At the most fundamental level, a human brain is a network of about 100 billion (i.e., $\sim 10^{11}$) neurons, and about $10^{15}$ connections, called synapses. Neurons are the brain's elementary information processing units. That a typical neuron has thousands or even tens of thousands of synaptic connections to other neurons has been argued to be crucial for the brain's ability to engage in highly complex information processing tasks.

A popular "first order approximation" computational view of this intricate network of interconnected neurons, is that of the brain as an *associative memory* [1]. An associative memory can be used for storage and retrieval of patterns; for simplicity, we will assume those patterns are Boolean/binary-valued vectors. While not all neurons in

© Springer International Publishing AG 2016
G.A. Ascoli et al. (Eds.): BIH 2016, LNAI 9919, pp. 61–71, 2016.
DOI: 10.1007/978-3-319-47103-7_7

a human or animal brain are used for storing such patterns, it is reasonable to assume that a considerable fraction of the neurons do. It then makes sense to pose the question: what is the overall *memory capacity* of the brain? That is, *how many distinct patterns* can be stored into and retrieved from (the pattern storage/memory part of) the brain? Estimates of the actual memory capacity of a human brain broadly vary, and generally fall in the range from 1 TB (terabyte) up to 1,000 TB; in comparison, the entire US Library of Congress (i.e., all volumes in it together) contain about 10 TB of data [2].

While functioning of human brain as a memory device is highly complex and multi-faceted (and requires neuroscience expertise way beyond our own), a "mathematically clean" if largely over-simplified associative memory model of the brain can be useful in getting the ballpark estimate of the brain's memory capacity – as well as help us address several other important quantitative aspects of possible behaviors of brains viewed as large-scale networks of interconnected neurons (see Sect. 3). Another useful aspect of such "mathematically clean" models is that it becomes much easier to mathematically and computationally formulate important questions about a variety of quantitative properties of brains viewed as distributed, networked computational devices; answers to thus formulated questions will then provide some guidance as well as, in a sense, lower bounds on the complexity of the "real" brains' behavior.

Let's take a closer look at some numbers related to human brain; for simplicity, let's assume that about 10% of the brain's neurons are used for storing binary patterns. That is, some 1 GB ($10^9$) simple processing units store patterns of 0s and 1s, where a 1 corresponds to an active or firing neuron, and a 0 to a non-firing one. How do we define a pattern that has been "memorized"? One reasonable assumption, in tune the brain-as-an-associative-memory paradigm, is to consider only those patterns that, if slightly perturbed, can be recovered [1]. In addition to resilience to small perturbations, the stored or "memorized" patterns should be *persistent* as opposed to of a temporary, transient nature. These requirements suggest identifying only recurrent or stable configurations of the underlying "network of neurons" as being memorized – in contrast to temporary or transient configurations.

Throughout this paper, we will assume that (i) time is discrete (so, the system moves from its configuration at time t to in general some other configuration at time t + 1); and further that (ii) the dynamics of the systems/networks we study are deterministic (in particular, this assumption implies that, given the system's configuration at time t, there is a unique "next-step" configuration at time t + 1). *Recurrent configurations* of a (deterministic) dynamical system or, equivalently for our purposes, a complex network with deterministic dynamics, come in two varieties: namely, as the "fixed points" and the temporal cycles. A *fixed point configuration* (FP for short) is a tuple of all nodes' values or states such that, when all the nodes are updated either in parallel or sequentially according to the Hopfield or other Boolean Network's update rules, each node's state remains unchanged. A *temporal cycle* (TC) is a finite sequence of global configurations $C_1, C_2, \ldots, C_k = C_1$; once the dynamics of a network reaches such temporal cycle, it "stays there" in a sense that each configuration in such a temporal cycle keeps getting revisited with some fixed (time) periodicity. (Note that the fixed periodicity, as well as "no straying away" from the cycle once the network's dynamics has reached a cycle configuration, are both direct consequences of the assumed *determinism of network's dynamics.*) FP, CC and other important types of configurations of a discrete dynamical system are formally defined in Sect. 2.

Assuming our associative memory (that is, the part of the brain that stores binary patterns) is a network of some $10^9$ binary-valued nodes, the above discussion of *recurrent configurations* of such a network provides a natural and compelling notion of "memorized patterns" – namely, those network configurations that are *recurrent*. Moreover, for certain types of such discrete networks' dynamics, temporal cycles (of non-fixed-point variety) are either impossible, or else very rare and, from a statistical standpoint, basically can be ignored; see, e.g., [3–5]. In such situations, the pattern storage capacity of a discrete network boils down to the problem of determining (exactly or at least approximately) the number of that network's "fixed point" configurations. It is precisely this *fixed point enumeration problem* that we study and relate to the problem of estimating storage capacity of an associative memory.

The rest of the paper is organized as follows. In Sect. 2, we formally introduce Discrete Hopfield Nets as our associative memory model. We then briefly overview most relevant prior arts on DHNs, with an emphasis on the quantitative properties of DHN dynamics. In Sect. 4, we present our main results related to the computational complexity of enumerating stable configurations of a DHN and related models of Boolean Networks, followed by those results' interpretations in the context of associative memories. Last but not least, we summarize the key insights from our work and outline some interesting directions for future research.

## 2  Boolean Networks and Discrete Hopfield Nets: Background

The mathematical model of associative memory we adopt is that of *Discrete Hopfield Networks* (DHNs) [5, 6]. In the DHN model, both time and each node's or neuron's state are discrete. We will refer to the basic processing units of a DHN interchangeably as to a *node* (when complex network view is adopted) or a *neuron* (esp. when discussing associative memories and implications of various DHN properties incl. our results presented here for the computational neuroscience). Similarly, we will refer to the links connecting the nodes as connections or synapses. From a *connectionist computing* standpoint, DHNs can be viewed as a particular kind of recurrent neural networks. From the broader computer science and discrete dynamical systems standpoints, DHNs can also be viewed as a subclass of Boolean (or Binary) Networks; we cf. adopt this latter view.

**Definition 1:** *A Boolean Network* (also called *Boolean Network Automaton*, or BNA for short) is a directed or undirected graph so that each node in the graph has a state, 0 or 1; and each node periodically updates its state, as a function of the current states of (some or all of) its neighboring nodes (possibly, but not necessarily, including itself). A BNA dynamically evolves (or, equivalently, computes) in discrete time steps. If the node $v_i$ has $k$ neighbors $v_{i1}, ..., v_{ik}$ (where this list of neighbors may or may not include $v_i$ itself), then the next state of $v_i$ is determined by evaluating a Boolean-valued function $f_i(v_{i1}, ... v_{ik})$ of $k$ Boolean variables. Function $f_i$ is called *local update function* or *transition rule* (for node $v_i$).

Several comments are in order. First, in general, different nodes $v_i$ may use different local update functions $f_i$. This applies to *Discrete Hopfield Nets* (defined below), as well as many other classes of Boolean Networks including those originally introduced by Kauffman in the context of systems biology [7, 8], and also several related models proposed in the context of modeling large-scale distributed computing and various cyber-physical infrastructures [9–12]. Classical *Cellular Automata* (CA) can then be viewed as a special case of BNA, where all the nodes use the same local update rule $f_i$. (We note, however, that the underlying graphs in BNA are almost always assumed to be finite, whereas CA have been extensively studied in both finite and infinite settings.) The individual node updates can be done either synchronously in parallel, or sequentially, one at a time (and if so, either according to the fixed update ordering, or in a random order). While other communication models are worth considering (see [4]), the above three possibilities have been studied the most. In this paper, we will focus entirely on the parallel, perfectly synchronous node updates. This means, the next state of the node $v_i$ is determined according to

$$v_i^{t+1} \leftarrow f_i\left(v_{i1}^t, \ldots, v_{ik}^t\right) \tag{1}$$

The tuple of all $f_i$'s put together, $F = (f_1, \ldots, f_n)$, denotes the *global map* that acts on the configurations of a BNA. When all $f_i$ are identical, the notation in the literature is often abused so that no differentiation is made between the local transition function, acting on a state of a single node, and the global map $F$, acting on entire configurations of a cellular or network automaton (that is, on all the nodes).

**Definition 2:**  A *Discrete Hopfield Network* (DHN) is made of n binary-valued nodes. Associated to each pair of nodes $(v_i, v_j)$ is (in general, real-valued) their weight, $w_{ij}$. The weight matrix of a DHN is defined as $W = [w_{ij}]_{i,j\,=\,1..n}$. Each node also has a fixed real-valued threshold, $h_i$. A node $v_i$ updates its state $x_i$ from time step t to step t + 1 according to a (binary-valued) *linear threshold function* of the form

$$x_i^{t+1} \leftarrow \text{sgn}\left(\sum w_{ij} \cdot x_j^t - h_i\right)$$

where the summation is over j = 1, ..., n; $h_i$ is the threshold that the weighted sum needs to reach or exceed in order for the node's state to update to +1; to break ties, we define $\text{sgn}(0) = +1$.

The default notation in most of the literature on Hopfield nets, is that the binary states of an individual node are $\{-1, +1\}$. In this paper, however, we adopt the Boolean values $\{0,1\}$ for the states of our Hopfield Network nodes, in order to be able to discuss DHNs and our results about them in the broader context of Boolean Networks (see, e.g., [7, 8]) without the need for cumbersome "translations". (Of course, the "0" in Boolean Networks should be interpreted as the "−1" in Hopfield Nets and vice versa, as the choice of labels for the nodes' binary values is a matter of mere syntax and inconsequential for any of our results or their interpretations.)

In most of the Hopfield Nets literature, two additional assumptions are made, namely, that (i) the diagonal elements of weight matrix W are all zeros: $w_{ii} = 0$; and

(ii) the weight matrix is symmetric, $w_{ij} = w_{ji}$ for all pairs of nodes i,j. We will adopt (ii) throughout (although it does not affect the main results and insights from them discussed in the next section). As for (i), we will consider two possibilities on the nodes' "memory" (of their own current state, as a part of the local transition rule): either $w_{ii} = 0$ for all nodes $v_i$, or else $w_{ii} = 1$ for all $v_i$. The main results in the next section will hold under either the *memoryless* ($w_{ii} = 0$) or *memory* ($w_{ii} = 1$) assumption. Moreover, in the memory case, our results can be readily extended to more general weighing $w_{ii}$ of how is a node's state at time t + 1 affected by its own state at time t; these variations will be discussed in detail in an expanded version of the present paper.

A BNA is called *dense* if the underlying graph on which it is defined is dense. Similarly, a DHN is dense if its weight matrix W is dense, i.e., informally if W contains many non-zero entries. The natural interpretation of a zero weight $w_{ij}$ in a DHN is that the corresponding nodes i and j do not directly affect each other. (That is, change of state of the i$^{th}$ node does not immediately affect the state of the j$^{th}$ node, and vice versa). In contrast, we call a BNA *sparse* if the underlying network topology (that is, the graph structure) is sparse; similarly, we call a DHN sparse if the weight matrix W is a sparse matrix. For our purposes, sparseness will mean O(1) neighbors per node (alternatively, non-zero weights per row of W), on average; that implies, the total number of edges in the underlying graph (equivalently, non-zero entries in W) is of the order O($n$) where $n$ is the number of nodes. Further, we say a Boolean Network or a Hopfield Network is *uniformly sparse* if every node is required to have only O(1) neighbors (that is, every row/column in W has only O(1) non-zero entries). So, for example, a star or a wheel graph on $n$ nodes would be sparse (the avg. node degree being O(1) in each case), but neither of them would be uniformly sparse (as the center of the star/wheel is adjacent to all other nodes, and hence has $\Theta(n)$ neighbors).

Recall, BNA and DHN are deterministic discrete dynamical systems, i.e., for any given current configuration $C^t$, there is a unique next-step configuration $C^{t+1}$. We conclude this section on the core background about Boolean Automata and DHNs by defining the types of a BNA or DHN *global configurations* (that is, tuples capturing the states of all nodes in a network; see Sect. 1) we are particularly interested in:

**Definition 3:** A (global) configuration of a cellular or network automaton or a discrete Hopfield net is a vector $(x_1, \ldots, x_n) \ \varepsilon \ \{0,1\}^n$, where $x_i$ denotes the state of the i$^{th}$ node. Equivalently, configuration can be thought of as a function $\gamma: V \rightarrow \{0,1\}$, where V denotes the set of nodes in the underlying graph of a CA, BNA or DHN.

**Definition 4:** A *fixed point* (FP) is a configuration such that, once a cellular or network automaton or DHN reaches that configuration, it stays there forever. A *cycle configuration* (CC) is a global state that, once reached, will be revisited infinitely often with a fixed, finite temporal period of 2 or greater. A *transient configuration* (TC) is a global configuration that, once reached, is never going to be revisited again. In particular, FPs can be viewed as a special (or perhaps, "degenerate") type of temporal cycles – those with periodicity 1.

**Definition 5:** Given two configurations C and C' of a CA, BNA or DHN, if F(C) = C' we say that C' is the *successor* of C and that C is a *predecessor* of C'. That is, C' is obtained from C by a single application of the global map F.

**Definition 5 (Continued):** If the dynamics of a CA/BNA/DHN is deterministic (which we assume throughout), then each configuration has the unique successor. However, a configuration may have 0, 1 or more predecessors. A configuration with no predecessors is called *Garden of Eden*. Lastly, configuration A is an *ancestor* of configuration C, if starting from A, the dynamics reaches configuration C after finitely many time steps (equivalently, if there exists $t \geq 1$ such that $F^t(A) = C$).

In particular, a predecessor is a special type of ancestor. Further, "fixed points" are the only type of configurations such that each is its own predecessor. Similarly, each cycle configuration is its own ancestor. In contrast, a transient configuration can never be its own ancestor: once a deterministic system leaves a TC, it never revisits it again.

# 3   Related Work: Dynamical Properties of Discrete Hopfield Networks

Hopfield Networks were originally introduced in [5] with a two-fold motivation: statistical physics on one hand, and connectionist computational models inspired by biology, on the other. Soon after the model was proposed, its huge promise for solving a broad range of combinatorial and optimization problems in computer science, operations research and other areas was realized [6]. Hopfield nets have also been extensively studied from a complex dynamical system viewpoint: researchers have posed kinds of questions about the Hopfield model that were previously studied in the contexts of classical Cellular Automata and Kauffman's Boolean Networks [7].

Among classical dynamical system problems about DHN (and more broadly, BNA in general) are those pertaining to the existence and number of various types of configurations, such as the stable/FP configuration and temporal cycles; the size of a FP's or cycle's "basin of attraction"; the reachability of various states (esp. those of recurrent variety); the typical vs. worst-case speed of convergence to a recurrent/stable configuration if the network starts from an arbitrary initial configuration, etc. Seminal work on the worst-case behavior with respect to these aspects of network dynamics, specifically in the context of DHNs, is found in [13–15], where [13] specifically focuses on the hardness of counting all fixed points of a DHN. More recently, interest in Hopfield Nets viewed as associative memories has reemerged, with several mostly simulation-based studies of the storage capacity of various architectures (that is, types of underlying graphs) and learning rules [16, 17]. In [17] some insights are offered into what types of (relatively sparse) underlying graphs provide the highest memory capacity (that is, tend to have the greatest number of FPs). We remark that it was independently discovered by us over a decade ago, that some very sparse BNA with simple local update rules indeed can have exponentially many (w.r.t. the number of nodes, $n$) stable configurations. These insights came out of our work on the enumeration problems about FPs, Gardens of Eden, predecessors of an arbitrary configuration, etc., originally studied in the context of two particular classes of BNA called *Sequential and Synchronous Dynamical Systems* [11, 12]. However, our original motivation came from the theory of large-scale, agent-based simulation of various cyber-physical and socio-technical systems, rather than biology. Our specific focus was in characterizing the computational complexity of the enumeration problems about such systems' dynamics, for a range of sparse graph structures and classes of update rules [12, 18–20]. We summarize our main insights next, and (re-)interpret hardness of counting a DHN's stable configurations in the context of computational neuroscience - specifically, in terms of associative memories' storage capacity.

## 4  On the Complexity of Enumerating Stable Configurations in Discrete Hopfield Nets and Other Boolean Network Automata

We now state our main results, and then briefly discuss their implications. We recall that the storage capacity of an associative memory is defined as the number of patterns (binary vectors) that can be stored to and retrieved from the memory; and that these patterns correspond to the stable configurations of the underlying DHN. Due to space constraints, we briefly introduce the key computational complexity concepts. A decision or optimization or enumeration problem is tractable, if it can be solved in the number of steps that is *polynomial* in the size of the problem's description. (For simplicity, we will treat the number of nodes $n$ as the "problem size"; for a detailed discussion on when this is or is not justifiable, see [12].) Otherwise, the problem is intractable, that is, any deterministic algorithm to solve it, presumably takes super-polynomial, which in practice usually means *exponential* (or worse), number of steps w.r.t. the input size. The most important class of decision problems (those with a YES/NO or TRUE/FALSE answer) that are presumed intractable are the **NP**-hard problems; a subset of these problems for which, if we guess a solution (or a little birdie whispers it to our ear), that solution can be *verified* in polynomial time, are called **NP**-complete. Many classical problems about logic, graphs, combinatorial optimization etc. are known to be **NP**-complete.

Now, enumeration or counting problems are intuitively more challenging than the decision problems, as one needs to determine not merely whether a solution exists, but actually how many distinct solutions a given problem has. The enumeration analogue of the **NP**-hard and **NP**-complete decision problems are called the **#P**-hard (resp., **#P**-complete). Some classical examples: whether a Boolean 3CNF formula is satisfiable (i.e., whether a solution satisfying the formula exists) is a paradigmatic **NP**-complete problem, whereas how many satisfying truth assignments (solutions) a given 3CNF formula has, is a **#P**-complete problem. The enumeration or counting versions of virtually all known **NP**-complete decision problems from logic, graphs, combinatorics etc. (for which the counting problem formulation makes sense) have been established to be **#P**-complete. What is more interesting, however, is that a number of important decision problems solvable in polynomial time actually have **#P**-complete counting analogues. Some examples include Monotone CNF Boolean formulae (with only *AND* and *OR* operators, i.e., no *negation*), 2CNF formulae (with each clause having only 2, as opposed to 3 or more, literals) and many others. (Some of those, specifically sparse

Monotone 2CNF formulae, have been extensively used in our prior work, including to establish formal proofs of some of the main computational complexity properties of BNA and DHN discussed below.)

**Theorem 1:** Determining the storage capacity of an associative memory implemented as a *sparse* (in the sense, sparse-on-average) DHN with memory is, in the worst-case, computationally intractable: specifically, it is **#P-complete** to determine the exact number of stable configurations of a sparse discrete Hopfield network.

This result (in the context of certain classes of BNA defined on the *star graphs*) was originally proved by us in [12]. Complexity of counting FPs on the classes of BNA investigated in that paper readily translates to the DHN context. The construction of the original proof assumed BNA/DHN with memory (meaning, each node's next state depends on its own current state, that is, in the weight matrix, all $w_{ii} = 0$). For star graphs, the memory assumption is critical (as a periphery node's update rule then takes two arguments, $x_i \leftarrow f(x_C, x_i)$ where $x_C$ denotes the central node of the star; whereas, in a memoryless model, one has $x_i \leftarrow g(x_C)$ where g is a Boolean function of a *single* Boolean variable). However, the argument in [12] can be slightly modified and applied to e.g. wheel graphs, which are also very sparse on average, so that the worst-case complexity of enumerating patterns remains intractable for the memoryless DHNs (with $w_{ii} = 0$ along the main diagonal of weight matrix W), as well. Note that, for a memoryless DHN defined over a wheel, each peripheral node updates according to a linear threshold Boolean-valued function of three Boolean variables, of the general form $x_i \leftarrow f(C, x_{i-1}, x_{i+1})$, giving us the sufficient "degrees of freedom" to establish the same worst-case complexity akin to that for DHNs (defined over stars or wheels) with memory. (For details on the star graphs, see [12]; details on the wheel graphs will be provided in an extended version of the present paper.)

Furthermore, the result from Theorem 1 can be further strengthened, by requiring that the underlying graph (equivalently, DHN's weight matrix W) *be uniformly sparse*:

**Theorem 2:** The problem of enumerating all stable configurations of a uniformly sparse Hopfield Net is in general **#P**-complete.

That is, even if we require that each "neuron" in a DHN is connected, and hence its state depends upon, only a handful of other neurons, determining the number of that DHN's fixed point configurations is in general computationally intractable. Moreover, we have shown that the constant "hidden inside the O(1)" can be made really small – in particular, our hardness result holds in Hopfield Nets with memory even when each neuron is restricted to have no more than three neighbors [18].

The main technical result above has immediate, and we argue far-reaching, implications for the central problem of the storage capacity of associative memories:

**Corollary:** Determining the storage-capacity of an associative memory implemented as a uniformly sparse DHN is, in the worst-case, provably computationally intractable. That is, other than for very small numbers of nodes or "neurons" $n$, we cannot determine within reasonable time and computational resources, how many patterns that associative memory can store.

One immediate implication of the above results is that at least some properties of associative memories and by extension human or animal brains, actually do not require high interconnectedness among the neurons in order to exhibit complex behavior. (Implicit in this statement is an ontological assumption, that if some well-defined quantitative property of a system cannot be established using a feasible amount of time and computational resources, then that property can be reasonably considered to be "complex".) Specifically, the total number of possible dynamics, and (closely related to it) the total number of stable configurations of a Hopfield network, are in general computationally intractable. In particular, given a description of an associative memory (that is, the graph structure and the local node update rule(s) of the DHN that implements that associative memory) of a non-trivial size, we cannot tell what is that memory's storage capacity. Similarly, several other aspects that can be naturally formulated as combinatorial counting problems, are also provably computationally intractable – even for the underlying networks that are uniformly sparse, i.e., such that each "neuron" is connected to a small number of other neurons (such as, to only 3 or 4 other neurons, depending on the specific assumptions about the update rules [18, 19]).

## 5 Summary and Future Work

This paper briefly discusses the storage capacity of associative memories. After motivating the problem's importance, we suggest a possible, mathematically rigorous if oversimplified from a neuroscience perspective, formulation of the problem. Then, using tools and methodology from both the study of (discrete) dynamical systems and theoretical computer science, we show that our formulation of the memory capacity problem, in general, is demonstrably computationally intractable – shedding some light, for example, on why are the estimates (or, perhaps more appropriately, "guestimates") on the memory capacity of our own, human brains varying so widely among the neuroscience and brain science communities – after decades of intensive theoretical, experimental and simulation-based research on human (and advanced animal) brains and memory. We remark, our computational complexity results outlined (and re-interpreted) in this paper were originally obtained in decidedly non-neuroscience contexts (see [11, 12, 18–20]); however, these results can be readily (with some minor technical "tweaks" where necessary) adapted to, and re-interpreted in, the context of quantifying the storage capacity of associative memories.

There are a number of lines of interesting future work we would like to pursue. Due to space constraints, we mention just two. First, we would like to compare-and-contrast the worst-case behavior vs. the average, or "typical", behaviors of various types of BNA and Hopfield Networks, esp. when biologically relevant constraints are imposed on the underlying graph structures (or "network topologies"). Systematic investigation along those lines would combine theoretical methodology (cf. focusing on worst-case behavior) with extensive computer simulations (to capture "typical" behavior). Second, we would like to investigate further the main qualitative differences in possible dynamics, related to stable configurations and other properties of interest, between memory and memoryless DHN models, defined over *the same* types of underlying graphs. It is already known that, in several cases, important differences exist; we would like to capture and summarize the most salient, pervasive among those differences in a unified and systematic manner across a broad variety of biologically plausible Boolean Networks and Discrete Hopfield Networks.

# References

1. McEliece, R.J., et al.: The capacity of the Hopfield associative memory. IEEE Trans. Inf. Theory **33**(4), 461–482 (1987)
2. http://www.human-memory.net/
3. Tosic, P.T., Agha, G.: Characterizing configuration spaces of simple threshold cellular automata. In: Sloot, P.M., Chopard, B., Hoekstra, A.G. (eds.) ACRI 2004. LNCS, vol. 3305, pp. 861–870. Springer, Heidelberg (2004)
4. Tosic, P.: Cellular automata communication models: comparative analysis of parallel, sequential and asynchronous CA with simple threshold update rules. Int. J. Nat. Comput. Res. (IJNCR) **1**(3), 66–84 (2010)
5. Hopfield, J.J.: Neural networks and physical systems with emergent collective computational abilities. Proc. Natl. Acad. Sci. (USA) **79**, 2554–2558 (1982)
6. Hopfield, J.J., Tank, D.W.: Neural computation of decisions in optimization problems. Biol. Cybern. **52**, 141–152 (1985)
7. Kauffman, S.A.: Emergent properties in random complex automata. Phys. D: Nonlinear Phenom. **10**(1–2), 145–156 (1984)
8. Graudenzi, A., et al.: Dynamical properties of a Boolean model of a gene regulatory network with memory. J. Comput. Biol. **18**(10), 1291–1303 (2011)
9. Mortveit, H., Reidys, C.: Discrete sequential dynamical systems. Discret. Math. **226**(1–3), 281–295 (2001)
10. Barrett, C., et al.: Reachability problems for sequential dynamical systems with threshold functions. Theor. Comput. Sci. **295**(1–3), 41–64 (2003)
11. Barrett, C., et al.: Gardens of Eden and fixed points in sequential dynamical systems. In: Discrete Mathematics & Theoretical Computer Science (DMTCS) (Discrete Models: Combinatorics, Computation, and Geometry), vol. AA, pp. 95–110 (2001)
12. Tosic, P.: On the complexity of counting fixed points and gardens of Eden in sequential and synchronous dynamical systems. Int. J. Found. Comput. Sci. (IJFCS) **17**(5), 1179–1203 (2006). World Scientific
13. Floreen, P., Orponen, P.: On the computational complexity of analyzing Hopfield nets. Complex Syst. **3**, 577–587 (1989)
14. Floreen, P., Orponen, P.: Attraction radii in binary Hopfield nets are hard to compute. Neural Comput. **5**, 812–821 (1993)
15. Orponen, P.: Computational complexity of neural networks: a survey. Nord. J. Comput. **1**, 94–110 (1996)
16. Wu, Y., et al.: Storage capacity of the Hopfield network associative memory. In: Proceedings of 5th International Conference on Intelligent Computation Technology and Automation, pp. 330–336, January 2012
17. Davey, N., Calcraft, L., Adams, R.: High capacity, small world associative memory models. Connect. Sci. **18**(3), 247–264 (2006)
18. Tosic, P.: On the complexity of enumerating possible dynamics of sparsely connected Boolean network automata with simple update rules. In: Discrete Math & Theoretical Comp. Sci. DMTCS (Post-Proceedings Automata-2010, 16th International Workshop Cellular Automata & Discrete Complex Systems), pp. 125–144 (2010)

19. Tošić, P.T., Agha, G.: On computational complexity of counting fixed points in symmetric Boolean graph automata. In: Calude, C.S., Dinneen, M.J., Păun, G., Pérez-Jímenez, M.J., Rozenberg, G. (eds.) UC 2005. LNCS, vol. 3699, pp. 191–205. Springer, Heidelberg (2005)
20. Tošić, P.T.: On modeling and analyzing sparsely networked large-scale multi-agent systems with cellular and graph automata. In: Alexandrov, V.N., van Albada, G.D., Sloot, P.M., Dongarra, J. (eds.) ICCS 2006. LNCS, vol. 3993, pp. 272–280. Springer, Heidelberg (2006)

# Investigations of Human Information Processing Systems

# Human Emotion Variation Analysis Based on EEG Signal and POMS Scale

Youjun Li[1,2,3,4(✉)], Haiyan Zhou[1,2,3,4], Jianhui Chen[1,2,3,4],
Jiajin Huang[1,2,3,4], Meng Chen[2], Yan Liu[2], and Ning Zhong[1,2,3,4,5]

[1] Beijing Advanced Innovation Center for Future Internet Technology,
Beijing, China
lyj@ncut.edu.cn, zhong@maebashi-it.ac.jp
[2] International WIC Institute, Beijing University of Technology, Beijing, China
[3] Beijing International Collaboration Base on Brain Informatics and Wisdom
Services, Beijing, China
[4] Beijing Key Laboratory of MRI and Brain Informatics, Beijing, China
[5] Department of Life Science and Informatics,
Maebashi Institute of Technology, Maebashi, Japan

**Abstract.** Emotion is considered as a critical aspect of human brain behavior. In this paper, we investigate human normal emotion variation for a long period without stimuli. Eight subjects participated in the experiment for seven days. The EEG signal and POMS scale of the subjects were collected in the experiment. After data collection and preprocessing, Pearson correlation analysis and multiple linear regression analysis were carried out between EEG features and POMS emotion components. The results of Pearson correlation analysis show that the correlation coefficient of EEG features and POMS emotion component range from 0.367 to 0.610 at 0.01 significant levels. Based on this, multiple linear regression models are built between POMS emotion components and EEG features. With these models, the POMS scales of the subjects can be predicted such that the $R^2$ between the prediction scale and real scale ranges from 0.329 to 0.772; the emotion of 'Depression-Dejection' has the lowest $R^2$ (0.329); and the 'Negative Emotion' has the highest $R^2$ (0.772).

## 1 Introduction

Emotion, in everyday speech, is any relatively brief conscious experience characterized by intense mental activity and a high degree of pleasure or displeasure [1, 2]. Emotion is considered as a critical aspect of human brain behavior. Researches on human emotion have increased significantly over past two decades with contributions in many fields including psychology, neuroscience, endocrinology, medicine, history, sociology, and even computer science.

The development of wearable biosensor and mobile communication technology make it possible to conveniently record human's bio-signal for a long period. In this study, we adopted a kind of wearable EEG belt and mobile devices to record subjects' EEG signal and POMS scale [3]. A system based on wearable EEG belt and Android APP is built to collect EEG signal and POMS scale. We designed and carried

G.A. Ascoli et al. (Eds.): BIH 2016, LNAI 9919, pp. 75–84, 2016.
DOI: 10.1007/978-3-319-47103-7_8

out experiments to collect data by using the data collection system. With the data analysis, results present high correlation between EEG features and POMS emotion component scales. Furthermore, multiple linear regression models are built to predict subjects' POMS emotion variation.

The rest of the paper is organized as follows: Sect. 2 discusses related work. Section 3 presents how to design experiments and collect data. Section 4 describes how to analyze the collected data and gives preliminary results. Section 5 provides concluding remarks.

## 2 Related Work

### 2.1 POMS Scale in Emotion Variation Study

As a traditional emotion assessment tool, the POMS scale has been widely accepted in the field of psychological research. The POMS 2™ is a self-report measure that allows for the quick assessment of transient, fluctuating feelings, and enduring affect states. As multi-dimensional and comprehensive assessment, the POMS assessment has proven itself a valuable measure of affective mood style fluctuations in a wide variety of populations. The long form of the POMS consists of 65 adjectives that are rated by subjects on a 5-point scale. Six emotion factors are derived from the POMS, including Anger-Hostility, Confusion-Bewilderment, Depression-Dejection, Fatigue-Inertia, Tension-Anxiety and Vigor-Activity. The POMS short versions contain a subset of 35 items from the full-length versions. The short versions provide an efficient means for determining the need for additional assessment or services. Total Mood Disturbance (TMD for short) is a function of these six scale scores, which represents the disturbance of the subject. The higher the value of TMD, the less peaceful of the emotion is.

Beili Zhu et al. studied the Model of POMS Scale for Chinese [4]. The whole experiment indicates that POMS scale suits Chinese to measure their emotion states. In this study, the POMS scale is employed to record the long period variation of the subjects' emotion states.

### 2.2 Emotion Analysis Based on EEG Signal

Former studies [5, 6, 14, 15] on emotion mainly focus on the detection and assessment of the different emotion by monitoring and analyzing the behavioral indicators and physiological signal in a short time (no more than one day) with stimuli from different kinds of pictures, music, or videos. For example, DEAP [7], an open dataset records the EEG data of the subjects with stimuli of videos. In such experiment, the EEG signals of 32 participants are recorded. Each subject watches 40 one-minute long videos. With such dataset, significant correlates are found between the participant ratings and EEG frequencies. In another study, Chen and colleagues proposed an EEG-based emotion assessment system to analyze the gender-specific correlations between EEG features and two emotional dimensions [8, 9]. In their study, negative correlations are found between female EEG signal and arousal/valence, and positive correlations are found between male EEG signal and arousal/valence, in which DEAP dataset is also used as their material.

Traditional EEG analysis methods usually employ statistics, linear and non-linear analysis methods to extract EEG features from EEG signal. For different experiment objectives, people extract different EEG features. With different features, people can study emotion from different aspects. For example, with the frequency-domain analyses method, features (such as the absolute power of the different sub-bands, the relative power of the different sub-bands) were extracted from EEG signal in several classic non-overlapping frequency bands. With these features, different sub-bands can reflect different affects related activities [10]. Entropy is proposed to calculate the information of the EEG signal, such as Shannon entropy, spectral entropy, and Kolmogorov entropy [11]. In [11], Kolmogorov entropy was calculated to analyze EEG signal at various sleep stages. C0-complexity is a description of time sequences randomness. In [12], the coefficient of variation and the fluctuation index of IMFs were extracted by EMD method as features for recognition of ictal EEG.

However, few studies have investigated on how human emotion changes during a long period, such as several weeks, even months. It is more important to study human's emotion variation in everyday life for a long period. For example, in the clinical study of mental health, the hospitalized patients' emotion variation during his/her hospital staying is very important for medical staffs to improve the antidiastole level and to identify the therapeutic effect. Another example is that the students' emotion variation is very important for the evaluation of the courses' attraction during remote education. In these contexts, no designed stimuli are taken and the observation must sustain a long period (at least 7–14 days). The key questions are how to evaluate human emotion variation in a large time granularity and how to evaluate human normal emotion variation without artificial stimuli. In this study, we collect subjects' resting state EEG signal (without artificial stimuli) for a long period.

## 3 Experiment and Data Collection System

### 3.1 Experiment Protocol and Design

Before the start of the experiment, we provide subjects with documentation detailing the experimental protocol, subject consent procedures, and subject recruitment. In the approval, it is necessary to explicitly describe every type of data collected from the subjects as well as the equipment used in the study. Particular interest is to make sure the protocol protecting the individual's right to maintain their health information privacy. The subjects involved in this experiments are fully notified the protocol. For studying the emotion variation of normal people, we plan to recruit 30 subjects for the study. By the time of writing, eight subjects have finished the experiment.

The procedure of the experiment is as follows. Once a subject agrees to take part in the experiment by signing the informed consent, he/she is asked to provide the information about demographic, physical history and physical examination. After that, the study begins. The content of the experiment is to record subject's resting state EEG signal. Due to the limitation of the reality (such as the battery capacity of the EEG belt), the experiment cannot last for a whole day. Therefore, the EEG signal is recorded twice a day. Every morning (about 9:00–10:00) and evening (about 19:00 to 20:00), the EEG signal is recorded by the data collection system which is deployed in a smart phone as an APP. Another content of the experiment is to record subject's POMS scale. The POMS scale collection software is also designed as an APP deployed in the smart phone. Each subject can take a self-evaluation with that APP conveniently. The self-evaluation is fulfilled once a day in the evening just after the EEG testing. The data is stored in the phone temporarily. After the whole day's experiment finished, the collected data stored in the phone is transferred to a data server with Wi-Fi signal.

## 3.2    Data Collection System

EEG signal often refers to the recording of the brain's natural electrical activity in a short period of time (10–20 min). The EEG signal is usually recorded from multiple electrodes placed on the scalp. The 10–20 international system is used as the standard naming and positioning scheme for EEG measurements. In this study, a wearable EEG belt, NeuroSky B3 belt, is employed to collect EEG signal with two dry electrodes. The EEG belt chooses Fp1 as a testing electrode to collect EEG signal for the reason of that the frontal lobe is without hair covering and easy to recognize. A1 is chosen as a reference electrode. In this study, the objective of the experiment is to capture the resting state EEG signal of the subjects, which means the subjects are required to close their eyes, keep relax and stay in a quiet environment. Therefore, the noisy signal caused by muscle activations and eye blinking has been reduced to a minimum degree. In this section, a data collection system based on EEG wearable belt, smart phone/pad and Android APPs is introduced. The structure of the system is shown in Fig. 1.

As shown in Fig. 1, the system can be divided into two parts. The part below the dotted line corresponds to the data collection, and the part up to the dotted line corresponds to the data analysis. Data collection system is composed of three components.

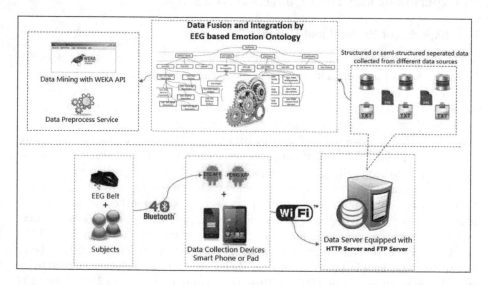

**Fig. 1.** Structure of data collection system

From left to right, they are bio-sensor devices (wearable EEG belt), data collection devices (Android based smart phone or pad), collection software (APPs), and data integration server. The EEG signal was sent from the EEG belt by Bluetooth signal.

At the time of writing this paper, a total number of 112 EEG signal files and 56 POMS scale files have been collected. The experiments were carried out from 2015-7-15 to 2015-7-21. Eight subjects (7 male, 1 female) participated in the experiments. The age of the subjects is between 23 and 26 years old. All of them are graduated students in school. All subjects and their families have no psychiatric history.

## 4 Emotion Variation Analysis by EEG Signal and POMS Scale

Before feature extraction from EEG signal, the data must be de-noised. Artifacts must be corrected before further analysis [13]. In this study, db5 wavelet was employed to decompose the raw EEG signal, and soft threshold filtering method was adopted to remove the artifacts from the raw data. Normal EEG signal is between 10–100 μV in amplitude and fall in the range of 0.5–50 Hz. The activity below or above this range is mostly the noisy signal, and should be removed [13].

After that, six EEG features were extracted from the de-noised data. The features include coefficient of variation (Cn), fluctuation index (Fn), power spectral entropy (SE), C0-complexity (C0), beta and theta power rate (BT) and the power of the EEG signal (P).

In this subsection, three parts are introduced. First, as an indicator of the emotion variation, subjects' TMD scales are calculated and analyzed. After that, correlation analysis is researched between POMS scale and EEG features. Third, multiple linear regression analysis is done between EEG features and POMS scale to build an emotion variation prediction model.

### 4.1 Subjects' TMD Scale Statistics and Survey

As the summary of the daily emotion state, the POMS scales are collected by evaluating and recording the subjects after dinner in the evening (around 19:00–19:30). In our system, each subject's POMS scale is recorded in a text file. The APP consists of 40 questions, which ask about the subject's daily emotion state. Each answer includes four options. For example, the answer for the question about the depression emotion consists: 'Not at all', 'A little', 'Depress', 'Very Depress'. Each option corresponds to an integer from zero to three. In order to reduce the subject's memory effect, we randomize the order of the questions. Any emotion question that took the subject less than 1 s to respond to would appear again in the following test.

With the POMS scales, subjects themselves can evaluate significant outcomes. TMD and other component emotion scales are counted with the given formula of POMS. The formula to count the TMD value can be expressed as:

$$TMD = N_s - P_s + 100 \tag{1}$$

where $N_s$ means the sum of the negative emotion evaluated value and $P_s$ means the sum of the positive emotion evaluated value.

Using the statistics of POMS, we can objectively trend a subject's emotion variation over time. The statistics of subjects' TMD is presented in Fig. 2 by using the box and whisker plot of subjects' TMD values, where boxes have lines at the lower quartile, median, and upper quartile values. We can see two points from Fig. 2: the first is that all subjects' TMD values changed during seven days, which means we captured subjects' emotion variation by POMS scale; Another point is that the degree of the subjects' TMD variations is different, which means the emotion variation of the subjects is different. For example, subjects 1, 4, 5, 6, and 7 have a great variation. However, subjects 2 and 3 have little emotion variation. The emotion of subject 8 almost did not change during the experiment period.

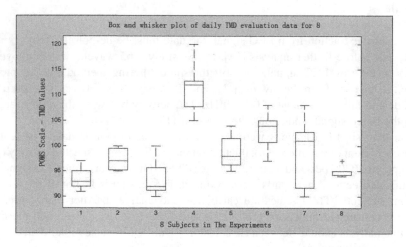

**Fig. 2.** Box and whisker plot of daily TMD evaluation data for eight subjects for seven days

## 4.2  Correlation Analysis Between EEG Signal and POMS Scale

Table 1 shows the results of the correlation analysis between EEG signal features and POMS scale. From Table 1, we can see that four types of EEG features are extracted and analyzed, and only the results with significant correlations (** means at 0.01 level, and * means at 0.05 level) were presented in the table. Firstly, with the analysis result, we can see that most of the emotion has significant correlation with the EEG features. Secondly, some of the POMS component scale has significant correlation with more than one EEG features. For example, the 'Vigor-Activity' has significant correlation with C0, SE and C3 at 0.01 levels, and with F1 and GL1 at 0.05 levels.

## 4.3  Regression Analysis of the People's Emotion Variation

In order to find the relationship between EEG signals and people's emotion variation, all extracted EEG features are used for a regression analysis with the POMS scales. SPSS is employed for such analysis. Six types of EEG features (about 23 EEG features) are chosen as entered independent variables. POMS component scales and TMD are

**Table 1.** Pearson correlation analysis result between POMS scale and EEG features

| POMS component scale and TMD | EEG features which have significant correlation with the component scale at 0.01 level | EEG features which have significant correlation with the component scale at 0.05 level |
|---|---|---|
| Tension-anxiety | C0: P = .610**, S = .000<br>SE: P = .449**, S = .001<br>... | F1: P = .287*, S = .046<br>F2: P = .317*, S = .026<br>... |
| Anger-hostility | F1: P = .575**, S = .000<br>F2: P = .389**, S = .006<br>... | C1: P = .318*, S = .026<br>C2: P = .288*, S = .045<br>... |
| Depression-dejection | C3: P = .453**, S = .001 | F3: P = .290*, S = .043 |
| Vigor-activity | C0: P = .525**, S = .000<br>SE: P = .370**, S = .009<br>... | F1: P = .279*, S = .038<br>GL1: P = .291*, S = .030 |
| Confusion-bewilderment | C0: P = .450**, S = .001<br>SE: P = .367**, S = .010<br>... | C1: P = -.283*, S = .049 |
| Ego | F2: P = .392**, S = .005<br>F3: P = .565**, S = .000<br>... | B-T: P = .341*, S = .010<br>F4: P = .341*, S = .010<br>... |
| Fatigue-inertia | F3: P = .409**, S = .004<br>C3: P = .602**, S = .000<br>... | C3: P = .295*, S = .039<br>... |
| TMD | C3: P = .512**, S = .000 | C2: P = .306*, S = .022 |

EEG features presented in this table only are the features, which have significant correlation with the POMS component, including coefficient of variation (C1–C5) and fluctuation index (F1–F5), power (GL1–GL5) of the 5 IMFs, and beta-theta sub-band power rate (B–T). P means Pearson correlation coefficient. S means signification.

chosen as dependent variables. Multivariate regression method is employed to analyze the linear relation between variables. The stepwise method is adopted to choose the independent variables. The stepwise rule is that the F value of the entered independent variables must under 0.05. The independent variables with F value upper than 0.1 are eliminated. The results are summarized along with their $R^2$, standardized coefficients and Sig. (P) as shown in Table 2.

As we can see from Table 2, different emotion components, negative emotion, positive emotion and TMD were analyzed separately. The $R^2$ of the relation is between 0.329 and 0.772. The emotion of 'Depression-Dejection' has the lowest $R^2$ (0.329), and the 'Negative Emotion' has the highest $R^2$ (0.772). The standardized coefficients raw gives the chosen independent variables (EEG features) and the standardized coefficients. The Sig. raw gives the Sig. values (P) to the corresponding independent variables. In addition, we can see from Table 2 that the EEG features extracted from IMFs have high correlation with the emotion variation. Therefore, most of the coefficients are composed by these EEG features.

The emotion variation model built by the multiple linear regression analysis results will be expressed as

**Table 2.** The results of multivariate regression analysis between EEG features and POMS scales

| POMS scales component | Multivariate regression analysis results | | |
|---|---|---|---|
| | R2 | Standardized coefficients | Sig. (P) |
| Tension-anxiety | 0.684 | C0: 1.807 | 0.000 |
| | | F2: −1.320 | 0.000 |
| Anger-hostility | 0.690 | C1: 3.325 | 0.000 |
| | | F1: −2.844 | 0.000 |
| | | GL1: 0.283 | 0.004 |
| Depression-dejection | 0.329 | C1: 2.360 | 0.001 |
| | | F1: −1.949 | 0.004 |
| Ego | 0.659 | C3: 0.846 | 0.000 |
| | | C5: −0.441 | 0.000 |
| Fatigue-inertia | 0.556 | C3: 0.887 | 0.000 |
| | | B-T: −0.367 | 0.004 |
| Negative emotion | 0.772 | C3: 1.055 | 0.000 |
| | | C4: −0.619 | 0.000 |
| Positive emotion | 0.682 | C3: 0.875 | 0.000 |
| | | C5: −0.239 | 0.010 |
| TMD | 0.713 | C3: 0.931 | 0.000 |
| | | C4: −0.749 | 0.043 |

$$E_i = c_1 f_1 + c_2 f_2 + \ldots + c_{n-1} f_{n-1} + c_n f_n \tag{2}$$

where $E_i$ represents the emotion components of the POMS, the summary of the negative or positive emotion and the TMD scale; $c_n$ represents the standardized coefficients corresponding to the $f_n$ which means the chosen EEG features. Taking the variation of TMD as an example, with the multiple linear analysis result in Table 2, the TMD calculated model built by EEG features can be expressed as

$$E_{TMD} = 0.931 \times C_3 - 0.749 \times C_4 \tag{3}$$

Next, we compare the TMD values calculated by the built model and from POMS scales as shown in Fig. 3. From Fig. 3, we can see that the full line is the TMD values calculated from the POMS component scales, and the dotted line is the TMD values calculated by the emotion variation model expressed by Formula (2). Two TMD values exhibit higher correlation as shown in Fig. 3. Pearson correlation analysis is employed to analyze the correlation of two TMD values. The result shows that two TMD values have a correlation at 0.01 levels, and the Pearson correlation coefficient is 0.775. The other emotion's variation model also can be built with this method. Since the emotion of subject 8 has little variation during 7 days, we only analyzed the data of other seven subjects.

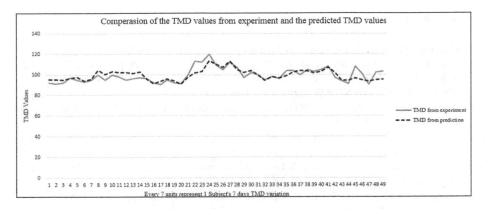

**Fig. 3.** The comparison of POMS TMD values and evaluated TMD values

## 5 Concluding Remarks

In this study, we proposed a new method to study the normal emotion variation of human with resting state EEG signal and POMS scale. Experiments were designed to collect the relative data. Eight subjects participated in the experiment for seven days. The result represents that each emotion component has high correlation with the extracted EEG features. The Pearson correlation coefficient of EEG features and POMS emotion component is between 0.367–0.610 at 0.01 significant level. Multiple linear regression analysis builds regression model between EEG features and POMS emotion components (TMD as an example). With the regression model, we predict subjects' TMD variation. The result shows that the predicted TMD value and the real TMD value have a correlation at 0.01 levels, and the Pearson correlation coefficient is 0.775.

Although we can announce that a long period human emotion variation can be predicted with EEG signal, some limitations of this research must be thought of. Further studies should be carried out in the future. For example, the number and the type of the participants are no enough. There are only eight subjects (7 male and 1 female). The difference of their age is not so big. In addition, the level of their education experience is similar. Therefore, in the future work, we will collect more subjects to validate our methods and the model. Another point worth noting is that with the results of correlation analysis between EEG features and POMS emotion components, we find that some EEG features have high correlation with many different emotion components. The reason for that will be studied in the future work.

**Acknowledgement.** This work was partly supported by the National Basic Research Program of China under grant no. 2014CB744600, by the International Science & Technology Cooperation Program of China under grant no. 2013DFA32180, by the National Natural Science Foundation of China grant no. 61272345, by the Beijing Key Laboratory of Magnetic Resonance Imaging and Brain Informatics, and by the Beijing Municipal Commission of Education.

# References

1. Cabanac, M.: What is emotion? Behav. Process. **60**(2), 69–83 (2002)
2. Schacter, D.L.: Psychology, 2nd edn. Worth Publishers, New York (2011). p. 310. ISBN 978-1-4292-3719-2
3. MULTI-HEALTH SYSTEMS. http://www.mhs.com/
4. Zhu, B.: Brief introduction of POMS scale and its model for China. J. Tianjin Inst. Phys. Educ. **10**(1), 35–37 (1995)
5. Su, Y., Hu, B., Xu, L., Cai, H., Moore, P., Zhang, X., Chen, J.: EmotionO+: physiological signals knowledge representation and emotion reasoning model for mental health monitoring. In: Proceedings of 2014 IEEE International Conference on Bioinformatics and Biomedicine (BIBM 2014), pp. 529–535 (2014)
6. Wang, D., Miao, D., Xie, C.: Best basis-based wavelet packet entropy feature extraction and hierarchical EEG classification for epileptic detection. Expert Syst. Appl. **38**(11), 14314–14320 (2011)
7. DEAP data set online web index. http://www.eecs.qmul.ac.uk/mmv/datasets/deap/
8. Chen, J., Hu, B., Moore, P., Zhang, X., Ma, X.: Electroencephalogram-based emotion assessment system using ontology and data mining techniques. Appl. Soft Comput. **30**, 663–674 (2015)
9. Muhl, C., Soleymani, M., Lee, J.S., Yazdani, A., Ebrahimi, T., Pun, T., Nijholt, A., Patras, I.: DEAP: a database for emotion analysis using physiological signal. IEEE Trans. Affect. Comput. **3**(1), 18–31 (2012)
10. Chanel, G., Kierkels, J.J.M., Soleymani, M., Pun, T.: Short-term emotion assessment in a recall paradigm. Int. J. Hum. Comput. Stud. **67**, 607–627 (2009)
11. Acharya, R., Faust, U.O., Kannathal, N., Chua, T., Laxminarayan, S.: Non-linear analysis of EEG signal at various sleep stages. Comput. Methods Programs Biomed. **80**, 37–45 (2005)
12. Li, S., Zhou, W., Yuan, Q., Geng, S., Cai, D.: Feature extraction and recognition of ictal EEG using EMD and SVM. Comput. Biol. Med. **43**(7), 807–816 (2013)
13. Khatwani, P., Tiwari, A.: A survey on different noise removal techniques of EEG signal. Int. J. Adv. Res. Comput. Commun. Eng. **2**(2), 1091–1095 (2013)
14. Iacoviello, D., Petracca, A., Spezialetti, M., Placidi, G.: A real-time classification algorithm for EEG-based BCI driven by self-induced emotions. Comput. Methods Programs Biomed. **122**(3), 293–303 (2015)
15. Tsuchiya, S., Morimoto, M., Imono, M., Watab, H.: Judging emotion from EEGs based on an association mechanism. Proc. Comput. Sci. **60**, 37–44 (2015)

# Visual Information Processing Mechanism Revealed by fMRI Data

Jinpeng Li[1,2], Zhaoxiang Zhang[1,2,3], and Huiguang He[1,2,3(✉)]

[1] Research Center for Brain-Inspired Intelligence, Institute of Automation,
Chinese Academy of Sciences, Beijing, China
huiguang.he@ia.ac.cn
[2] University of Chinese Academy of Sciences (UCAS), Beijing, China
[3] Center for Excellence in Brain Science and Intelligence Technology,
Chinese Academy of Sciences, Beijing, China

**Abstract.** The functional Magnetic Resonance Imaging (fMRI) data of both the ventral pathway and the dorsal pathway on the visual cortex in a classification task was analyzed. We found that the classification performance improved hierarchically from lower-level regions to higher-level regions in both pathways, which partly verified the visual pathway theory proposed in cognitive neuroscience. Moreover, the LO (Lateral Occipital), V3a and V3b fMRI data were good classification basis no worse than the widely-used features such as GIST, HOG and LBP. It indicated that imitating the activity patterns of visual cortex to design new feature-extraction algorithms might be favorable. Finally, the performance of V3a and V3b voxels were very close to that of LO voxels. Consequently, in the design of brain-like intelligence systems, we should consider the coordination mechanism between the two pathways rather than focusing on the ventral pathway alone. The relationship of human visual pathway and deep learning structure was also discussed tersely.

**Keywords:** Visual cortex · Ventral pathway · Dorsal pathway · fMRI · Classification · Representation

## 1 Introduction

The mechanism of human visual system has long been an attractive research topic, and still under research by enthusiastic scholars. The research mainly involves biology, psychology, cognitive neuroscience and pattern recognition algorithms, thus it forms a comprehensive research field. The understanding of human visual cortex is not supposed to be merely a fundamental research issue concerning medical anatomy or biology, for the benefits it brings to the development of artificial intelligence (AI) and various engineering techniques are beyond measure. The understanding of visual system will in turn instruct us to design more brain-like algorithms (e.g. new deep learning models) to accomplish pattern recognition tasks.

The visual cortex across the brain is believed to be hierarchically organized by different function-specialized regions and could be further divided into two pathways according to different functions, i.e. the ventral pathway and the dorsal pathway [1].

© Springer International Publishing AG 2016
G.A. Ascoli et al. (Eds.): BIH 2016, LNAI 9919, pp. 85–93, 2016.
DOI: 10.1007/978-3-319-47103-7_9

The former one is tightly related to object identification, while the latter one mainly deals with object localization. In 1970s, Hubel and Wiesel realized from their empirical observations that the activity mode of the neurons located in V1 resembled Gabor wavelet filters, and different neurons corresponded to different frequencies and orientations [2, 3]. Their work successfully explained the computational characters in the primary cortex V1, which was the shared "entrance" of both the ventral and dorsal pathway. Encouraged by the success of the shallow V1 model, researchers began to try deeper models under the hope of describing downstream areas and proposed the HMAX model to imitate the activity patterns of the ventral pathway [4]. The basic HMAX structure consisted of four layers. The first layer was formed by Gabor filters. The second layer performed max-pooling. The third layer extracted the output of the second layer and operated template matching, and the forth layer was another pooling layer. The multi-layer HMAX model was capable of explaining the computational characters of V1 and V2, but had trouble extending to higher cortical areas such as V4 and IT (Inferior Temporal) [5]. In 1990s, researches turned to a more direct approach. The central methodology was to collect response data to various stimulus at multiple region-of-interests ROIs and used statistical fitting techniques to find model parameters that produced the observed stimulus-response relationship. However, they soon realized that multilayered networks fitted to neural data in higher areas such as V4 ended up overfitting the training data and predicting comparatively small amounts of explained variance on novel testing images [6]. Thus the features extracted from such models were not good classification basis. The reasons might include such two following aspects: (1) the data amount was not large enough to provide a precise representation of connections between regions, and (2) the process of image identification in the visual cortex could not be easily explained by the simple cascaded ventral pathway V1-V2-V4-IT. There were countless coupled and cross-pathway connections between the ventral and dorsal pathways, so the mechanism of object identification cannot be simply described by a single pathway. The contributions of the dorsal pathway should not be neglected, so the complex synergistic effects of the dorsal pathway (e.g. V3a and V3b areas) should also be included into the models. We should study the activity patterns of ROIs located along the dorsal pathway as well as ventral ones when designing new feature-extraction algorithms.

The instruments for visual cortex research differs according to diverse application fields, in which fMRI is suitable for cerebral cortex imaging. The fMRI technology measures the Blood Oxygen Level Dependent (BOLD) in the brain vessels, which is tightly related to image-understanding process. Simultaneously, fMRI is able to offer us a deep and precise insight into different ROIs at a time resolution of less than one second and a space resolution in millimeter. With the help of fMRI and distributed pattern analysis method, researchers were able to investigate where and how complex natural scene information was encoded and discriminated by the brain [7, 8].

In this paper, we analyzed fMRI data for both the ventral pathway V1-V2-V4-LO and the dorsal pathway V1-V2-V3-V3a-V3b in a natural image classification task, and the results were instructive.

## 2   Data and Task

In order to explore the organization and function of the visual cortex, as well as to identify which areas are involved in object recognition process, the classification accuracy (based on BOLD values of each region) is introduced as the analyzing tool and evaluation criterion. BOLD is a direct measurement of the cerebral cortex activities, so the better the image is encoded by cortex regions, the higher classification accuracy of the BOLD-based classifiers will acquire.

The data set contained the fMRI responses of 1750 natural photographs, and the stimulus included animals, buildings, food, humans, indoor scenes, manmade objects, outdoor scenes, and textures. During the experiment, the subject looked at a sequence of natural photographs displayed on a screen, and at the same time, the BOLD responses of multiple cortex regions were recorded by fMRI scanning synchronously. The experiment used flashing technique to enhance the signal-to-noise ratio of voxel responses. The fMRI responses for each image were recorded according to the stimulus design shown in Fig. 1. Seven ROIs were considered, including V1, V2, V3, V3a, V3b, V4 and LO, and their overall tridimensional distribution on the occipital lobe was shown in Fig. 2(a). In Fig. 2(b), two different paths were illustrated, in which V1, V2, V4, LO belonged to the ventral pathway, and V1, V2, V3, V3a, V3b belonged to the dorsal pathway. In order to optimize the data structure, several steps for preprocessing were performed, i.e. the alignment was performed manually and the data were temporally interpolated to account for differences in slice time acquisition [9]. Peak BOLD responses to each of the 1750 images were then estimated from the preprocessed data and stored. The responses for each voxel were z-scored, so for a given voxel the units of each "response" were standard deviations from that voxel's mean response [9]. Notice that in an fMRI map, the voxel numbers of each ROI was different according to the researchers' selection, as is shown in Table 1.

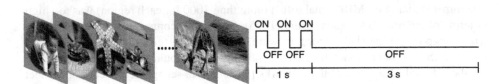

**Fig. 1.** Stimulus design. Every image was shown in a 1 s–3 s schedule. During the first 1 s, the same image flashed three times (each time for 200 ms) to stimulate the brain's corresponding response patterns to the maximum, and the following 3 s was grey background, then the next picture was shown.

The dataset was originally contributed by Gallant et al. at UC Berkeley [9, 10]. For more detailed information about the data set, or download it for research purpose, log on to the website (https://crcns.org/data-sets/vc/vim-1/about-vim-1).

In order to perform classification task, we tagged the output labels for the 1750 fMRI maps by hand. We selected 1575 samples (90 %) for supervised training and 175 samples (10 %) for validation.

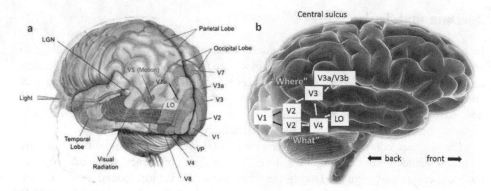

**Fig. 2.** The distribution and voxel number of ROIs. (a) The brief structure of human visual system (https://quizlet.com/11094814/neuro-3-vision-2-chp-6-flash-cards/). The visual information is first collected by the retina and transmitted to the Lateral Geniculate Nucleus (LGN), then get into the visual cortex mainly located at the Occipital Lobe (OL) via the visual radiation. Henceforth, the brain extracts complex features in a highly-nonlinear way and begins the understanding process. (b) The two visual pathways. The dorsal pathway deals with the "where" problem and the ventral pathway deals with the "what" problem. The double sided arrows indicate that the information flow in both pathways are bidirectional rather than unidirectional, and there are connections between the two channels.

**Table 1.** The voxel numbers considered in seven ROIs.

| ROIs | V1 | V2 | V3 | V3a | V3b | V4 | LO |
|---|---|---|---|---|---|---|---|
| Voxel number | 1294 | 2036 | 1973 | 484 | 314 | 701 | 928 |

## 3    Experiments and Results

The dimensionality of fMRI signal (often more than 1000 for each region) was too high in terms of the limited sample amount (1575). So the full-connected shallow networks with backpropagation (BP) algorithm were not favorable (generally to implement a model with full-connection networks, the training cases should be at least ten times the number of total parameters of the networks [5]. Our data set apparently could not meet such strict requirement). In order to efficiently perform classification with small sample amount and high-dimensional features, we chose SVM classifiers and performed PCA before classification.

All the results in our work were obtained by three-fold cross-validation and shown in the form of mean ± SD.

### 3.1    The Rising Trend of Performance Along Both Pathways

We found that there were distinguishable differences among each ROI's performance along both pathways, and there were some regular patterns or distinct trends that acted in accordance with cognitive neuroscience findings. The results were summarized in

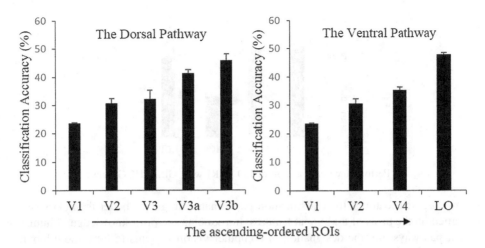

**Fig. 3.** Performance trend along both pathways. (a) The ventral pathway (four ROIs). (b) The dorsal pathway (five ROIs).

Fig. 3. In the ventral pathway V1-V2-V4-LO, the performance was 23.6 %, 30.7 %, 35.2 % and 47.8 % respectively. The dorsal pathway V1-V2-V3-V3a-V3b showed a similar trend that classification accuracy improved as the level of ROIs advanced, and the performance was 23.6 %, 30.7 %, 32.2 %, 41.3 %, and 45.9 % respectively. Apparently, there was a common phenomenon in both pathways that classification performance improved significantly as visual information passed on from lower areas to higher areas. Among all the ROIs considered, LO (47.8 %) played the best, followed by V3b (45.9 %) at the top of the dorsal pathway in this experiment.

## 3.2 LO fMRI Data Contains Substantial Information of Images

The visual tasks (usually classification) have long been a difficult challenge to modern computer science. Numerous algorithms aimed at representing images were previously proposed [11, 12]. They were designed quite statistical and mathematical for computer calculation, but far from imitating the way the brain worked. Unsurprisingly, if our goal was simply classification accuracy, the opinions diverged as to whether more biological detailed models would ultimately be needed [13].

In order to show the superiority of the brain over traditional feature-extraction methods in image representation, we extracted 512-D GIST features (unlike SIFT who aimed at giving pictures local and regional descriptions, GIST aimed at offering global and overall features), 576-D HOG features and 256-D LBP features for each of the 1750 natural photographs, and designed SVM classifiers accordingly. The results were summarized in Fig. 4. It turned out to be that in this task, LBP (48.4 %) was slightly better than LO fMRI (47.8 %), LO fMRI played better than GIST (46.8 %), while HOG (42.1 %) played the worst.

Therefore, if we designed deep models that could eventually simulated the response activities of voxels located at LO or V3b (and even-higher areas) to imitate the way the

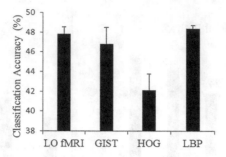

**Fig. 4.** Performance comparison of LO fMRI with GIST, HOG, and LBP.

brain-extracted features, the classification performance might be better than classifiers designed on the basis of traditional features. Introducing the prior knowledge of human visual pathways into the designation of computer vision systems to form more bionic visual models for various tasks was commendable. The brain is undoubtedly more effective than human-assigned feature-extraction approaches.

### 3.3 The Dorsal Pathway Contributes to Object Identification

The relatively high performance of LO was natural, because modern neuroscience had found numerous evidences of the specific function of ventral pathway in object recognition. However, we found that the performance of V3a and V3b (41.3 % and 45.9 % respectively) were not far from LO. The results indicated that the dorsal pathway (including V3, V3a and V3b at least) also contributed to object identification.

We also performed canonical correlation analysis (CCA) [12] to seek for the correlationship of V3a and V3b with other ROIs. The results were shown in Fig. 5. CCA algorithm linearly mapped two sets of variables to new spaces respectively, and then

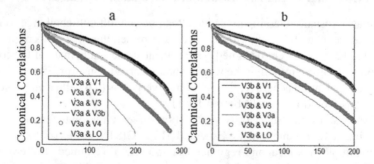

**Fig. 5.** The correlationship of V3a and V3b with other regions measured by CCA. (a) The canonical correlation of V3a and other regions. There was a relatively strong correlationship between V3a and V2, as well as with V3. (b) The same analysis was performed on V3b, and the result demonstrated that relatively strong correlationship existed between V3b and V2, as well as with V3. Both the figures show that the activity patterns of V3a and V3b were tightly related to V2 and V3 voxels. It should be mentioned that V4 and LO also had relatively good correlationship with the two regions.

maximized the correlationship of two sets of mapped data. Therefore, CCA was an appropriate method to evaluate the linear correlationship of two given variables. Here voxel activities of different regions were considered as variable sets, and the linear unoriented correlationship (the strongest relationship) of V3a and V3b with other regions was thus excavated. The introduction of CCA aimed at analyzing unoriented functional connectivity of ROIs rather than the oriented effective connectivity, and was often done by electroencephalograph.

Simultaneously, the recent findings in deep learning also confirmed our speculation. In 2012, Krizhevsky et al. built the famous convolutional neural network and won the ImageNet competition [14]. It marked the beginning of the dominance of deep neural networks in computer vision. In the past four years, error rates had dropped further, roughly matching (or even exceeded) human performance in the domain of visual object classification [13]. In order to give the high performance a physiological explanation and improve recent deep model structure, researchers tried to compare the state-of-art deep neural networks with the visual pathway to see how much they match in architecture. For example, Eickenberg et al. extracted the outputs of all layers after rectified linear units (ReLU) of OverFeat (2013). They used L2 penalized linear regression to fit a predictive model to each voxel of the measured brain activity after spatial smoothing and subsampling. They found that the outputs of some layers e.g. the fourth or fifth convolutional layer were able to predict the activities of V3a and V3b voxels at relatively high accuracy. It implied that there were some internal relationships between network layers and the two ROIs. Consequently, if the deep networks were confirmed to be "brain-like" (some scholars are working on the interesting topic, such as Kriegeskorte [13], Cambridge and DiCarlo [5], MIT), then we might come to the conclusion that V3a and V3b played an important role in object recognition. Moreover, the role of V3a and V3b in the real visual pathway might be similar with the corresponding layers in the deep network.

Although building the one-to-one correspondence between deep network layers and visual pathway regions is not accessible now (the existing deep models can only roughly imitate the visual system), yet deep networks are still regarded as best models of human visual system till today.

# 4  Discussion

The results demonstrates that the accuracy increases along the path V1-V2-V4-LO, which is the main part of the 'ventral pathway'. The ventral path mainly solves the problem of object recognition, so the outcome is not surprising. The increasing trend of accuracy corresponds to the fact that as we track the information stream in the human visual system, the representations of the stimulus grow more and more abstract and global for comprehension. Along the entire visual path, the higher functional areas assemble the information delivered by lower ones to form more comprehensive and integrated representations. Notice that V1 is the "entrance" of the ventral pathway, and the whole information of any given image is "stored" in V1, so the representations of this region are intuitively expected to perform the best. However, we find that the following regions all perform better in classification task, which indicates that the visual information is deeply hidden in V1 with high nonlinearity, so the SVM classifiers are unable to excavate the essence of the data. But that is exactly why the ventral visual pathway exists. The V1 information is further transmitted in a highly nonlinear way among the cascaded cortex regions. In this process, the nonlinearity is decoded gradually, making the representations change from wide and shallow to deep and narrow [5]. The mechanism of vision can be described as a nonlinear data miming (DM) process.

The results also demonstrates that the prediction accuracy of LO based classifiers rivals the traditional-feature-based classifiers. Image classification is difficult because it's hard to excavate the deep statistical essence (features) of the data. The features should possess enough distinguishing ability between different samples, but represent similar samples as close as possible. Our work shows brain cortex regions have such characteristics no less than traditional features do. Therefore, we can design new brain-like feature-extraction methods to simulate the activity patterns of visual cortex regions (especially higher regions).

The dorsal pathway also shows its contribution to object recognition process, although it was traditionally believed to be tightly related to localization problems and not effective in object recognition. In fact, there are many complex connections between ventral neurons and dorsal neurons, and the contributions of dorsal regions in recognition tasks should not be neglected.

The relationship between visual pathway and deep neural networks is confusing but interesting. They are similar in the hierarchically-connected structure (some scholars even matched up the layers and regions), and the basic element of artificial neural network imitates the real nerve cell, and the convolutional networks even simulates the local receptive field character. They are different because the brain is a deep and complex recurrent neural network [13], which could not be fully described by the current feed-forward deep models. Moreover, it is physiologically unlikely that the visual cortex learns exactly by BP algorithm, because true biological postnatal learning in humans may use a large amount of unsupervised data. However, the deep networks are still regarded as the best models of the brain and have achieved great success in various fields, such as speech recognition and machine translation [13]. Our results verified that there are "information pyramids" in our visual system, including the ventral pathway as well as the dorsal pathway. There's a commonly addressed question that, why our visual system (and the deep networks) are hierarchically organized? Previous studies have shown that three-layer shallow BP network can approximate continuous functions with arbitrary precision by adding a sufficient number of hidden units and suitably setting the weights [15], but why a "multi-layer pyramid" structure is needed? The reason depth matters is that deep models can represent many complex functions more concisely [13], because they are endowed with more powerful nonlinear feature-extraction ability.

Almost all researches that try to bind deep learning and visual pathway together are limited to analyzing how much they match, but until today, there's no effective way to improve deep learning structure by the foreknowledge of the visual cortex (e.g. redesign convolutional filters for each layer in accordance with corresponding cortex regions and even weight updating algorithm). This direction deserves much further research. Based on classification accuracy and previous evidences in the OverFeat network, we find that V3a and V3b located at the dorsal pathway are also involved in object recognition process. V3a and V3b have their own important status in visual information encoding, consequently, if we want to redesign each layer (or layers) by different ROIs' activity characteristics, not only the regions of the ventral pathway should be included, but also the ROIs of the dorsal pathway should be considered.

**Acknowledgements.** This work was supported by National Natural Science Foundation of China (61271151, 91520202) and Youth Innovation Promotion Association, Chinese Academy of Sciences (CAS).

# References

1. Kruger, N., Janssen, P., Kalkan, S., Lappe, M., Leonardis, A., Piater, J., Wiskott, L.: Deep hierarchies in the primate visual cortex: what can we learn for computer vision? IEEE Trans. Pattern Anal. Mach. Intell. **35**(8), 1847–1871 (2013)
2. Hubel, D.H., Wiesel, T.N.: Receptive fields of single neurones in the cat's striate cortex. J. Physiol. **148**(3), 574–591 (1959)
3. De Valois, K.K., De Valois, R.L., Yund, E.W.: Responses of striate cortex cells to grating and checkerboard patterns. J. Physiol. **291**, 483 (1979)
4. Riesenhuber, M., Poggio, T.: Hierarchical models of object recognition in cortex. Nat. Neurosci. **2**(11), 1019–1025 (1999)
5. Yamins, D.L., DiCarlo, J.J.: Using goal-driven deep learning models to understand sensory cortex. Nat. Neurosci. **19**(3), 356–365 (2016)
6. Gallant, J.L., Connor, C.E., Rakshit, S., Lewis, J.W., Van Essen, D.C.: Neural responses to polar, hyperbolic, and Cartesian gratings in area V4 of the macaque monkey. J. Neurophysiol. **76**(4), 2718–2739 (1996)
7. Schmah, T., Hinton, G.E., Small, S.L., Strother, S., Zemel, R.S.: Generative versus discriminative training of RBMs for classification of fMRI images. In: Advances in Neural Information Processing Systems, 1409–1416 (2008)
8. Walther, D.B., Caddigan, E., Fei-Fei, L., Beck, D.M.: Natural scene categories revealed in distributed patterns of activity in the human brain. J. Neurosci. **29**(34), 10573–10581 (2009)
9. Kay, K.N., Naselaris, T., Prenger, R.J., Gallant, J.L.: Identifying natural images from human brain activity. Nature **452**(7185), 352–355 (2008)
10. Kay, K.N., Naselaris, T., Gallant, J.L.: fMRI of human visual areas in response to natural images (2011). CRCNS.org
11. Wang, X., Han, T.X., Yan, S.: An HOG-LBP human detector with partial occlusion handling. In: 2009 IEEE 12th International Conference on Computer Vision, pp. 32–39. IEEE Press (2009)
12. Cruz-Mota, J., Bogdanova, I., Paquier, B., Bierlaire, M., Thiran, J.P.: Scale invariant feature transform on the sphere: theory and applications. Int. J. Comput. Vis. **98**(2), 217–241 (2012)
13. Kriegeskorte, N.: Deep neural networks: a new framework for modeling biological vision and brain information processing. Ann. Rev. Vis. Sci. **1**, 417–446 (2015)
14. Krizhevsky, A., Sutskever, I., Hinton, G.E.: Imagenet classification with deep convolutional neural networks. In: Advances in Neural Information Processing Systems, pp. 1097–1105 (2012)
15. Schäfer, A.M., Zimmermann, H.-G.: Recurrent neural networks are universal approximators. In: Kollias, S.D., Stafylopatis, A., Duch, W., Oja, E. (eds.) ICANN 2006. LNCS, vol. 4131, pp. 632–640. Springer, Heidelberg (2006)

# Research About Alpha EEG Asymmetry and Self-consciousness in Depression

Xiaomeng Ma[1,2,3,4], Minghui Zhang[1,2,3,4], Jialiang Guo[1,2,3,4],
Haiyan Zhou[1,2,3,4(✉)], Jie Yang[5], Lei Feng[5], and Gang Wang[5]

[1] Beijing Advanced Innovation Center for Future Internet Technology,
Beijing University of Technology, Beijing 100124, China
zhouhaiyan@bjut.edu.cn
[2] The International WIC Institute, Beijing University of Technology, Beijing, China
[3] The Beijing International Collaboration Base on Brain Informatics and Wisdom
Services, Beijing, China
[4] The Beijing Key Laboratory of MRI and Brain Informatics, Beijing, China
[5] Mood Disorders Center and China Clinical Research Center for Mental Disorders,
Beijing Anding Hospital Capital Medical University, Beijing, China

**Abstract.** Depressive disorders shows an alpha EEG asymmetry with higher activation in the left anterior brain. This phenomenon might be associated with the strengthened negative activities in the right side of the brain, especially the information related to self-concept. However, it is absent of direct evidence to support the relationship between the alpha EEG asymmetry and self-concept, and it is not clear what the variation of the correlation between the two factors in depressive disorders. To investigate the issues, we collected the resting EEG data with eye-closed and the self-consciousness level data to compare the relationship between alpha EEG asymmetry and self-concept in depression patients and healthy controls. Results show that both the two groups have strong correlations between the self-consciousness and alpha asymmetry in the brain, but differed in the correlation patterns. Depressions show that self-consciousness is correlated with the more anterior alpha EEG asymmetry in the brain, while the healthy group correlate with the more posterior alpha asymmetry. These results indicate that the impairment of the correlation between self-concept and alpha asymmetry in depressive disorders might be a biomarker of the disease to be considered in future study.

## 1 Introduction

In recent years, with the rapid development of the society, people with depression are gradually increasing. At present, depression is not only the most common mental illness but also one of the most harmful illnesses. Depression is expected to grow to be human's second largest burden of disease in 2020 just fail behind the coronary heart disease. Moreover, depression is easy to relapse. However, the pathology of depression is not clear now. More and more researches are

© Springer International Publishing AG 2016
G.A. Ascoli et al. (Eds.): BIH 2016, LNAI 9919, pp. 94–103, 2016.
DOI: 10.1007/978-3-319-47103-7_10

concentrated in relationship between the neural mechanism and psychological behavior in depressive disorders to provide biomarkers.

Depressive disorders shows a kind of negative bias during cognition [1]. It reported that the underlying automatic cognitive biases could affect the onset, maintenance and recurrence of depressive symptoms (Beck 1976, 1987; Ingram and Ritter 2000; Teasdale 1983). Negative bias means that depressions tend to choose the negative information [2]. Studies have indicated that the negative bias of depression appears in many aspects of information processing [3]. For examples, studies have shown that patients with depression have obvious negative bias to emotional faces (Joormann and Gotlib, 2007; Elaine Fox et al., 2004) [4]. When the depressive patients were shown the positive and negative pictures, they pay more attention to the negative ones [4]. Similarly, depressive disorders memorized the negative word better than the positive ones (Reza et al. 2009). Furthermore, individuals with depression have a tendency to interpret information negatively (Berna et al., 2011).

In addition, the negative bias is more obvious when the information is self-related [5]. Negative self-views are one of the defining features of depression. The symptoms of Major Depressive Disorder include the feelings of worthlessness, according to the Diagnostic and Statistical Manual of Mental Disorders (DSM-IV; American Psychiatric Association, 1994), and the negative associations with self. Freud defined depression as anger turned inward, and psychodynamic theorists argued that depression was marked by excessive self-criticism (Blatt 1974). Aaron Beck's cognitive model of depression provided a cognitive triad, which was defined as negative views of the self, the future, and the world (Beck 1976). Later theorists had argued that negative views of the world and the future were limited to one's world and one's future, and could be conceptualized as specific kinds of self-views (Haaga et al. 1991). The reformulated helplessness theory of depression also assigns an important role to internal attributions, or self-blame, for negative events (Abramson et al. 1978). Nolen-Hoeksema's response styles theory of depression highlights the role of a specific form of self-reflection known as rumination in the development of depression (Nolen-Hoeksema, 1991). The hopelessness theory of depression deemphasized the role of internal attributions but argued that one proximal cause of depression is inferring negative consequences about the self in response to negative life events (Abramson and Alloy 1989). In addition to these theoretical views, substantial empirical evidence suggests that depression is marked by negative associations with the self [5]. Relative to their non-depressed counterparts, depressed individuals report more negative views of themselves on self-report measures, make more pessimistic predictions for themselves than for others, and respond to self-reflection with more negative mood and thinking. Depressed individuals are also more likely to blame themselves when negative events happen to them [6].

Except for the negative bias in cognition, depression shows an alpha EEG asymmetry in the brain activity [7]. The alpha EEG asymmetry is defined as the difference in alpha activity comparing the right hemisphere to the left hemisphere in the brain, especially in the resting EEG activities [8]. By comparing to the healthy individuals, depressive disorders present greater activation in the left than that in the right side of the brain, suggesting a weakened left alpha activity since increased alpha activation means weak activity in the brain). Researches have shown that current and remitted depression are associated with increased left (versus right) alpha activity (Allen et al. 1993; Debener et al. 2000; Gotlib et al. 1998; Henriques and Davidson 1991; Mathersul et al. 2008; Rosenfeld et al. 1996). Davidson proposed that the alpha asymmetry might be associated with the negative and positive system. In this hypothesis, the activity in the left side is related to the positive motivation, while the right side is related to the negative motivation [8]. Less activity in the left hemisphere in depression might suggest an decreased positive processing strategy during cognitive processing (Coan and Allen 2003; Sutton and Davidson 1997; Coan and Allen 2004; Harmon-Jones and Allen 1998).

However, it is not clear what is the relationship or connection between self-consciousness and alpha EEG asymmetry in depression? To investigate this issue, we collected both the data of self-consciousness level and alpha asymmetry EEG from the depressive and healthy individuals in this study. First, the direct relationship of the two factors was examined; and then, the different correlation patterns was compared between the depressive and healthy groups. We hypothesized that there would be a strong correlation between the self-consciousness and alpha EEG asymmetry, and the correlation patterns could be different between the depressive group and the healthy controls.

## 2 Materials and Methods

### 2.1 Participants

Participants were 36 males and females, including 18 (9 males and 9 females) participants diagnosed as patients with depression by two experienced psychiatrist(aged 18–64, M = 43.44 y, SD = 13.27 y) and 18 (9 males and 9 females) participants came from nearby residents (aged 21–61, M = 43.19 y, SD = 13.03 y). For depressed participants, the enter criteria are included: right-handed; ages are between 18 to 65; not taking any anti depressive and other psychiatric medicine before 2 weeks; no neurological and other psychiatric disorders (such as schizophrenia, mood disorders) or serious body disease; no serious suicidal ideation and behavior; no alcohol addiction or drug addiction. And for normal participants, the enter criteria are: right-handed; ages are between 18 to 65; no neurological disorders or serious body disease; no alcohol addiction or drug addiction. There were no statistical difference between the depression and healthy groups in gender, age and education years. This research program was reviewed by the ethics committee of Beijing An-ding Hospital, Capital Medical University, Beijing, China. All subjects participated voluntarily and signed the informed consent form.

## 2.2   Self-consciousness Assessment

The Self-Consciousness Scale (SCS) (Fenigstein et al. 1975) was used to assess the structure and level of self-consciousness. There are three different dimensions were included in SCS: private self-consciousness, public self-consciousness, and social anxiety [9]. Private self-consciousness is conceived as one's tendency to attend to or think about the covert and hidden aspects of the self (such as inner thoughts and feelings) that are not easily known by others. Public self-consciousness refers to a person's tendency to attend to or think about his or her overt and publicly displayed aspects of the self (such as overt behavior and expressive qualities), which easily can be known and examined by others. As for social anxiety, it refers to discomfort in the presence of other people. In contrast to the private and public self-consciousness, which are related to the process of self-focused attention, social anxiety was regarded as the reaction or by-product of self-consciousness, particularly public self-consciousness. There are 23 items were included in SCS with 10 items measuring the private self-consciousness, 7 items measuring the public self-consciousness and 6 items measuring social anxiety. Responses were recorded using a five-point Likert scale ranging from strong disagreement (0 = very false for me) to strong agreement (4 = very true for me).

## 2.3   EEG Data Acquisition and Analysis

The EEG data were recorded with 64 Ag/AgCl electrodes, which were positioned according to the extended 10/20 system and digitized with a sampling rate of 500 Hz (Brain Products GmbH). The TP9 and TP10 electrodes served as the reference, respectively. Vertical and horizontal electrooculogram (EOG) data were recorded from two additional channels to monitor eye movements. The impedance for all electrodes was maintained below 5 K, and the online filter band was 0–100 Hz.

EEG data were analyzed by using Brain Vision Analyzer. First of all, we established Raw Data, History and Export three folders and imported the original data to Raw Data folder; Second, open the Raw Data folder, set the new reference electrode, and here we used TP9 TP10 two channels as new reference electrodes. Then the original data pretreatment, including: Removed eye noise, try to remove noise that due to the moving of eyes; Removed the artifact, that is to say that remove noise because of a experimental equipment or participants in the process of the disturbance; Filter, which based on the analysis of signal frequency, waveform bandwidth set properly, filter out unwanted signal; Segments, namely according to the logo will be extracted for further analysis of EEG signals, in here, the time is 4 min. Fast Fourier transform, the FFT, so will the EEG from time domain to frequency domain, the transformed unit for voltage density; Average, the FFT data on average; Exported division frequency data, this article used alpha waves, its spectrum is 8–13 Hz, namely the output voltage of the frequency band density values. Taken ln for each channel voltage and got some values. And then we used the value of left side to minus the value of right side. We had 64 electrodes, removed two reference electrodes, two eyes, and other data that is not good, in the end we got 26 electrode pair values. Finally all data into SPSS to statistical analysis.

## 2.4   Statistical Analysis

There were 26 alpha EEG asymmetry values. We analyzed the correlation between 26 alpha EEG asymmetry values and private self, the correlation between 26 alpha EEG asymmetry values and public self and the correlation between 26 alpha EEG asymmetry values and social anxiety.

## 3   Results

### 3.1   Results of Depression Group

**Correlation of Alpha Asymmetry and Private Self.** As shown in Fig. 1, there is a significant correlation between private self-consciousness and alpha asymmetry in the electrode pair of CP6-CP5 (r = 0.484, P = 0.042).

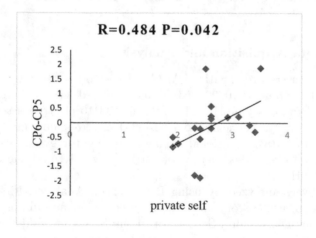

**Fig. 1.** The correlation of alpha asymmetry and private self in depression group

**Correlation of Alpha Asymmetry and Public Self.** There is no significant correlation between private self-consciousness and alpha asymmetry in any electrode pairs.

**Correlation of Alpha Asymmetry and Social Anxiety.** As shown in Fig. 2, there is a significant correlation between social anxiety and alpha asymmetry in the electrode pair of C6-C5 (r = 0.482, P = 0.043), FC6-FC5 (r = 0.535, P = 0.022) and FT8-FT7 (r = 0.581, P = 0.012).

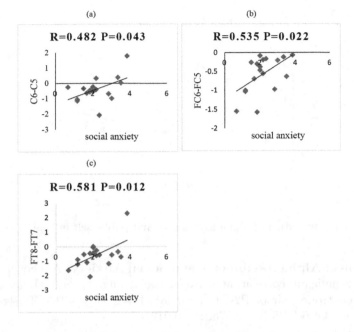

Fig. 2. The correlation of alpha asymmetry and social anxiety in depression group

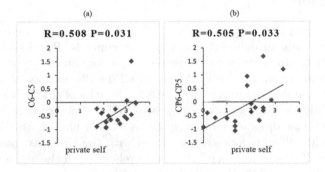

Fig. 3. The correlation of alpha asymmetry and private self in heathy group

## 3.2   Results of Heathy Group

**Correlation of Alpha Asymmetry and Private Self.** As shown in Fig. 3, there is a significant correlation between private self-consciousness and alpha asymmetry in the electrode pair of C6 C5 ($r - 0.508$, $P = 0.031$) and CP6-CP5 ($r = 0.505$, $P = 0.033$).

**Correlation of Alpha Asymmetry and Pubic Self.** As shown in Fig. 4, there is a significant correlation between public self-consciousness and alpha asymmetry in the electrode pair of P8-P7 ($r = 0.517$, $P = 0.028$).

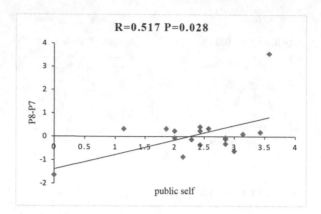

**Fig. 4.** The correlation of alpha asymmetry and public self in heathy group

**Correlation of Alpha Asymmetry and Social Anxiety.** As shown in Fig. 5, there is a significant correlation between social anxiety and alpha asymmetry in the electrode pair of P2-P1 (r = 0.488, P = 0.040), CP4-CP3 (r = 0.506, P = 0.032) and CP6-CP5 (r = 0.578, P = 0.012).

## 4    Discussion

By collecting alpha EEG asymmetry and self-consciousness, we investigated the relationship of them in depression and healthy controls. Results show that in the depression group, private self-consciousness is significantly correlated with the alpha asymmetry in the electrode pair of CP6-CP5, and social anxiety correlated with the alpha asymmetry in the electrode pairs of C6-C5, FC6-FC5 and FT8-FT7. While for the heathy group, private self-consciousness is significantly correlated with the alpha asymmetry in the electrode pair of C6-C5 and CP6-CP5; and public self-consciousness correlated with the alpha asymmetry in the electrode pairs of P8-P7 and social anxiety correlated with the alpha asymmetry in the electrode pairs of P2-P1, CP4-CP3 and CP6-CP5.

The results show that there are different correlation patterns in the depression and healthy groups. In the depression group, the correlations are located in the more anterior regions of the frontal and temporal junction area in the brain, which are closed to the salient network (SN). While in the health group, more posterior parietal and occipital regions are correlated with self-consciousness, which are closed to the default mode network (DMN). SN is a network that is sensitive to semantic content in comparisons of semantic tasks more than rest control tasks [10]. The semantic sensitivity might be related to the rapid evaluation of the surrounding information to find the most relevant and irrelevant stimulus. SN is also suggested to be related to the classification of external stimuli and internal events to switch to the related processing system (Sheline et al. 2009). While DMN is related to the self-referential processing and cognitive resource allocation Wei et al. 2015). The different correlation pattern

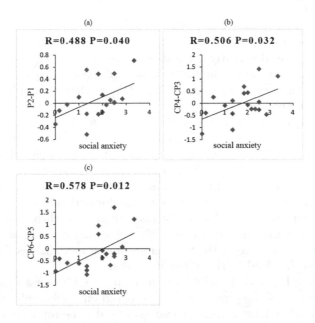

**Fig. 5.** The correlation of alpha asymmetry and social anxiety in heathy group

of self-consciousness and alpha asymmetry between the depression and health groups suggest a differential self-construal or impairment of cognition control in depression.

Another point should be noted is related to the structure of self-consciousness. The results suggest that the most significant different correlation in the depression and health is associated with the social anxiety. In several recent reviews, it has been proposed that an attentional bias for mood-congruent information is a primary feature of anxiety (Dalgleish and Watts 1990; Mathews 1990; Williams et al. 1988). Beck (Beck et al. 1986; Beck et al. 1979) and Bower (1981, 1987) predict that mood-congruent biases operate throughout cognitive processes, including perception, attention and memory, in both anxiety and depression [11]. Several probe detection studies have provided evidence of an attentional bias for threat information in anxiety (e.g. Broadbent and Broadbent 1988; MacLeod 1986; Mogg et al. 1992). This result prove that social anxiety has a strong relationship with negative bias in cognition. So, it accord with the theory that attentional bias exist in anxiety and provided a new direction and mechanism for the study of depression.

Self-consciousness is a unique psychological system, which has the character-istics of consciousness, sociality, activity, identity and so on. Self-consciousness is often associated with shyness and embarrassment, in which case a lack of pride and low self-esteem can result in a positive context, self-consciousness may affect the development of identity, for it is during periods of high self-consciousness that people come the closest to knowing themselves objectively [12]. Self-consciousness affects people in varying degrees, as some people are constantly self-monitoring or self-involved, while others are completely oblivious about themselves. Different levels of self-consciousness affect behavior, as it is common for people to act differently when they "lose themselves in a crowd". Being in a crowd, being in a dark room, or wearing a disguise creates anonymity and temporarily decreases self-consciousness [12]. This can lead to uninhibited, sometimes destructive behavior.

A large number of Chinese and western studies focused on the types of self, mostly think of the same type self-reference processing should have the same neural mechanisms [13]. Some scholars divided self into individual self and collective self while some divided self into physical self and psychological self in these studies [14]. And the scholars use stimulations include self and non-self stimulation to activate differences between behavior and nervous to inspect self-effect. The differences of these different studies, to discuss self-processing, mainly is the stimulus materials and methods. Different stimulus material induced different types of self and may activate different neural mechanisms. This may be the main reason that lead to the different results.

There is still a lot of work to be done in the future. First of all, the sample is limited. The results of the present study are based on a relatively small sample size of non-clinical undergraduates. These data need to be replicated with larger nonclinical samples and clinical samples to improve the reliability of these results. Second, it needs more investigation to help localize the EEG data in the brain. In that case, we could do more exploration and understand more about the connection between alpha symmetry and self-consciousness.

**Acknowledgments.** This work was supported by the National Basic Research Program of China (2014CB744600), International Science and Technology Cooperation Program of China (2013DFA32180), National Natural Science Foundation of China (61272345), and also supported by Beijing Municipal Commission of Education, Beijing International Collaboration Base on Brain Informatics and Wisdom Services and Beijing Key Laboratory of Magnetic Resonance Imaging and Brain Informatics.

# References

1. Beck, A.T., Burns, D.: Cognitive therapy of depressed suicidal outpatients. In: Cole, J.O., Schatzberg, A.F., Frazier, S.H. (eds.) Depression, pp. 199–211. Springer US, Heidelberg (1978)
2. Beck, A.T.: Cognitive models of depression. J. Cogn. Psychother. **1**(1), 5–37 (1987)
3. Teasdale, J.D.: Negative thinking in depression: cause, effect, or reciprocal relationship? Adv. Behav. Res. Ther. **5**(83), 3–25 (1983)
4. Fox, E., Russo, R., Dutton, K.: Attentional bias for threat: evidence for delayed disengagement from emotional faces. Cogn. Emot. **16**(3), 355–379 (2002)
5. Haaga, D.A., Dyck, M.J., Ernst, D.: Empirical status of cognitive theory of depression. Psychol. Bull. **110**(110), 215–236 (1991)
6. Crandell, C.J., Chambless, D.L.: The validation of an inventory for measuring depressive thoughts: the Crandell cognitions inventory. Behav. Res. Ther. **24**(4), 403–411 (1986)

7. Allen, J.J., Iacono, W.G., Depue, R.A., Arbisi, P.: Regional electroencephalographic asymmetries in bipolar seasonal affective disorder beforeand after exposure to bright light. Biol. Psychiatry **33**(8/9), 642–646 (1993)
8. Coan, J.A., Allen, J.J., McKnight, P.E.: A capability model of individual differences in frontal EEG asymmetry. Biol. Psychol. **72**(2), 198–207 (2006)
9. Burnkrant, R.E., Page, T.J.: A modification of the Fenigstein, Scheier, and Buss Self-consciousness Scales. J. Pers. Assess. **48**(6), 629–637 (1985)
10. Wei, M., Qin, J., Yan, R., Bi, K., Liu, C., et al.: Association of resting-state network dysfunction with their dynamics of inter-network interactions in depression. J. Affect. Disord. **174**, 527–534 (2015)
11. Dalgleish, T., Watts, F.N.: Biases of attention and memory in disorders of anxiety and depression. Clin. Psychol. Rev. **10**(5), 589–604 (1990)
12. Mitchell, J.P., Banaji, M.R., Macrae, C.N.: The link between social cognition and self-referential thought in the medial prefrontal cortex. J. Cogn. Neurosci. **17**, 1306–1315 (2005)
13. Wicklund, R.A.: Objective self-awareness. Adv. Exp. Soc. Psychol. **8**, 233–275 (1975)
14. Nathaniel, B.: The Psychology of Self-Esteem. Nash Publishing Corp. p. 42, (1969). 0–8402-1109-0
15. Coan, J.A., Allen, J.J.: Frontal EEG asymmetry and the behavioral activation and inhibition systems. Psychophysiology **40**(1), 106–114 (2003)
16. Andrews-Hanna, J.R., Reidler, J.S., Sepulcre, J., Poulin, R., Buckner, R.L.: Functional-anatomic fractionation of the brain's default network. Neuron **65**(4), 550–562 (2010)

# The Situation Model in Text Reading: Evidence from an Eye Movement Study

Xiaofeng Lu[1,2,3,4], Mi Li[1,2,3,4(✉)], Shengfu Lu[1,2,3,4], Jiying Xu[1,2,3,4], and Jia Xue[1,2,3,4]

[1] Beijing Advanced Innovation Center for Future Internet Technology,
Beijing University of Technology, Beijing 100024, China
limi@bjut.edu.cn
[2] International WIC Institute, Beijing University of Technology,
Beijing 100024, China
[3] Beijing International Collaboration Base on Brain
Informatics and Wisdom Services, Beijing, China
[4] Beijing Key Laboratory of MRI and Brain Informatics, Beijing, China

**Abstract.** Understanding and processing of information in text reading have been the core content of the reading psychological research, and it is a hot topic of great concern in cognitive science community. In this study, we used eye tracking to investigate the cognitive mechanisms during peoples reading of narratives and statistical information, and we explored the differences in behavior of people during their reading of different text information from the human cognitive behavior. This study confirmed previous view that the natural process of text reading is a dual processing process of coherent reading and focus reading, and different material characteristics might trigger different information processing activities. We found that the construction of situation model contributed to text reading, which provided some evidences for the situation model from fixation point distribution.

## 1 Introduction

Text reading is a unique cognitive activity of human, which is an important way for human to get information. Understanding and processing of information in text reading have been the core content of the reading psychological research. Text reading not only helps us to reveal the nature and law of human cognitive activity, but also provides psychological basis for the development of machine reading, artificial intelligence, etc. Thus, it is an important topic of great concern in cognitive science community.

For text reading, Van Dijk and Kintsch (1983) proposed the concept of situation models for narrative understanding, namely, people will establish a corresponding mental representation of the scene described in the text when they are reading it, and these dynamic representations is called situation models [1]. Readers will integrate the knowledge of characters, events, objective described in the text before, to build a more detailed characterization of the text [2]. When

G.A. Ascoli et al. (Eds.): BIH 2016, LNAI 9919, pp. 104–113, 2016.
DOI: 10.1007/978-3-319-47103-7_11

the reader construct such a situation model, he will start from constructing the mental representation based on initial text information and priori knowledge of the reader, follow-up information is then mapped to the established developing model, which allows readers to be able to do some more complex reasoning about the described events. That is, As the described events unfold the reader has to continuously update his or her mental representation, such as characters move to new locations, objects are left behind, events are no longer operative lost objects are found again, and so on [3]. Therefore, the situation model is mental representation of people, things, places, time and behavior described in the text, not of the words, phrases, clauses, sentences and paragraphs of a text. Situation model mentors the reading comprehension and memory together with the word level and sentence level processing.

Text comprehension researchers typically identify at least five dimensions of situations, also known as five dimensions: the space, time, causation, intentionality and protagonist. Protagonist and intentionality constitute the main body of situation model, Readers appear to be intensively engaged in keeping track of protagonists during comprehension whereas the amount of focus on objects appears to be more dependent on contextual cues. To achieve a proper understanding of the situation described by a text, the reader needs to know when the described events took place both relative to each other and relative to the time at which they were narrated. Spatial information has received a relatively large amount of attention in the text-comprehension literature as the nonlinear nature of space provides an interesting mismatch with the linear nature of language. Researchers have carried out some experimental researches in each dimension, and achieved a lot [3–5].

There has been a controversial theory about the specific constructing and updating mechanism of situation model in the processing of text reading. There are two most typical theories, one is the here-and-now hypothesis of constructivist assumption, the other is the memory-based text processing view.

The here-and-now hypothesis of constructivist assumption considers that reading is a process during which readers constantly active their background knowledge initiatively corresponding to the current contents of the text, and during which readers integrate current information and prior information to construct and update the situation model. When they read the protagonist information, the readers examine the sentence only with the current, updated model. In this process, the background knowledge before the updated will not be automatically, negatively reactivated. This theory emphasizes the initiative and strategic aspect of situation model constructing and updating [6–8]. The memory-based text processing view considers that readers will not construct and update the situation model initiatively and actively during the text processing, and the current reading information activates the text information associated with this information in long-term memory through the "resonance" approach non-strategically, passively and quickly, which triggers the constructing and updating situation model [9–11].

Reading is an important aspect of the human visual pattern recognition. From information theory view, text reading can be seen as the process of information decoding. The text signal was converted into nerve signal through the retina and sent to the central nervous system to be handled, while at the same time, in return, the central nervous system control the eye movement via the motor nerve, made it gather information in a more appropriate the manner and rate. Although it is difficult to detect brain activity using objective methods during the reading process directly, it is possible to study the brain's information processing though the recording and analysis of the eye movements during the reading process, which is controlled by the brain [12].

Late 19th early 20th century, psychologists began using a simple eye movement recording technology to investigate eye movement in graphics scanning and text reading, and the relationship between eye movement and the visual information processing. In the mid-20th century, the researchers developed a number of eye movement recording technology for psychological research, but these eye movement recording technology existed shortcomings such as big error, operational difficulties and big burden to eyes etc. After the mid-20th century, the introduction of camera technology, especially the use of computer technology, promoted the development of high-precision eye tracker, which greatly promoted the eye movement studies in international psychology and application in related disciplines.

Recently, eye movement technology has been applied to the interface evaluation, web design and other research fields gradually. For example, a study focused on the impact of space and location information to the interface layout design [13]. Our group using eye tracking investigated the visual behavior during peoples information search on pages and the effect of floating ads to visual search behavior [14], the visual characteristics of visual search and browse on web pages [15], and the impact of web pages of information overload on visual search quantitatively, they used eye tracking technology to study the visual search behavior of the user on the page of information overload [16]. The present study focused on the differences when people reading different types of texts from eye movement perspective, to identify the user's different working conditions and psychological load based on eye movement trajectories and other indexes, which will help us understanding the human mental state and provide some eye movement evidences for the situation model.

## 2    Methods

### 2.1    Participants

The participants were 30 (15 females and 15 males) undergraduate or graduate students from various majors of Beijing University of Technology with an age range from 22 to 27 (M = 24.1, S.D. = 1.0). All participates were right-handed had normal or corrected-to-normal vision, native Chinese speakers, had not participated in a similar experiment. After the experiment, we checked the quality and accuracy of data records, and excluded 8 subjects data which were not recorded accurately (data not collected or eye positioning had large deviations).

## 2.2   Experimental Materials

There are 2 types of experimental materials (Fig. 1), narrative text and statistical information text. Each type has 40 texts, and each text is constituted of 3 sentences. The narrative texts were selected from Aesop's Fables, Aesop's Fables is a classic narrative works, there are many studies using Aesop's Fables as the experimental material domestically and overseas. So we selected some of the fragments from it and adapted, and made it a shorter form to match the length with statistical information. We wiped off a number of uncommon words and grammar that were not commonly used, and made it did not contain people and other social information. Statistical information was made by our own based on certain criteria, and its form is the corresponding relationship between project name and their values. We used 40 common statistical events in everyday life (including fruits, vegetables, furniture, stationery, household appliances, food, clothing, transportation, sports, musical instruments, commodities, culture, sports, beverages, jewelry and seafood etc.). Narrative Text $(34.2 \pm 3.0)$ and statistical information texts $(34.4 \pm 2.1)$ had no significant difference in number of words $[F(1, 78) = 0.15, p > 0.05]$.

We made all stimuli materials into pictures in order to import them into the eye tracker easily, the text font is Times New Roman, font size 20, line spacing of 2 lines, color is white, the background is black, the text is located in the center of the background, pictures size is $1024 \times 768$.

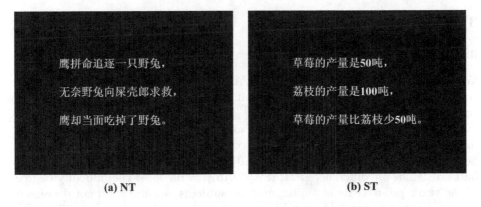

Fig. 1. An example of experimental materials. (a) NT: An example of narrative texts (meaning that an Eagle was chasing a hare, presently the hare had to beg a beetle to aid her, but the eagle seized the hare and ate her up; (b) ST: An example of statistical text (meaning that the production of strawberry is 50 tons, the production of litchi is 100 tons, and the production of strawberry is 50 tons less than that of litchi.)

## 2.3  Experimental Environment and Procedure

Eye movements were recorded at the rate of 120 HZ by Tobii T120 eye-tracker, which had a 17 inch LCD monitor with resolution set to 1024 × 768 pixels and at the refresh rate of 60 HZ.

Experimental procedure was divided into two stages: the first stage was practice, its purpose was to make subject familiar with the experimental procedure and the key press. Practice contains 4 narrative tasks and 4 statistical information tasks, all tasks were randomly presented. The second stage was formal experiment, and it was divided into four parts (session1, session2, session3, session4), each section contains 20 tasks (10 narrative tasks and 10 statistical information tasks), and all tasks were randomly presented in each session. Subjects can have a rest after the completion of a session and then proceed to the next session.

We called a task one trial, each trial's lasting time was 14 s, and each session took approximately $20 \times 14$ s $= 4$ min 40 s. If one session lasted too long, the subjects might move their heads because of unable to remain seated or visual fatigue, and experimental data records would be not accurate. Therefore, in the course of the experiment, subjects were asked to keep their heads fixed and read each text carefully.

The sentences were presented one after another: first, we presented the first sentence of the text; second, the first sentence stayed on the screen and we presented the second sentence, last, three sentences were presented on the screen together. At the end of each reading task, subjects need to answer a question depending on the text (left button "Space" refers to right, right button "Enter" refers to wrong).

## 3  Results

### 3.1  Accuracy and Reaction Time

We did the analysis of variance (ANOVA) on the accuracy and reaction time. As shown in Table 1, there were no significant differences between two types of texts on the accuracy and reaction time. First, the subjects participated in the experiment carefully and the accuracy of answering two types of texts was higher, more than 92 % on average, so it can be considered experimental data was valid; Second, because the story text $(34.2 \pm 3.0)$ and statistics text words $(34.4 \pm 2.1)$ had no significant difference $[F(1, 78) = 0.15, p = 0.70]$, so the difficulty degree of the two types of texts is similar, and the subjects' accuracy did not decreased or reaction time became longer because a certain kind of text was difficult to understand.

### 3.2  Analysis of Eye Movement Indexes

We conducted variance test to five eye movement indexes of the third stimuli, namely saccade distance (means the distance between two consecutive fixation

**Table 1.** Accuracy and reaction time of reading two types of text (*mean ± SD*)

|                    | NT            | ST             | F(1, 21) | p-value |
|--------------------|---------------|----------------|----------|---------|
| Accuracy (%)       | 92.31 ± 5.04  | 93.43 ± 7.36   | 0.36     | 0.55    |
| Reaction time (s)  | 2.09 ± 0.34   | 2.09 ± 2.09    | 0.01     | 0.93    |

NT: narrative text, ST: statistical text.

point), pupil diameter, fixation count, fixation duration and mean fixation duration. Table 2 shows the comparison results for the 5 eye movement indexes of the two type tasks, the results showed: 4 indexes had no significant difference in the reading of two types of text, including pupil diameter, total fixation duration, fixation count and mean fixation duration, in which the difference in the saccade distance was significant $[F(1, 21) = 26.90, p < 0.000]$.

Pupil diameter can reflect the changes in people's mental activity objectively, and its changes also reflect the psychological load's changes. The pupil diameter dilates with an increasing mental load, while the pupil diameter constricts with a decreasing mental load. Fixation duration refers to the sum of all fixation time of a certain area; fixation count refers to the number of fixation points in a certain area, average fixation duration refers to the average values of all fixation point in a certain area. These parameters had no significant difference, indicating that there was no difference in mental workload when subjects were reading two types of texts. These further indicated that there was no significant difference between two types of text in the grammar, words etc., and subjects' fixation duration and fixation count did not increase because a certain text was difficult to understand.

**Table 2.** Eye movement indexes of reading the third sentence (*mean ± SD*)

|            | NT             | ST              | F(1, 21) | p-value   |
|------------|----------------|-----------------|----------|-----------|
| PD(mm)     | 4.28 ± 0.61    | 4.27 ± 0.59     | 0.01     | 0.94      |
| SD(pixel)  | 95.33 ± 7.94   | 113.90 ± 15.22  | 26.9     | < 0.000   |
| FD(s)      | 1.82 ± 0.31    | 1.80 ± 0.28     | 0.07     | 0.79      |
| FC         | 7.13 ± 1.33    | 1.80 ± 0.28     | 0.72     | 0.40      |
| MFD(s)     | 0.22 ± 0.04    | 0.22 ± 0.06     | 0.17     | 0.69      |

NT: narrative text, ST: statistical text, PD: pupil diameter, SD: saccade distance, FD: total fixation duration, FC: fixation count, MFD: mean fixation duration.

## 3.3 Fixation Point Distribution Maps

Fixation point distribution maps were superimposed by many fixation points of many subjects, it was also called heat maps (Fig. 2). It can reflect which part is the most interesting part in the stimuli directly and clearly. As shown in Fig. 2, the more warm colors (red) indicated the higher degree of concern.

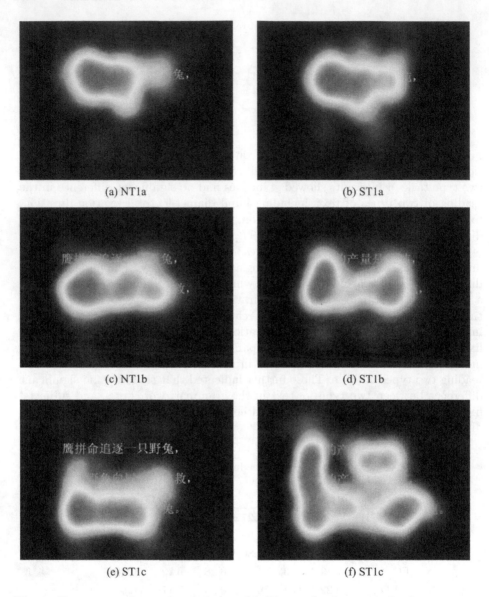

(a) NT1a                                   (b) ST1a

(c) NT1b                                   (d) ST1b

(e) ST1c                                   (f) ST1c

**Fig. 2.** Heat maps of two types of text, (a) (b) are the first stimuli of narrative 1 (NT1a) and the first stimuli of statistical information 1 (ST1a), (c) (d) are the second stimuli (NT1b and ST1b), (e) (f) are the third stimuli (NT1b and ST1b). (Color figure online)

From fixation point distribution maps, the fixation point is continuous when subjects were reading the first sentence, indicating that subjects were reading sentence continuously. When subjects were reading the second sentence, fixation point of narrative was mostly continuous, while fixation point of statistical information had a significant jump. Subjects gazed more for key words in a sentence, and skipped over the less important information. Furthermore, subjects had backsight in both texts at the first sentence, while backsight in statistical information back was more obvious, and subjects looked back on the key words largely. When subjects read the third sentence, the fixation points of narrative were mostly continuous, while fixation points of statistical information still had obvious jump, subjects gazed more on the key words. There was less backsight in narrative than in statistical information, therefore, subjects' saccade distance in statistical information was significantly greater than narrative.

## 4    Discussion

In our study, subjects' eye movement behavior from the perspective of eye movement during text reading, and found that two types of reading behavior had significant difference. Our hypothesis was that subjects would construct a situation model during narrative reading, while the construction of situation model would take some time, and subjects needed to look back previous information constantly in order to complete the construction of situation model, therefore, reading time of narrative was longer and backsight count was more than statistical information. However, in this study we found the opposite result, the experimental results showed that situation model help the understanding and memory of text.

The results of this study corresponded with dual processing theory of text reading. The basic view of dual-processing theory of text reading was that, the natural process of text reading was a dual process of coherent reading and focus reading [17]. The theory states that, in the natural reading process, which process subjects taken was mainly caused by character of reading materials (including forms or information character). Different material characters might trigger different information processing activities. Readers would take different processing activities alternatively according to the nature character of the content and form. In text reading there was processing activities put forward by minimum assumptions theory and memory-based text processing view, which was to maintain local coherence and to activate the information in long-term memory through the "resonance" approach, it was passive, negative, and its purpose was to maintain the coherence of the information, which was called "coherent reading processing". There was also processing activities put forward by constructivist theory, which was related to the target integration caused by target behavior, or the follow-construction around the protagonist, it was a proactive, positive construction process, which fully reflected the subjectivity and strategic aspect of the reading process, and it was called "focus reading process". We can see from the eye movement trajectory graph and fixation point distribution map of this study, subjects mostly used coherent reading and jump reading coherent mode when they read narrative, and it was a dual processing process of "coherent reading processing" and "focus reading processing". While for statistical information, although it was not narrative text, and there was no space, time, causality, intentions, protagonist and other information, but subjects' reading pattern was similar with this theory, and it was mostly a "focus reading processing". We can see from the analysis of the results, subjects' fixation points fell mostly on some crucial phrase when read statistical information, and we can also obtained the corresponding conclusion from the statistical analysis results of saccade distance.

Construction of situation model helped the understanding and memory of text. The construction would take some time, but when the model was constructed by the subjects, the information can be more easily understood and deposited into their long-term memory. It was a process of integration processing when subjects read the third sentence, and it was easier for subjects to extract previous information because of the role of situation model, and made a conclusion thought the integration with current information, so subjects hardly needed to look back the previous information. While subjects read statistical information, there was no situation model to construct, and it was hard for subjects to remember the information read before. The memory of prior information needed to be done through working memory, but working memory had a certain range, and it was hard for subjects to remember the information out of the range of working memory. When subjects read the last sentence of the text, which was an information integration process, although subjects were able to remember the information newly read, it was difficult to remember the information earlier, so subjects needed to look back more to complete the integration processing of the entire text, showing different modes compared with narrative reading.

## 5    Conclusions

This study investigated the differences of eye movement pattern between narrative reading and statistical information reading, and found situation model helped understanding and memory of the text. Our results confirmed the previous dual processing theory in text reading, and provided some evidence from the perspective of eye movement. The results might be related to the design of the experimental materials, and narrative and statistical information were designed into a short form. There was no complex plot in narratives, and it might be easier for subjects to remember the narrative. Future research could try to use more complicated narratives, and further discussed eye movement pattern differences between narrative reading and statistical information reading.

**Acknowledgements.** This work was supported by the National Basic Research Program of China (2014CB744600), the Beijing Natural Science Foundation (4164080), the Beijing Outstanding Talent Training Foundation (2014000020124G039), the National Natural Science Foundation of China (61420106005), the Grant-in-Aid for Scientific Research (C) from Japan Society for the Promotion of Science (26350994), the Beijing Municipal Science and Technology Project (D12100005012003), the Beijing Municipal Administration of Hospitals Clinical Medicine Development of Special Funding (ZY201403).

# References

1. van Dijk, T.A., Kintsch, W.: Strategies of Discourse Comprehension. Academic Press, San Diego (1983)
2. Zwaan, R.A., Radvansky, G.A.: Situation models in language comprehension and memory. Psychol. Bull. **123**, 162–185 (1998)
3. Zwaan, R.A., Madden, C.J.: Updating situation models. J. Exp. Psychol. Learn. Memory Cogn. **30**, 289–291 (2004)
4. Zwaan, R.A., Magliano, J.P., Graesser, A.C.: Dimensions of situation model construction in narrative comprehension. J. Exp. Psychol.: Learn. Memory Cogn. **21**, 386–397 (1995)
5. Zwaan, R.A., Lanfston, M.C., Graesser, A.C.: The construction of situation models in narrative comprehension: an event-indexing model. Psychol. Sci. **6**, 292–297 (1995)
6. Bower, G., Morrow, D.: Mental models in narrative comprehension. Science **247**, 44–48 (1990)
7. Graesser, A.C., Singer, M., Trabasso, T.: Constructing inferences during narrative text comprehension. Psychol. Rev. **101**, 371–395 (1994)
8. Singer, M., Graesser, A.C., Trabasso, T.: Minimal or global inference during reading. J. Memory Lang. **33**, 421–441 (1994)
9. Mckoon, G., Ratcliff, R.: Memory-based language processing: psycholinguistic research in the 1990s. Annu. Rev. Psychol. **49**, 25–42 (1998)
10. OB'rien, E.J., Albrecht, J.E., Rizzella, M.L., Halleran, J.G.: Updating a situation model: a memory-based text processing view. J. Exp. Psychol. Learn. Memory Cogn. **24**, 1200–1210 (1998)
11. Yarkoni, T., Speer, N.K., Zacks, J.M.: Neural substrates of narrative comprehension and memory. NeuroImage **41**, 1408–1425 (2008)
12. Sun, F.C., Stark, L.: Visual information processing: eye movements during reading Chinese and English. ACTA Biophys. Sin. **4**, 1–6 (1998)
13. Terenzi, M., Nocera, F., Action, F.: Not only semantics: underlies expected location for interface elements. In: The 4th Italian Symposium on Human Computer Interaction (2005)
14. Li, M., Yin, J., Lu, S., Zhong, N.: The effect of information forms and floating advertisements for visual search on web pages: an eye-tracking study. In: Zhong, N., Li, K., Lu, S., Chen, L. (eds.) BI 2009. LNCS (lnai), vol. 5819, pp. 96–105. Springer, Heidelberg (2009)
15. Li, M., Zhong, N., Lu, S.F.: Exploring visual search and browsing strategies on Web pages using the eye-tracking. J. Beijing Univ. Technol. **37**, 773–779 (2011)
16. Li, M., Lu, W.X., Lu, S.F., Song, Y.Y., Yin, J.J., Zhong, N.: Strategy and processing mode of visual search under information overload on Web pages: an eye-tracking study. J. Beijing Univ.Technol. **38**, 390–395 (2012)
17. Mo, L., Wang, R.M., Leng, Y.: The bi-processing theory of text comprehension and experimental evidences. Acta Psychol. Sin. **44**(5), 569–584 (2012)

# Alterations in Emotional and Salience Responses to Positive Stimuli in Major Depressive Disorder

Yang Yang[1,2,4,5], Lei Feng[6,7], Kazuyuki Imamura[2],
Xiaojing Yang[3,4,5], Huaizhou Li[3,4,5], Gang Wang[1,6,7], Bin Hu[8],
Shengfu Lu[1,3,4,5], and Ning Zhong[1,2,3,4,5(✉)]

[1] Beijing Advanced Innovation Center for Future Internet Technology,
Beijing University of Technology, Beijing, China
yang@maebashi-it.org, zhong@maebashi-it.ac.jp
[2] Maebashi Institute of Technology, Maebashi, Japan
[3] International WIC Institute, Beijing University of Technology, Beijing, China
[4] Beijing International Collaboration Base on Brain Informatics and Wisdom
Services, Beijing, China
[5] Beijing Key Laboratory of MRI and Brain Informatics, Beijing, China
[6] Mood Disorders Center, Beijing Anding Hospital,
Capital Medical University, Beijing, China
[7] China Clinical Research Center for Mental Disorders, Beijing, China
[8] Ubiquitous Awareness and Intelligent Solutions Lab,
Lanzhou University, Lanzhou, China

**Abstract.** To find out the influences on the emotionality and attentional deployment caused by depression, we recruited 19 MDD patients and 19 healthy controls, and implemented a task-state fMRI experiment using a distraction task paradigm. Our results showed relatively decreased brain activation in the right precuneus and left DLPFC, in the MDD group compared with the healthy group across the positive, neutral, and negative task conditions. During only the positive condition, decreased subcortical responses and concurrently reduced brain activation in the salience network were found only in MDD patients. Further brain-symptom analysis demonstrated significant correlation between alterations in the key region of the salience network and the depressive severity of the patients. Our findings suggest a crucial role of aberrant salience processes (especially in the anterior insulae) in the abnormal perception of positive stimuli in MDD patients, which is likely to be the underlying pathology of the anhedonia.

## 1 Introduction

As a hallmark symptom of MDD, the anhedonia was defined in DSM-IV-TR (American Psychiatric Association, 1994) as diminished interest or pleasure in response to stimuli that were previously perceived as rewarding during a pre-morbid

---

Y. Yang and L. Feng—These authors contributed equally to this work.

G.A. Ascoli et al. (Eds.): BIH 2016, LNAI 9919, pp. 114–123, 2016.
DOI: 10.1007/978-3-319-47103-7_12

state. Because the capacity to feel pleasure is a critical step during the normal processing of rewards, anhedonia has been greatly implicated in the reward deficits of MDD patients [1]. Neuroimaging studies, especially functional magnetic resonance imaging (fMRI) studies, have played an important role in revealing brain abnormalities in major depressive disorder (MDD) [2]. However, previous findings are still ambiguous to tell the underlying mechanism of anhedonia.

Several brain areas showing alterations in MDD patients have been indicated, including cortical, subcortical, (para) limbic, and midbrain regions that mediate cognition, emotion, as well as metabolism. Most of these areas are associated with emotional and reward processing. A number of neurobiological models of MDD have been proposed to interpret the observed alterations in the patients, such as the limbic-cortical model that suggests the association of over-activity in limbic areas traditionally linked to emotional processing and inadequate inhibition by prefrontal areas in MDD patients [3]; the corticostriatal model that highlights the subcortical structures in information processing and their dysfunction associated with symptoms such as psychomotor retardation [4]; furthermore, an increasing emphasis has been put on the relationship between the default mode network (DMN) and depressive symptoms where patients were reported to present increased self-reflective rumination [5]. Although each of the hypothesized models can be supported by abundant neuroimaging evidence, a consensus about the neural pathology of the depressive anhedonia has not been achieved.

As a newly proposed hypothesis, Uddin [6] indicates that abnormally functioning in the salience system associated with detection of behaviourally relevant stimuli of the outward environment is a key factor to many neuropsychiatric disorders, such as schizophrenia, autism, and depression. Alterations in the salience network comprised of the anterior parts of insular and cingulate cortices might result in misappropriated salience detection and altered attentional processes. Abnormalities in recognition of reward or positive stimuli have been identified in MDD patients. For instance, depressed patients showed decreased perceptual sensitivity to positive words and pictures, but exhibited increased vigilance towards negative information [7]. Therefore, emerging evidence suggests the relationship between the biased attentional processing and the morbid processes on reward or positive stimuli in MDD patients.

In the present study, we employed a distraction task paradigm to examine the responses to affective images and attentional control of MDD and healthy cohorts. We hypothesized that abnormal emotionality in MDD patients may be implicated in altered attentional activities.

# 2 Materials and Methods

## 2.1 Participants

Nineteen right-handed MDD outpatients (8 males and 11 females) from Beijing Anding Hospital, China, and 19 healthy controls (HC) matched for gender, age, and years of education with MDD patients recruited from community participated in our experiment. Clinically trained and experienced raters (T. Tian and B. Fu) performed diagnostic assessments for all the participants, by means of the DSM-IV-based Mini

**Table 1.** Demographic and clinical characteristics of MDD patients and healthy controls.

| Characteristics | MDD patients (n = 19) | Controls (n = 19) | p-Value |
|---|---|---|---|
| Gender (male:female) | 8:11 | 8:11 | 1 |
| Mean age (years) | 33.8 ± 10.5 | 33.3 ± 9.9 | 0.88 |
| Education level (years) | 14.1 ± 3.2 | 13.9 ± 3.6 | 0.89 |
| HDRS-17 total score | 15.8 ± 8.0 | - | - |
| PHQ-9 | 11.3 ± 6.2 | 3.9 ± 3.1 | 0.00 |
| QIDS | 11.4 ± 5.6 | 4.3 ± 3.5 | 0.00 |

Abbreviation: HDRS-17: Hamilton Depression Rating Scale 17 Items; PHQ-9: Patient Health Questionnaire 9 Items; QIDS: Quick Inventory of Depressive Symptomatology.

International Neuropsychiatric Interview 6.0 (MINI 6.0) [8]. Clinical symptom severity of depression was evaluated for only patients using Hamilton Depression Rating Scale 17 items (HDRS-17). The demographics and clinical characteristics of participants are presented in Table 1. The following criteria were applied to exclude participants who are unsuitable for our fMRI experiment: (1) depressive patients with any mania episode or history of any comorbid major psychiatric illness on Axis I or Axis II; (2) concurrent serious medical illness or primary neurological illness; (3) history of head injury resulting in loss of consciousness; (4) abuse of or dependence on alcohol or other substances; (5) and contraindication for MRI. All subjects signed the informed consent and this study was approved by the Ethics committee of Beijing Anding Hospital, Capital Medical University.

## 2.2    Experimental Design

Participants were displayed with pictures and then required to solve mental arithmetic problems presented as overlays on the pictures. Three types of pictures were applied, with positive (e.g., joyful, exciting), neutral, and negative (e.g., aversive) valences, respectively, corresponding to three task conditions. As distractors, 2-digit simple mental addition and subtraction problems without carrying and borrowing were employed to avoid ceiling and floor effects. The difficulty level of such arithmetic problems was verified to be appropriate for attracting attention of both MDD and healthy groups by performing a pre-experiment. All the visual stimuli were presented in a block-designed pattern.

Each trial consisted of an emotion induction phase and a distraction phase. During the induction phase (2000 ms), a valenced picture was displayed. Participants passively viewed the picture to elicit an initial emotional response. During the distraction phase (4000 ms), participants needed to shift attention from the picture to an arithmetic problem, and then decide whether the displayed solution was correct or incorrect by pressing two response keys using the left and right thumbs. The accuracy and reaction time of each response were recorded. Incorrect displayed solutions deviated by ±1 or ±10 from the correct solutions in 50 % of all the trials. The frequency of occurrence of each number was balanced and the proportion of each arithmetic operation was 50 %

for all conditions. Twelve successive trials with same task condition constituted a task block. Blocks of three conditions were mixed and counterbalanced, and every two task blocks were separated by a rest block. Data were acquired in three functional runs with a total of 36 trials for each type of task.

## 2.3   MRI Data Acquisition

All the participants were scanned by using a 3.0 T MRI system (Siemens Trio Tim; Siemens Medical System, Erlanger, Germany) and a 12-channel phased array head coil. To limit head motion and reduce scanning noise, foam padding and headphone were employed. 192 slices of structural images with a thickness of 1 mm were acquired by using a T1 weighted 3D MPRAGE sequence (TR = 1600 ms, TE = 3.28 ms, TI = 800 ms, FOV = 256 × 256 mm$^2$, flip angle = 9°, voxel size = 1 × 1 × 1 mm$^3$). Functional images were collected through a T2 gradient-echo EPI sequence (TR = 2000 ms, TE = 31 ms, flip angle = 90°, FOV = 240 × 240 mm$^2$, matrix size = 64 × 64). Thirty axial slices with a thickness of 4 mm and an interslice gap of 0.8 mm were acquired.

## 2.4   Data Preprocessing

The preprocessing of fMRI data was performed with SPM12 software (Wellcome Trust Centre for Neuroimaging, London, UK, http://www.fil.ion.ucl.ac.uk) based on MATLAB platform (MathWorks, Natick, MA). The first two images were discarded to allow the magnetization to approach dynamic equilibrium. Temporal and spatial corrections were performed on the functional images to eliminate influences from slice-timing differences and rigid body motion. Patients with head movement exceeding 3 mm or 3° were rejected. The high resolution anatomical image was co-registered with the mean image of the EPI series and then spatially normalized to the MNI template. After applying the normalization parameters to the EPI images, all volumes were resampled into 3 × 3 × 3 mm$^3$. Then the normalized task-state images were smoothed with an 8-mm FWHM isotropic Gaussian kernel.

## 2.5   Functional MRI Analysis

Statistical analysis was performed on the preprocessed data with SPM12. After specifying the design matrix, each participant's hemodynamic responses induced by the trials were modeled with a box-car function convolved with a hemodynamic function. The parameters for the effects of the positive task (PT), neutral task (NEUT), and negative task (NT) which displayed pictures with respective valences were estimated. Contrast images were constructed individually based on the general linear model (GLM). Due to the involvement of two factors in the present study, the group-level analysis was implemented based on a 2 by 3 factorial design with factors of "Group" (2 levels) and "Condition" (3 levels). Main effects of "Group" and "Condition" were analyzed to confirm whether differences in brain activation pattern exist between MDD patients and healthy controls (HC), and among PT, NEUT, and NT. Interaction was also examined for the two factors. Further inspections for the simple effects could be computed following a significant interaction, by which comparisons between groups under either emotion state would be allowed. Thresholds were set at a voxel-level $p < 0.005$, cluster size $> 1242 \ mm^3$, corresponding to a corrected $p < 0.05$ as determined by AlphaSim correction.

Finally, the mean percentage BOLD signal change acquired from each region of interest (ROI) was extracted by a 6 mm-radius sphere for each subject, and correlated with the symptom scores of depression to investigate the interaction between altered brain functions and severity of clinical symptoms. SPSS 19.0 software (SPSS, Chicago, IL, USA) was used for the statistical analyses.

# 3 Results

## 3.1 Behavioral Results

We carried out two-way analyses of variance on the accuracy (ACC) and reaction time (RT) by specifying the 3 task conditions as within-group factor and the 2 groups as between-group factor. In the MDD group, the average ACC was $86.84 \pm 11.51$ % (mean $\pm$ SD) for the positive task (PT), $85.96 \pm 15.94$ % for the neutral task (NEUT), and $85.75 \pm 12.46$ % for the negative task (NT). In the HC group, the average ACC was $92.25 \pm 7.49$ % for the PT, $92.98 \pm 6.10$ % for the NEUT, and $90.94 \pm 5.23$ % for the NT. Only the main effect of group was significant, with the F (1, 108) = 8.897, p = 0.004. MDD patients showed significantly lower ACC than the healthy subjects.

In the MDD group, the average RT was $2461.96 \pm 463.03$ ms for the PT, $2467.21 \pm 498.99$ ms for the NEUT, and $2500.29 \pm 485.92$ ms for the NT. In the HC group, the average RT was $2391.31 \pm 375.99$ ms for the PT, $2405.70 \pm 346.38$ ms for the NEUT, and $2452.68 \pm 384.96$ ms for the NT. Neither main effect nor interaction reached significance.

## 3.2 fMRI Results

The group-level analysis based on factorial design exhibited significant main effects of group and condition, as well as significant interaction between group and condition. Post hoc 2-sample t-tests were implemented to examine brain activation differences of emotional responses and attentional control between MDD and HC groups under different emotional state. In the positive condition, MDD patients showed only decreased brain activation in the left anterior insula (AI), right orbital part of inferior frontal gyrus around the AI, dorsal part of anterior cingulate cortex (dACC), left precuneus, bilateral angular gyri (AG), bilateral dorsolateral prefrontal cortices (DLPFC), and bilateral thalamus extending to putamen, caudate nuclei, pallidum, and other subcortical areas (see Fig. 1). In the neutral condition, decreased brain activations were observed in the right precuneus and left DLPFC in MDD patients compared with healthy subjects (see Fig. 2A). In the negative condition, MDD group showed a similar pattern as in neutral condition with only decreased activation in the right precuneus and

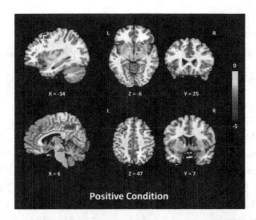

**Fig. 1.** Regions showing significant group differences revealed by positive condition. The color bar indicates t-values from the post hoc t-test analysis. (Color figure online)

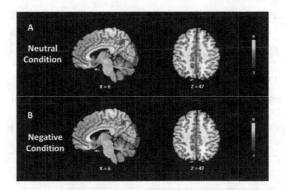

**Fig. 2.** Regions showing significant group differences revealed by neural and negative conditions respectively. The color bars indicate t-values from the post hoc t-test analyses. (Color figure online)

left DLPFC (see Fig. 2B). All the regions with significant activation are listed in Table 2. No increased activation was found for MDD patients in either condition.

### 3.3   Brain-Symptom Associations

According to the aforementioned results of fMRI analyses, more prominent discrepancies in brain activation between the MDD and HC groups can be found during the positive condition. Particularly, the salience network that consists of AI and dACC showed significant group differences during only positive condition. Therefore, we further focused on the BOLD signal in salience-related regions. In the MDD group, the mean percentage BOLD signal change of the right AI during the positive task exhibited significant negative correlations with the total score of Hamilton Depression Rating

**Table 2.** Regions with decreased activation elicited by contrasts of MDD versus HC in positive condition, neutral condition, and negative condition, respectively.

| Region | BA | Cluster | Peak MNI x | y | z | T-score |
|---|---|---|---|---|---|---|
| *Positive task* | | | | | | |
| L. Insula | 47/13 | 87 | −36 | 24 | −12 | −3.86 |
| R. IFGorb/Insula | 47 | 44 | 42 | 51 | −12 | −4.21 |
| R. dACC | 32 | 43 | 6 | 27 | 36 | −3.24 |
| R. Thalamus | | 73 | 12 | −3 | 0 | −4.56 |
| L. Thalamus | | 69 | −3 | −3 | 0 | −4.57 |
| L. DLPFC | 8/6 | 54 | −33 | 9 | 57 | −4.39 |
| R. DLPFC | 8/6 | 45 | 36 | 18 | 54 | −4.47 |
| L. Precuneus | 7 | 168 | 3 | −54 | 42 | −4.29 |
| L. AG | 40 | 54 | −45 | −63 | 30 | −3.40 |
| R. AG | 40 | 52 | 42 | −57 | 54 | −3.54 |
| *Neutral task* | | | | | | |
| R. Precuneus | 7 | 78 | 6 | −57 | 39 | −3.56 |
| L. DLPFC | 8/6 | 50 | −33 | 18 | 42 | −3.52 |
| *Negative task* | | | | | | |
| R. Precuneus | 7 | 45 | 3 | −60 | 42 | −3.63 |
| L. DLPFC | 6 | 52 | −33 | 6 | 57 | −3.59 |

Abbreviation: IFGorb, orbital portion of inferior frontal gyrus; dACC, dorsal part of anterior cingulate cortex; DLPFC, dorsolateral prefrontal cortex; AG, angular gyrus; L, left; R, right; BA, Brodmann area.

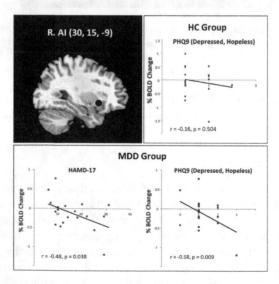

**Fig. 3.** Correlations between the percent BOLD change of AI and clinical data.

Scale 17 Items (r = −0.48, p = 0.038) and the subscore for feeling down, depressed or hopeless of 9-item Patient Health Questionnaire (r = −0.58, p = 0.009), suggesting that patients with more severe MDD symptoms show lower BOLD signal change when engaging in positive task. No other significant correlation was found between other task-induced brain activation and clinical data in MDD patients. In the HC group, no significant correlation was found between fMRI results and clinical data. Results of the brain-symptom associations are shown in Fig. 3.

## 4  Discussion

As post hoc results of the group-level analyses, only significantly decreased activation was revealed by comparing MDD patients with HC subjects in all the three task conditions. Hypo-activity was found in the left DLPFC and precuneus across the three conditions in MDD group. The left DLPFC is well-known for its role in central executive of working memory and top-down voluntary modulation of positive and negative emotions [9]. Given that the decreased activation in the left DLPFC was consistent even during neutral task in this study, abnormalities in this region is more likely to associate with difficulties in active cognitive control, i.e., cognitive manipulation in mental calculation. This inference was borne out by the behavioral results which showed significantly lower accuracy in patients relative to healthy subjects. The precuneus, serving as a component of the default mode network (DMN) which is always deactivated during goal-oriented activities, is particularly critical for the facilitation of self-referential cognitive activity and autobiographical memory [10]. It has been evidenced that the self-projection related to personal past experience relies closely on the precuneus [10]. The relatively greater deactivation in precuneus might imply the endeavor to suppress depressive rumination while MDD patients attempted to control their attention. The general pattern of the hypo-activity across task conditions indicated the poor executive control and maladaptive rumination, especially difficulties in shifting from the DMN activity to the task-positive network activity in MDD patients during participating in distraction tasks.

As a hallmark clinical symptom, anhedonia rates highly in making a diagnosis of depression. Lack of reactivity to pleasurable stimuli within brain is conceived as a cardinal feature of anhedonia, reflected in the dysfunction of midbrain, striatum, and limbic areas [11]. Given the prior evidence indicating reduced response to positive stimuli and selective attention to negative stimuli in MDD patients [12], the abnormalities in the salience detection of positive stimuli is likely to contribute to the diminished pleasure. In the present study, concurrent hypo-activation was found in the reward-related subcortical areas and regions in charge of salience processing, suggesting an impaired incentive salience processing, that is, a possible neglect of positive stimuli in MDD patients. When allocating the attention from viewing pictures to arithmetic problems, multiple salient targets are supposed to elicit more increased activation in the salience-related regions. This pattern can be observed across the three conditions in HC subjects (see Fig. 4). However, positive pictures failed to induce activation in the bilateral insulae of MDD patients, even when the corresponding activation could be elicited by neutral pictures. Furthermore, the subsequent ROI

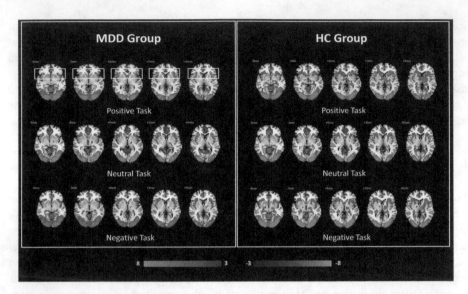

**Fig. 4.** Results of comparisons between each task condition and baseline (interval of two task blocks) for each group.

analysis demonstrated that patients with higher depressive symptom rates showed lower BOLD signal changes in the right anterior insula (AI) when evoked by positive stimuli. While the right AI is conceived as a critical note in the salience network for salience detection [6].

Taken together, it can be speculated that the abnormalities in reward processing related to the anhedonia of MDD patients are possibly caused by a morbid detection for the salience of positive stimuli. This task-based finding is consistent with previous resting-state study [13].

## 5    Conclusion

In conclusion, the present study applied a distraction task paradigm to examine the emotionality and attentional control of MDD and healthy cohorts. Across all the tasks, MDD patients showed poorer executive control and maladaptive rumination relative to healthy participants. Moreover, close relations were identified between salience processing and brain responses to positively valenced stimuli/rewards. Our findings suggest a crucial role of aberrant salience processes (especially in the anterior insulae) in the abnormal perception of positive stimuli in MDD patients, which is likely to be the pathology underlying the anhedonia.

**Acknowledgements.** This work was funded by National Basic Research Program of China (2014CB744600), International Science & Technology Cooperation Program of China (2013DFA32180), National Natural Science Foundation of China (61420106005, 61272345), and JSPS Grants-in-Aid for Scientific Research of Japan (26350994), and supported by Beijing Municipal Commission of Education, and Beijing Xuanwu Hospital.

# References

1. Der-Avakian, A., Markou, A.: The neurobiology of anhedonia and other reward-related deficits. Trends Neurosci. **35**, 68–77 (2012)
2. Diener, C., Kuehner, C., Brusniak, W., Ubl, B., Wessa, M., Flor, H.: A meta-analysis of neurofunctional imaging studies of emotion and cognition in major depression. NeuroImage **61**, 677–685 (2012)
3. Mayberg, H.S., Liotti, M., Brannan, S.K., McGinnis, S., Mahurin, R.K., Jerabek, P.A., Silva, J.A., Tekell, J.L., Martin, C.C., Lancaster, J.L., Fox, P.T.: Reciprocal limbic-cortical function and negative mood: converging PET findings in depression and normal sadness. Am. J. Psychiatry **156**, 675–682 (1999)
4. Bora, E., Harrison, B.J., Davey, C.G., Yucel, M., Pantelis, C.: Meta-analysis of volumetric abnormalities in cortico-striatal-pallidal-thalamic circuits in major depressive disorder. Psychol. Med. **42**, 671–681 (2012)
5. Sheline, Y.I., Barch, D.M., Price, J.L., Rundle, M.M., Vaishnavi, S.N., Snyder, A.Z., Mintun, M.A., Wang, S., Coalson, R.S., Raichle, M.E.: The default mode network and self-referential processes in depression. Proc. Natl. Acad. Sci. U.S.A. **106**, 1942–1947 (2009)
6. Uddin, L.Q.: Salience processing and insular cortical function and dysfunction. Nat. Rev. Neurosci. **16**, 55–61 (2015)
7. Henderson, S.E., Vallejo, A.I., Ely, B.A., Kang, G., Krain Roy, A., Pine, D.S., Stern, E.R., Gabbay, V.: The neural correlates of emotional face-processing in adolescent depression: a dimensional approach focusing on anhedonia and illness severity. Psychiatry Res. **224**, 234–241 (2014)
8. Sheehan, D.V., Sheehan, K.H., Shytle, R.D., Janavs, J., Bannon, Y., Rogers, J.E., Milo, K. M., Stock, S.L., Wilkinson, B.: Reliability and validity of the Mini International Neuropsychiatric Interview for Children and Adolescents (MINI-KID). J. Clin. Psychiatry **71**, 313–326 (2010)
9. Phillips, M.L., Ladouceur, C.D., Drevets, W.C.: A neural model of voluntary and automatic emotion regulation: implications for understanding the pathophysiology and neurodevelopment of bipolar disorder. Mol. Psychiatry **13**(829), 833–857 (2008)
10. Buckner, R.L., Carroll, D.C.: Self-projection and the brain. Trends Cogn. Sci. **11**, 49–57 (2007)
11. Pizzagalli, D.A., Holmes, A.J., Dillon, D.G., Goetz, E.L., Birk, J.L., Bogdan, R., Dougherty, D.D., Iosifescu, D.V., Rauch, S.L., Fava, M.: Reduced caudate and nucleus accumbens response to rewards in unmedicated individuals with major depressive disorder. Am. J. Psychiatry **166**, 702–710 (2009)
12. Asthana, H.S., Mandal, M.K., Khurana, H., Haque-Nizamie, S.: Visuospatial and affect recognition deficit in depression. J. Affect. Disord. **48**, 57–62 (1998)
13. Tahmasian, M., Knight, D.C., Manoliu, A., Schwerthoffer, D., Scherr, M., Meng, C., Shao, J., Peters, H., Doll, A., Khazaie, H., Drzezga, A., Bauml, J., Zimmer, C., Forstl, H., Wohlschlager, A.M., Riedl, V., Sorg, C.: Aberrant intrinsic connectivity of hippocampus and amygdala overlap in the fronto-insular and dorsomedial-prefrontal cortex in major depressive disorder. Front. Hum. Neurosci. **7**, 639 (2013)

# Pattern Classification and Analysis of Memory Processing in Depression Using EEG Signals

Kin Ming Puk[1]([✉]), Kellen C. Gandy[2], Shouyi Wang[1], and Heekyeong Park[2]

[1] Department of Industrial, Manufacturing, and Systems Engineering,
University of Texas at Arlington, 701 S Nedderman Dr, Arlington, TX 76019, USA
kinming.puk@mavs.uta.edu, shouyiw@uta.edu
[2] Department of Psychology, University of Texas at Arlington,
701 S Nedderman Dr, Arlington, TX 76019, USA
kellen.gandy@mavs.uta.edu, hkpark@uta.edu

**Abstract.** An automatic, electroencephalogram (EEG) based approach of diagnosing depression with regard to memory processing is presented. EEG signals are extracted from 15 depressed subjects and 12 normal subjects during experimental tasks of reorder and rehearsal. After preprocessing noisy EEG signals, nine groups of mathematical features are extracted and classification with support vector machine (SVM) is conducted under a five-fold cross-validation, with accuracy of up to 70 %–100 %. The contribution of this paper lies in the analysis and visualization of the difference between depressed and control subjects in EEG signals.

**Keywords:** Depression · Working memory · Long-term memory · EEG · Machine learning · Signal processing · Feature extraction · Feature selection · Classification · Support vector machine

## 1 Introduction

Depression, according to [2], is a term referring to a disabling and prevalent psychiatric illness, major depressive disorder (also known as clinical depression). Depressed patients tend to feel sad and pessimistic for a long period of time, and they are likely associated with low self-esteem and tendency to commit suicide, among other negative symptoms. It has been reported that depressed patients suffer from poor concentration and memory. For the sake of evaluating the effectiveness of memory retrieval, working memory (WM) and long-term memory (LTM) are the primary research interest in this work [6]. Techniques of brain signal analysis of EEG with classification framework in data mining is adopted in this regard. Indeed computer-aided diagnosis using EEG signals is a popular field of research. Classification framework consists of EEG preprocessing, feature extraction, feature selection and classifier. Depending on the disorder/disease and framework, classification accuracy may vary from 80 % [3] to 97 % [5]. Interested readers are referred to [3–5,10,11] for more details.

© Springer International Publishing AG 2016
G.A. Ascoli et al. (Eds.): BIH 2016, LNAI 9919, pp. 124–137, 2016.
DOI: 10.1007/978-3-319-47103-7_13

# 2   Experimental Design and Data Acquisition

**Participant.** Participants were recruited from the University of Texas at Arlington. Each participant completed a pre-screen questionnaire which included the Center of Epidemiological Studies Depression Scale (CES-D) for separating groups of individuals with high and low depressive symptomatology. Individuals who scored 25 or above qualified to be part of the high group, below 15 to be part of the low group, and 15–25 to be part of the moderate group. A total of 60 individuals - 20 with low depression, 20 with moderate depression, and 20 with high depression - were recruited for the purposes of this experiment. In this EEG analysis, only data from 15 high depression individuals (4 males, 11 females; Age: $20.3 \pm 3.21$) and low depression individuals (4 males, 8 females; Age: $20.5 \pm 2.66$) is used due to cleanliness of data and for the sake of binary classification (so that data from moderately depressed subjects is not used).

**Procedure.** Tasks of varying cognitive difficulty in semantic processing are designed with reference to [1]. During the entire experimental procedure, EEG signal is measured using the Brain Vision 32 channel system and recorded using the Pycorder software.

The assessment of working memory ("WM procedure") consists of "reorder" and "rehearsal". For reorder tasks, participants are instructed to mentally reorder the sequence of three pictorial items based on their physical weight in an arrangement from lightest to heaviest, with 1 representing the lightest item, 2 representing the mid-weight item, and 3 representing the heaviest item ("reorder"). For rehearsal tasks, participants were instructed to remember the sequence of three pictorial items based on their serial order from top to bottom, with 1 representing the top item, 2 representing the middle item, and 3 representing the bottom item ("rehearsal").

On the other hand, long-term memory is assessed by differentiating "new" from old images ("LTM procedure"). After the WM procedure, participants are asked to continue with LTM procedure by indicating whether each image appears using their right hand ("new"), followed by a confidence rating of that decision which ranged from 1 to 3, with 1 representing low confidence, 2 representing medium confidence, and 3 representing high confidence using their left hand.

# 3   Extraction and Classification of EEG Features

**Preprocessing of EEG Signals.** EEG data of 32 electrodes (FP1, FP2, F7, F3, Fz, F4, F8, FT9, FC5, FC1, FC2, FC6, FT10, T9, T7, C3, Cz, C4, T8, T10, CP5, CP1, CP2, CP6, P7, P3, Pz, P4, P8, Oz, Oz, O2; see Fig. 2) are imported into Matlab with software package "EEGLAB" [7]. EEG signals will then be re-referenced at channels T9 and T10 since these two channels are least influenced by cognitive processing, resampled from 1000 Hz to 256 Hz for reducing data size, and bandpass filtered at 1–35 Hz for removing unnecessary signal noise.

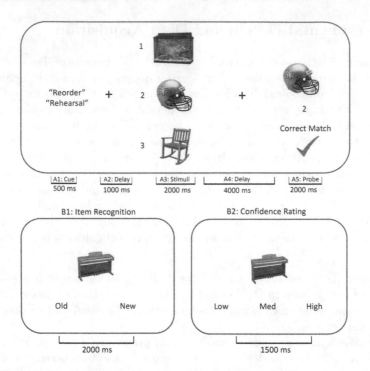

**Fig. 1.** (i) WM, Top: on rehearsal trials, participants are instructed to maintain the serial order of the three presented items (top to bottom), whereas on reorder trials, participants were instructed to mentally rearrange the items according to their physical weight (lightest to heaviest). (ii) LTM, Bottom: participants are instructed to recognize whether the image appeared in WM procedure or not.

**Epoching.** After preprocessing, EEG signal is partitioned into different epochs according to the experiment procedure for working memory and long-term memory. Each participant were shown 504 images, which correspond to 504 trials.

For working memory (Fig. 1), each trial (either reorder or rehearsal) consists of a cue on the center of the screen (A1, 500 ms), inter-stimulus interval (A2, 1000 ms), showing of the stimuli (A3, 2000 ms), delay (A4, 4000 ms) and probing for the answer (A5, 2000 ms). Therefore, EEG signal of 336 trials, with each trial lasting for 10500 ms (including baseline of 1000 ms before the start of each trial) are extracted for working memory.

As for long-term memory (Fig. 1), the procedure consists of item recognition (B1, 2000 ms) and rating the confidence of the recognition (B2, 1500 ms). Therefore, EEG signal of 168 trials, with each trial lasting for 4500 ms (including baseline of 1000 ms before the start of each trial) are extracted for long-term memory.

Please note that baseline removal can only be done after epoching with the availability of baseline signal.

**Artifact Removal.** Artifact is then removed from EEG signal with EEGLAB plugin - ADJUST (An Automatic EEG artifact Detector based on the Joint Use of Spatial and Temporal features) [9]. Artifact features including eye blinks, (vertical and horizontal) eye movements and generic discontinuities are accounted for. The four stages are (i) Epoched EEG signal is first decomposed into different independent components using independent component analysis (ICA); (ii) artifact features for each component are computed; (iii) the value of each artifact feature for each component is to be checked against threshold value computed by Expectation-Maximization [22] in order to determine whether that component is an artifact; and (iv) EEG signal is reconstructed using independent components which are not rejected.

**Feature Extraction.** Nine groups of mathematical features - statistical features, time-frequency features, signal power, Hjorth parameters, Hurst exponent, band power asymmetry and spectral edge frequency - are extracted from each trial of subjects as in [3,5,10]. These nine groups of features are extracted from EEG signal at each of the 30 channels (2 channels removed after rereferencing). They are then concatenated as a feature vector. This procedure is applied to all trials of EEG data for all participants. In the following, $X = \{x_1, x_2, ..., x_m\}$ denote a single-channel signal with $m$ time points.

(1) Statistical Features: Mean, variance, skewness, kurtosis at theta, alpha, beta and low gamma bands are computed. More specifically, mean is the averaged signal amplitude, variance measures the signal variability to the mean, skewness quantifies the extent to which the distribution leans to one side of the mean, and kurtosis measures the 'peakedness' of the distribution.

(2) Morphological features: Three morphological features at theta, alpha, beta and low gamma bands were extracted to describe morphological characteristics of a single-channel signal as in [11,23].

- Curve length is the sum of distances between any two pair of consecutive points. Intuition behind this feature is that curve length increase with the signal magnitude, frequency and amplitude variation. It is mathematically calculated as follows:

$$\frac{1}{m-1} \sum_{i=1}^{m-1} |x_{i+1} - x_i| \qquad (1)$$

- Number of peaks measures the overall frequency of a signal. It is mathematically calculated as follows:

$$\frac{1}{2} \sum_{i=1}^{m-2} \max(0, sgn(x_{i+2} - x_{i+1}) - sgn(x_{i+1} - x_i)) \qquad (2)$$

- Average nonlinear energy, according to [24], is sensitive to spectral changes and is calculated as:

$$\frac{1}{m-2} \sum_{i=2}^{m-1} x_i^2 - x_{i-1}x_{i+1} \qquad (3)$$

(3) Time-Frequency Features: Wavelet transform (WT) is a powerful tool to perform time-frequency analysis of signals. The fundamental idea of WT is to represent a signal by a linear combination of a set of functions obtained by shifting or dilating a particular function called mother wavelet [12]. The WT of a signal $X(t)$ is defined as:

$$C(a,b) = \int^R X(t) \frac{1}{\sqrt{a}} \Psi(\frac{t-b}{a}) dt \tag{4}$$

where $\Psi$ is the mother wavelet, $C(a,b)$ are the WT coefficients of the signal $X(t)$, $a$ is the scale parameter, and $b$ is the shifting parameter. Continuous wavelet transform (CWT) has $a \in R^+$ and $b \in R$ and discrete wavelet transform (DWT) has $a = 2^j$ and $b = k2^j$ for all $(j,k) \in Z$ given the decomposition level of $j$. Since CWT explores every possible scale $a$ and shifting $b$, it is generally a lot more computationally expensive than DWT. As a result, DWT is often used to perform time-frequency analysis of a signal at different decomposition levels [13]. The DWT coefficients provide a non-redundant and highly efficient representation of a signal in both time and frequency domain. At each level of decomposition, DWT works as a set of bandpass filters to divide a signal into two bands called approximations and details signals. The details (D) are the high-frequency components. Among different wavelet families, we employed Daubechies wavelet as it is frequently used in physiological signal analysis due to its orthogonality property and efficient filter implementation [14]. A 4-level discrete wavelet transform (DWT) decomposition was applied to the collected signals with the sampling rate of 256 Hz. Table 1 lists the decomposed signals D1, D2, D3 and D4, which roughly corresponded to the commonly recognized brain signal frequency bands theta, alpha, beta, and gamma, respectively.

**Table 1.** Frequency bands of signals by discrete wavelet decomposition.

| Decomposed level | Frequency range (Hz) | Approximate band |
|---|---|---|
| D1 | 4–8 | Theta |
| D2 | 8–12 | Alpha |
| D3 | 12–25 | Beta |
| D4 | 25–40 | Gamma |

After the four-level DWT decomposition, a set of wavelet coefficients can be obtained for each decomposed signals. To further decrease feature dimensionality, we employed a measure of wavelet coefficients called wavelet entropy (WE), which indicates the degree of multi-frequency signal order/disorder in the signals [25]. To obtain WE, the first step is to calculate relative wavelet energy for each decomposition level as follows:

$$p_j = \frac{E_j}{E_{total}} = \frac{E_j}{\sum_{j=1}^n E_j} \tag{5}$$

where $j$ is the resolution level, and $n$ is the number of decomposed signals ($n = 5$ in this study). $E_j$ is the wavelet power, the sum of squared wavelet coefficients, of decomposed signal $j$. The relative wavelet energy $p_j$ can be considered as the power density of the decomposed signal level $j$. Similar to Shannon entropy [26] for analyzing and comparing probability distributions, the WE is defined by

$$WE = -\sum_{j=1}^{n} p_j * ln(p_j) \tag{6}$$

WE characterizes the order/disorder of signals powers in the five brain signal frequency bands (theta, alpha, beta and gamma) during the experiment.

(4) Signal Power: Adopting the signal features used in a previous work [15], "band power" of EEG signals for each channel in commonly used frequency bands of brain signal including theta (4–8 Hz), alpha (8–12 Hz), beta (12–25 Hz), and gamma bands (25–40 Hz) is computed. On the other hand, "relative band power" at each channel is computed as the ratio of the band power of the individual band over the sum of band power of all four bands.

(5) Hjorth Parameters: Hjorth parameters, namely activity, mobility, and complexity, are frequently used in signal processing since its introduction by Bo Hjorth in 1970. These time-domain features are commonly used in brain signal analysis as in [5,16].

(6) Hurst Exponent: It is a statistical measure used to detect autocorrelation in time-series data such as EEG signal (usually notated as $H$). If the value of $H$ is 0.5, it indicates that the time-series data is a random series, whereas $H > 0.5$ indicates a trend reinforcing series [17].

(7) Band Power Asymmetry: Asymmetry of power in theta, alpha and beta bands between different regions (inter-hemispheric) and within the same region (intra-hemispheric) of the brain, as in Fig. 2, are computed as features [20].

(8) Spectral Edge Frequency: It measures the frequency below which a certain percentage of total power of the EEG time-series signal [18]. In this project, percentage values of 50 %, 90 % and 95 % are considered.

(9) Zero Crossing: It is the number of points where the sign of the EEG signal changes from positive to negative (or vice versa).

Table 2 summarizes the features extracted in this work.

**Feature Selection.** Feature selection method "minimal-redundancy-maximal-relevance criterion" (mRMR) [10] is used. mRMR aims at selecting a subset of feature set based on the statistical property of a target classification variable, subject to the constraint that the features are mutually dissimilar to each other but at the same time marginally similar to the target classification variable. Because of its first-order incremental nature, mRMR selects features very quickly without sacrificing classification performance. The number of features chosen in this classification study is 100.

**Table 2.** Summary of groups of mathematical features employed in this classification study

| No | Group name | Features (generated at 30 channels and 4 bands except for groups 2–3, 5–9) | Count |
|----|-----------|-----------------------------------------------------------------------------|-------|
| 1 | Statistical | Mean, variance, skewness, kurotsis (at each channel) | 120 |
| 2 | Morphological | Curve length, number of peaks, average nonlinear energy (at each channel) | 90 |
| 3 | Time-frequency | Wavelet entropy (power ratio of theta, alpha + low beta, beta and low gamma, alpha to beta ratio) | 180 |
| 4 | Signal power | Band power and relative band power | 240 |
| 5 | Hjorth | Activity, mobility, complexity (at each channel) | 90 |
| 6 | Hurst | - (at each channel) | 30 |
| 7 | Band power asymmetry | Asymmetry of inter-hemisphere and intra-hemisphere band power | 68 |
| 8 | Spectral edge frequency | Percentage values of 50 %, 90 % and 95 % (at each channel) | 90 |
| 9 | Zero crossing | - (at each channel) | 30 |

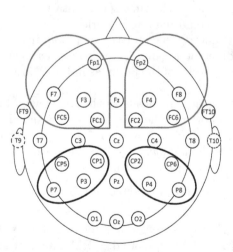

**Fig. 2.** Illustration of 4 groupings of channels (out of 32 according to 10–20 system) for inter- and intra-hemisphere band-power asymmetry. They correspond to left frontal, right frontal, left parietal and right parietal areas of the brain. T9 and T10 are not available after re-referencing.

**Classifier.** Support vector machine with radial basis function (RBF) kernel from Matlab (name of the function is fitcsvm) is used.

In binary classification, SVM basically seeks a separating hyperplane which maximizes the distance between two classes of data points in order to differentiate data point of one class from another. To ease the use of kernel trick, the dual formulation (7) of SVM is usually considered, in which $x$ is the feature vector (or data point in machine learning terminology) selected from the last step, and $y$ is the class of that feature vector:

$$\begin{aligned} \underset{\alpha}{\text{maximize}} \quad & \sum_{i=1}^{n} \alpha_i - \frac{1}{2} \sum_{i,j} \alpha_i \alpha_j y_i y_j K(x_i, x_j) \\ \text{subject to} \quad & \sum_{i=1}^{n} \alpha_i y_i = 0, \ i = 1, \ldots, n \\ & C \geq \alpha_i \geq 0, \ i = 1, \ldots, n. \end{aligned} \tag{7}$$

If $\sum_{i=1}^{l} \alpha y_i K(x_i^T x) + b \geq 0$ (where $l$ is the number of features), the data point is classified to be depressed subject; otherwise, it is classified to be control subject. The RBF kernel on two samples $x$ and $y$ is given by:

$$K(x, y) = exp(-\frac{||x - y||^2}{2\sigma^2}) \tag{8}$$

**Cross Validation.** Data will be divided into five (5) folds for cross validation (CV). In each fold of CV, 80 % of data are used for training the classification model by tuning the hyper-parameters with grid search (namely $C$ in Eq. (7) and $\sigma$ in Eq. 8 for SVM), whereas the remaining 20 % will be used for testing the trained model. Testing accuracy is the main measure of classification performance, which is calculated as the number of correctly predicted class of subjects in each trial (i.e. depressed or control) over the total number of trials available from all subjects in an epoch:

$$acc = \frac{\text{no. of correctly predicted class of subjects from all trials}}{\text{no. of trials available from all subjects in an epoch}} \tag{9}$$

## 4   Experimental Result and Analysis

Table 3 shows the accuracy of classifying subjects with high depression from those with low depression under different experimental tasks and epoches. The higher the accuracy, the greater the difference between the depressed and control subjects in performing experimental tasks. On the other hand, the epoch with high classification accuracy is investigated in order to better identify the difference between the two groups of subjects.

As mentioned before, each trial of WM procedure consists of a cue (A1), inter-stimulus interval (A2), showing of the stimuli (A3), delay (A4) and probing for the answer (A5). In these epoches, A3 is the time at which memory

**Table 3.** Classification accuracy with SVM for epoches in working memory (WM) and long-term memory (LTM). A means WM (A1: cue, A2: inter-stimulus interval, A3: stimuli, A4: delay, A5: probe), whereas B stands for LTM (B1: item recognition, B2: confidence rating).

|  | WM | | | | | LTM | |
|---|---|---|---|---|---|---|---|
|  | A1 | A2 | A3 | A4 | A5 | B1 | B2 |
| Reorder | 92 % | 100 % | 98 % | 86 % | 86 % | 73 % | 77 % |
| Rehearsal | 86 % | 91 % | 83 % | 86 % | 89 % | 86 % | 75 % |
| New | - | - | - | - | - | 57 % | 68 % |

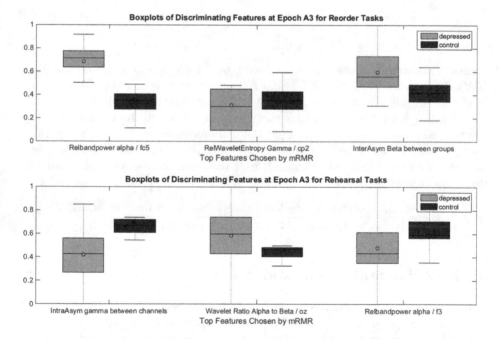

**Fig. 3.** Boxplot of Top 3 Features Used for Classification in Epoch A3. The top 3 features for reorder tasks are relative band power at beta (FC5), relative wavelet entropy of gamma band (CP2) and asymmetry inter-hemisphere band power at beta, whereas those for rehearsal tasks are asymmetry of intra-hemisphere band power at gamma, wavelet ratio of alpha to beta (Oz) and relative band power at alpha (F3).

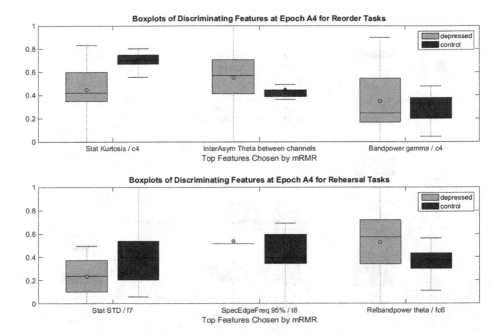

**Fig. 4.** Boxplot of Top 3 Features Used for Classification in Epoch A4. The top 3 features for reorder tasks are kurtosis (C4), asymmetry of inter-hemisphere band power at theta and band power at gamma (C4), whereas those for rehearsal tasks are standard deviation (F7), spectrum edge frequency at 95 % (T8) and relative band power at theta (FC6).

encoding takes place, and A4 is the time at which memory processing happens. As for long-term memory procedure, each trial consists of item recognition (B1) and rating the confidence of the recognition (B2). Therefore, B1 is the time at which retrieval of long-term memory takes place. Accuracy in "reorder" tasks is generally higher than those of "rehearsal" as a result of greater difficulty of cognitive processing required by "reorder" tasks [8]. Accuracy in "new" tasks is lowest among three kinds of tasks because of the same reasoning.

Epoches A3, A4 and B1 are worth investigating. It is because memory encoding and retrieval of working memory take place at epoches A3 and A4 respectively, whereas memory retrieval of long-term memory takes place at epoch B1. One way to investigate these epoches would be to consider the top 3 features (out of 100 selected by the mRMR algorithm) used for classification. There are 27 subjects, and therefore each feature (vector) under consideration consists of 27 values, with each one extracted from the EEG signal of one subject. Figures 3, 4 and 5 are the boxplots plotted with these 27 values of each feature.

An observation in this regard is that the higher the classification accuracy in that epoch, the farther the distance between the boxes of the depressed and control subjects. An example supporting this notion is epoch A3 for reorder

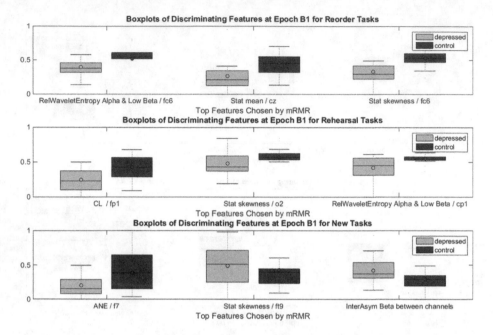

**Fig. 5.** Boxplot of Top 3 Features Used for Classification in Epoch B1. The top 3 features for reorder tasks are relative wavelet entropy at alpha and low beta (FC6), mean (Cz) and skewness (FC6), those for rehearsal tasks are curve length (Fp1), skewness (O2) and relative wavelet entropy at alpha and low beta (CP1), and those for new tasks are average non-linear energy (F7), skewness (FT9), and asymmetry of inter-hemisphere band power at beta.

tasks (Fig. 3), having accuracy of 98 %. Its top feature is relative band power at alpha band (FC5) - the box of depressed does not overlap with that of the control completely.

In addition to the above, topographical plots (Fig. 6) at epoches A3, A4 and B1 for theta (4–8 Hz) and alpha (8–12 Hz) bands are plotted with average EEG signal of trials after preprocessing. With topographical plots, activation in different frequency bands can be considered over the 30 EEG channels.

In epoch A3 (both theta and alpha bands), left prefrontal area is observed to have greater activation for control over depressed subjects for reorder task. Surprisingly, no distinct difference between depressed and control subjects can be found in epoch A4. Last but not least, there is stronger activation found in occipital area for control over depressed subjects at epoch B1 for new task.

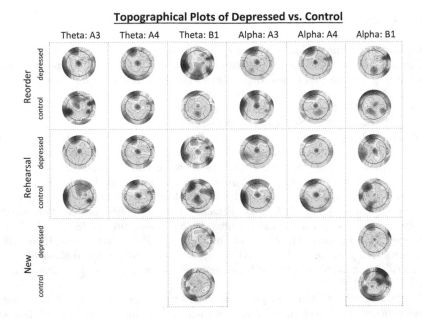

**Fig. 6.** Plots of relative topographical distribution of mean log power spectrum of theta and alpha bands at epoches A3 (showing of stimuli), A4 (Delay) and B1 (Item Recognition). These plots are generated with EEGLAB function "spectopo" and "topoplot".

## 5   Conclusion

This study investigated the difference of memory processing between depression and control groups using EEG signals. An extensive EEG feature study has been performed using the most popular techniques of feature extraction in the up-to-date literature. The popular technique of feature selection, minimal-redundancy-maximal-relevance criterion (mRMR), has been employed to identify the most discriminative EEG features among the two groups of subjects. Classification using support vector machine with RBF kernel showed that the depressed subjects indeed exhibited different patterns of brain activity in the processing of both working and long-term memory, with classification accuracies higher than 80 %. The top EEG features showed significantly different distributions between two groups of subjects. This preliminary data-driven study indicates that depression can affect a subject's memory processing considerably. In the future work, neural signatures of depression with regard to its effect to memory processing will be identified using advance data mining and machine learning techniques. The long-term goal of this study is to facilitate the understanding of neural mechanism of depression, and to develop better data-driven tools for diagnosis and treatment of depression in clinical practice.

# References

1. Ragland, J., Blumenfeld, R., Ramsay, I., Yonelinas, A., Yoon, J., Solomon, M., Carter, C., Ranganath, C.: Neural correlates of relational and item-specific encoding during working and long-term memory in schizophrenia. NeuroImage **59**, 1719–1726 (2012)
2. Loewenthal, K.: Depression. In: Leeming, D.A. (ed.) Encyclopedia of Psychology and Religion, pp. 1–5. Springer, Heidelberg (2016)
3. Hosseinifard, B., Moradi, M., Rostami, R.: Classifying depression patients and normal subjects using machine learning techniques and nonlinear features from EEG signal. Comput. Methods Programs Biomed. **109**, 339–345 (2013)
4. Li, Y., Fan, F.: Classification of schizophrenia and depression by EEG with ANNs. In: 2005 IEEE Engineering in Medicine and Biology 27th Annual Conference (2005)
5. Yuan, Q., Zhou, W., Li, S., Cai, D.: Epileptic EEG classification based on extreme learning machine and nonlinear features. Epilepsy Res. **96**, 29–38 (2011)
6. Baddeley, A., Eysenck, M., Anderson, M.: Memory. Psychology Press, Hove (2009)
7. Delorme, A., Makeig, S.: EEGLAB: an open source toolbox for analysis of single-trial EEG dynamics including independent component analysis. J. Neurosci. Methods **134**, 9–21 (2004)
8. Gandy, K.C.: An EEG investigation of memory in depression: the effect of cognitive processing. Master thesis, Department of Psychology, University of Texas at Arlington (2015)
9. Mognon, A., Jovicich, J., Bruzzone, L., Buiatti, M.: ADJUST: an automatic EEG artifact detector based on the joint use of spatial and temporal features. Psychophysiology **48**, 229–240 (2011)
10. Wang, S., Gwizdka, J., Chaovalitwongse, W.: Using wireless EEG signals to assess memory workload in the n-back task. IEEE Trans. Hum. Mach. Syst. **46**, 1–12 (2015)
11. Wang, S., Lin, C., Wu, C., Chaovalitwongse, W.: Early detection of numerical typing errors using data mining techniques. IEEE Trans. Syst. Man Cybern. Part A Syst. Hum. **41**, 1199–1212 (2011)
12. Addison, P.: The Illustrated Wavelet Transform Handbook. Institute of Physics Publishing, Bristol (2002)
13. Rosso, O., Martin, M., Figliola, A., Keller, K., Plastino, A.: EEG analysis using wavelet-based information tools. J. Neurosci. Methods **153**, 163–182 (2006)
14. Subasi, A.: EEG signal classification using wavelet feature extraction and a mixture of expert model. Expert Syst. Appl. **32**, 1084–1093 (2007)
15. Grimes, D., Tan, D., Hudson, S., Shenoy, P., Rao, R.: Feasibility and pragmatics of classifying working memory load with an electroencephalograph. In: Proceeding of the Twenty-Sixth Annual CHI Conference on Human Factors in Computing Systems - CHI 2008 (2008)
16. Oh, S., Lee, Y., Kim, H.: A novel EEG feature extraction method using Hjorth parameter. IJEEE **2**, 106–110 (2014)
17. Qian, B., Rasheed, K.: Hurst exponent and financial market predictability. In: IASTED Conference on Financial Engineering and Applications (2004)
18. Drummond, J., Brann, C., Perkins, D., Wolfe, D.: A comparison of median frequency, spectral edge frequency, a frequency band power ratio, total power, and dominance shift in the determination of depth of anesthesia. Acta Anaesthesiol. Scand. **35**, 693–699 (1991)

19. Peng, H., Long, F., Ding, C.: Feature selection based on mutual information criteria of max-dependency, max-relevance, and min-redundancy. IEEE Trans. Pattern Anal. Mach. Intell. **27**, 1226–1238 (2005)
20. Yuvaraj, R., Murugappan, M., Mohamed Ibrahim, N., Iqbal, M., Sundaraj, K., Mohamad, K., Palaniappan, R., Mesquita, E., Satiyan, M.: On the analysis of EEG power, frequency and asymmetry in Parkinsons disease during emotion processing. Behav. Brain Funct. **10**, 12 (2014)
21. Golinkoff, M., Sweeney, J.: Cognitive impairments in depression. J. Affect. Disord. **17**, 105–112 (1989)
22. Bruzzone, L., Prieto, D.: Automatic analysis of the difference image for unsupervised change detection. IEEE Trans. Geosci. Remote Sens. **38**, 1171–1182 (2000)
23. Wong, S., Baltuch, G., Jaggi, J., Danish, S.: Functional localization and visualization of the subthalamic nucleus from microelectrode recordings acquired during DBS surgery with unsupervised machine learning. J. Neural Eng. **6**, 026006 (2009)
24. Kaiser, J.: On a simple algorithm to calculate the 'energy' of a signal. In: International Conference on Acoustics, Speech, and Signal Processing, vol. 1, pp. 381–384 (1990)
25. Rosso, O., Blanco, S., Yordanova, J., Kolev, V., Figliola, A., Schrmann, M., Baar, E.: Wavelet entropy: a new tool for analysis of short duration brain electrical signals. J. Neurosci. Methods **105**, 65–75 (2001)
26. Shannon, C.: A mathematical theory of communication. Bell Syst. Tech. J. **27**, 379–423 (1948)

# A Comprehensive Feature and Data Mining Study on Musician Memory Processing Using EEG Signals

Kin Ming Kam[1]([✉]), James Schaeffer[2], Shouyi Wang[1], and Heekyeong Park[2]

[1] Department of Industrial, Manufacturing and Systems Engineering,
University of Texas at Arlington, Arlington, TX 76019, USA
kinming.kam@mavs.uta.edu, shouyiw@uta.edu
[2] Department of Psychology, University of Texas at Arlington,
Arlington, TX 76019, USA
james.schaeffer@mavs.uta.edu, hkpark@uta.edu

**Abstract.** There has been much interest in the beneficial effects of musical training on cognition. Previous studies have indicated that musical training was related to better working memory and that these behavioral differences were associated with differences in neural activity in the brain. However, it was not clear whether musical training impacts memory in general, beyond working memory. By recruiting professional musicians with extensive training, we investigated if musical training has a broad impact on memory with corresponding electroencephalography (EEG) signal changes, by using working memory and long-term memory tasks with verbal and pictorial items. Behaviorally, musicians outperformed on both working memory and long-term memory tasks. A comprehensive EEG pattern study has been performed, including various univariate and multivariate features, time-frequency (wavelet) analysis, power-spectra analysis, and deterministic chaotic theory. The advanced feature selection approaches have also been employed to select the most discriminative EEG and brain activation features between musicians and non-musicians. High classification accuracy (more than 95 %) in memory judgments was achieved using Proximal Support Vector Machine (PSVM). For working memory, it showed significant differences between musicians versus non-musicians during the delay period. For long-term memory, significant differences on EEG patterns between groups were found both in the pre-stimulus period and the post-stimulus period on recognition. These results indicate that musicians memorial advantage occurs in both working memory and long-term memory and that the developed computational framework using advanced data mining techniques can be successfully applied to classify complex human cognition with high time resolution.

## 1 Introduction

There has been much interest in the beneficial effects of musical training on cognition. Previous studies have indicated that musical training was related to better working memory and that these behavioral differences were associated

© Springer International Publishing AG 2016
G.A. Ascoli et al. (Eds.): BIH 2016, LNAI 9919, pp. 138–148, 2016.
DOI: 10.1007/978-3-319-47103-7_14

with differences in neural activity in the brain [1]. However, it was not clear whether musical training impacts memory in general, beyond working memory. By recruiting professional musicians with extensive training, we investigated if musical training has a broad impact on memory with corresponding electroencephalography (EEG) signal changes, by using working memory and long-term memory tasks with verbal and pictorial items. Behaviorally, musicians outperformed on both working memory and long-term memory tasks. A comprehensive EEG pattern study has been performed, including various univariate and multivariate features, time-frequency (wavelet) analysis, power-spectra analysis, and deterministic chaotic theory. The advanced feature selection approaches have also been employed to select the most discriminative EEG and brain activation features between musicians and non-musicians [2]. High classification accuracy (more than 95 %) in memory judgments was achieved using Proximal Support Vector Machine (PSVM) [3]. For working memory, it showed significant differences between musicians versus non-musicians during the delay period. For long-term memory, significant differences on EEG patterns between groups were found both in the pre-stimulus period and the post-stimulus period on recognition. These results indicate that musicians memorial advantage occurs in both working memory and long-term memory and that the developed computational framework using advanced data mining techniques can be successfully applied to classify complex human cognition with high time resolution.

## 2  Methodology

### 2.1  Data Acquisition and Experimental Settings

*Participants.* Initially, 36 musicians and non-musicians participated into the experiments. In those 36 participants, some of them were excluded based on behavioral observation and outlier analysis. If participants are failed to follow the instruction, they will be excluded. Two of them fell into this category and were excluded. Cook's D values of both short-term and long-term memory tests were calculated to identify outliers. Subsequently, four of them were excluded due to having negative Cook's D values on the long-term memory test. One participant achieved higher than 3 standard deviations so he was also excluded from the data. Finally, 29 subjects were remained for analysis. We had 14 professional musicians who have over 10 years of experience. Five of them were female. The average of experience is 22.9 years. We also had 15 participants without any musical training. They were marked as "non-musicians". Among them, eight were female. Informed consent was obtained from all participants in accordance with the experimental protocol approved by the University of Texas Institutional Review Board.

*Design of the Experiments.* The whole experiment was separated into two parts: 1. a study session Participants completed a study session followed by a test session involving words and pictures as stimuli. Stimuli were presented visually on a computer and all responses were made using the keyboard. During the study session, participants were presented with pairs of stimuli, one at a time. Each study trial began with a fixation cross (250 ms), the first stimulus (1000 ms), a blank screen (5000 ms), the second stimulus (2500 ms or until a response), and finally a blank screen (1000 ms). Upon presentation of the second stimulus, participants made a judgment of whether the second stimulus was the same as the first (Fig. 1a).

A few minutes following the study session, participants memory was tested. During this test session, stimuli presented during study were presented again along with new stimuli that had not been studied. Further, we only tested participants memory on stimuli that had only been presented once. Therefore, only stimuli presented on trials that were different during the study session (i.e. trials on which the second stimulus was different from the first) were presented during test. Each test trial began with a fixation (250 ms), followed by a stimulus (3000 ms or until a response), and then a blank screen (1250 ms). Upon presentation of the stimulus, participants made a memory judgment which included a rating of how confident they were in their memory (Fig. 1b). They were allowed to make three responses: *remember with low confidence*, *remember with high confidence*, or *new*.

Word and picture stimuli were blocked for both study and test phases, such that each participant was presented with a block of word trials followed by a

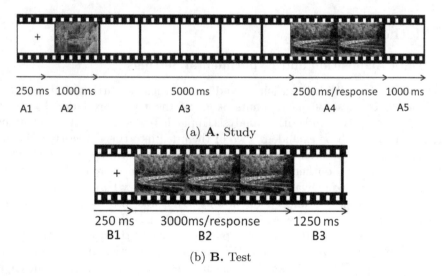

250 ms  1000 ms        5000 ms        2500 ms/response  1000 ms
A1      A2             A3             A4                A5

(a) **A.** Study

250 ms    3000ms/response    1250 ms
B1        B2                 B3

(b) **B.** Test

**Fig. 1.** Schematic of experimental paradigm. (A1 to A5) During study period, participants were asked to judge whether the second stimulus matched the first. (B1 to B3) During test period, participants made memory judgments to stimuli while rating their confidence. Low represents remember with low confidence, High represents remember with high confidence, and New represents a judgment where participants thought the stimulus was not studied.

block of picture trials (or vice versa). Whether or not participants were presented with words or pictures first was randomly determined for each participant.

*Types of Stimuli.* Participants were presented with pictures of complex scenes and words. During the study session, participants completed 96 trials of pictures (32 same, 64 different) and 96 trials of words (32 same, 64 different). Given that each trial contained two stimulus presentations, participants studied a total of 128 pictures and 128 words from different trials. These 248 studied stimuli were then used to test long-term memory during the test session. During the long-term memory task, participants completed 192 trials of pictures (128 studied, 64 new) and 192 trials of words (128 studied, 64 new).

*EEG Data.* EEG data were collected during both study and test sessions using the Brain Vision ActiChamp 32 channel system and recorded using the Pycorder software. Electrode positions followed the 10–20 system and included Fz, Cz, Pz, Oz, Fp1, Fp2, F3, F4, F7, F8, Fc1, Fc2, Fc5, Fc6, Ft9, Ft10, T7, T8, C3, C4, Cp1, Cp2, Cp5, Cp6, Tp9, Tp10, P3, P4, P7, P8, O1, and O2 according to standard 10/20 system. During recording, data were sampled at 1000 Hz and filtered between .01 and 100 Hz. Offline, data were high-pass filtered with a 0.1 Hz Butterworth filter, downsampled to 256 Hz, and referenced to the average of the mastoids (TP9 and TP10). Post-stimulus ERPs with a 1000 ms duration were extracted and were baseline-corrected with respect to a 200 ms prestimulus baseline. Visual inspection was then used to remove epochs that contained eye blinks and movement artifacts using a recently developed automatic ICA-based algorithm, called ADJUST [5].

## 2.2  Spatiotemperol Pattern Based Artifacts Removal

Brain signals often contain significant artifacts that lead to major problems in signal analysis, when the activity due to artifacts has a higher amplitude than the one due to neural sources. The common sources of artifacts include eye movements, muscle contractions, electric devices interference [4]. Independent Component Analysis (ICA) has been successfully applied for artifacts removal in many studies. The basic idea is to decompose the brain data into independent components, determine the artifacted components using pattern and source localization analysis, and reconstruct the brain signals by excluding those artifacted components. However, linking components to artifact sources (e.g., eye blinking, muscle movements) remains largely user-dependent. In this study, we employed ADJUST for signal artifact removal. ADJUST applies stereotyped artifact-specific spatial and temporal features to identify independent components of artifacts automatically. These artifacts can be removed from the data without affecting the activity of neural sources [5]. The data analysis in the following is based on the 'cleaned' data after artifact removal.

## 2.3    Signal Feature Extraction

We extensively investigated features from the collected physiological signals. Four groups of feature extraction techniques were employed to capture signal characteristics that may be relevant to assess memory workload. They were signal power, statistical, morphological, and wavelet features [6]. For a data epoch with $n$ channels, we first extracted features from signals at each channel, and then concatenated the features of all the $n$ channels to construct the feature vector of the data epoch. The feature extraction of four groups of signal features are listed in Fig. 2 [7] (Tables 1 and 3).

**Table 1.** Frequency ranges and the corresponding brain signal frequency bands of the four levels of signals by discrete wavelet decomposition.

| Decomposed level | Frequency range (Hz) | Approximate band |
|---|---|---|
| D1 | 32–64 | Gamma |
| D2 | 16–32 | Beta |
| D3 | 8–16 | Alpha |
| D4 | 4–8 | Theta |

## 2.4    Feature Vector Classification Using Proximal Support Vector Machine (PSVM)

*Classification Method.* In the experiments, we collected data from four difficulty levels (0-, 1-, 2-, 3-back). A popular binary classification technique, support vector machine (SVM), was employed to investigate the data separability at different mental workload levels. SVM techniques have been successfully applied in many classification problems [17–21]. The fundamental problem of SVM is to build an optimal decision boundary to separate two categories of data. Let $X$ denote a $n \times k$ dimensional feature vector for a multi-channel data session at certain difficulty level, where $n$ is the number of signal channels and $k$ is the number of features of each channel. To classify data between musicians and non-musicians, let $l$ denote the sample class label and $l = 1$ denotes musician, and $l = -1$ means non-musician.

Assume we have $p$ sessions of level one denoted by $S_1 = \{(X_1, l_1), (X_2, l_2), ..., (X_p, l_p)\}$, and $q$ sessions of level two denoted by $S_2 = \{(X_{p+1}, l_{p+1}), (X_{p+2}, l_{p+2}), ..., (X_{p+q}, l_{p+q})\}$. Each session is represented by a $n \times k$ dimensional feature vector. One can find infinitely many hyperplanes in $R^{n \times k}$ to separate the two data groups.

Standard SVM classifiers, such as Langragian Support Vector Machine (LSVM), usually require a large amount of computation time for training. Mangasarian and Wild [22] claims the Proximal SVM (PSVM) algorithm was about 10 to 20 times faster than LSVM. The formulation for the linear PSVM is described as follows:

$$\min_{\omega, \xi, b}\{\tfrac{1}{2}(\|\omega\|^2 + b^2) + \tfrac{1}{2}C\xi_i{}^T\xi_i : D(X^T\omega + be) = e - \xi_i\}, \qquad (1)$$

**Table 2.** 19 groups of features are considered. Sub-features are considered in some groups by means of considering various frequency bands and/or different statistics.

| F | Features (F) | Sub-features (f) |
|---|---|---|
| 1 | Basic statistics | Average; variance; skewness; kurtosis |
| 2 | Curve length [8, 9] | Curve length |
| 3 | Peak count | Peak count |
| 4 | Average nonlinear energy [10, 11] | Average nonlinear energy |
| 5 | Zero crossing | Zero crossing |
| 6 | Spectral edge frequency [12] | Spectral edge Frequency |
| 7 | Band power | 4 to 8; 8 to 13; 13 to 25; 25 to 40 (Hz) |
| 8 | Relative band power | 4 to 8; 8 to 13; 13 to 25; 25 to 40 (Hz) |
| 9 | Inter-regional asymmetry [13] | Left vs right channels; |
|   |   | Left groups: ([1 3 7], [4 5 6 9], [8 10 11 13]) vs |
|   |   | Right groups: ([27 28 30], [24 25 26 29], [18 20 21 23]) |
| 10 | Intra-regional asymmetry [13] | Left groups: ([1 3 7], [4 5 6 9], [8 10 11 13]) vs |
|   |   | Right groups: ([27 28 30], [24 25 26 29], [18 20 21 23]) |
| 11 | Hurst | Hurst |
| 12 | Hjorth | Activity, mobility, complexity |
| 13 | Barlow | Amplitude, frequency, SPI |
| 14 | Wavelet entropy [14–16] | Wavelet entropy, power ratio of theta, alpha+low beta, |
|   |   | Beta and low gamma, alpha to beta ratio |
| 15 | Brain rate | Brain rate |
| 16 | Wackermann | Sigma, Phi, Omega |
| 18 | Wavelet statistics | Max, mean, stdev of bands 4 to 8, 8 to 16, 16 to 32, 32 to 64 (Hz) |
| 19 | Range to variance ratio | Range to variance ratio |
| 20 | Network correlation | Network correlation |
| 21 | Approximate entropy | Approximate entropy |

where the traditional SVM inequality constraint is replaced by an equality constraint. This modification changes the nature of the support hyperplanes ($\omega^T X + b = \pm 1$). Instead of bounding planes, the hyperplanes of PSVM can be thought of as 'proximal' planes, around which the points of each class are clustered and which are pushed as far apart as possible by the term ($\|\omega\|^2 + b^2$) in the above objective function. It has been shown that PSVM has comparable classification performance to that of standard SVM classifiers, but can be an order of magnitude faster [22]. Therefore, we employed PSVM in this study.

*Training and Evaluation.* A classification problem generally follows a two-step procedure which consists of training and testing phases. During the training phase, a classifier is trained to achieve the optimal separation for the training data set. Then in the testing phase, the trained classifier is used to classify new samples with unknown class information. The N-fold cross-validation is an attractive method of model evaluation when the sample size is small. It is capable of providing almost unbiased estimate of the generalization ability of a classifier. For the 29 subjects, the total number of data samples (trials) for session A and B are 192 and 386 respectively. We designed a 2-fold cross-validation method to train and evaluate the SVM classifier [23].

To explore the differences of the responses of musicians and non-musicians under various events, we separate the data into five and three epochs for session

**Table 3.** Based on event labels, 12 and 21 conditions are defined for Group A and Group B respectively. All samples, Pictures only and Words only are considered. In these three subsets, we further split them into cases of Hit, Miss and Correct Rejection. In Group B, among those cases of Hit and Correct Rejection, we further split those subset by the responses, i.e. Low Confidence, High Confidence and New.

| \multicolumn{4}{c} Group A | | | | Group B | |
|----|----|----|----|----|----|
| CD | event | CD | event | CD | event |
| 1 | All samples | 13 | All samples | 25 | All samples & Low Confidence & Correct |
| 2 | Pictures | 14 | Pictures | 26 | All samples & High Confidence & Correct |
| 3 | Words | 15 | Words | 27 | All samples & New & Correct |
| 4 | All samples & Hit | 16 | All samples & Hit | 28 | Pictures & Low Confidence & Correct |
| 5 | All samples & Miss | 17 | All samples & Miss | 29 | Pictures & High Confidence & Correct |
| 6 | All samples & Correct Rejection | 18 | All samples & Correct Rejection | 30 | Pictures & New & Correct |
| 7 | Pictures & Hit | 19 | Pictures & Hit | 31 | Words & Low Confidence & Correct |
| 8 | Pictures & Miss | 20 | Pictures & Miss | 32 | Words & High Confidence & Correct |
| 9 | Pictures & Correct Rejection | 21 | Pictures & Correct Rejection | 33 | Words & New & Correct |
| 10 | Words & Hit | 22 | Words & Hit | | |
| 11 | Words & Miss | 23 | Words & Miss | | |
| 12 | Words & Correct Rejection | 24 | Words & Correct Rejection | | |

A and B respectively based on the test phases as shown in Fig. 1. In addition, A3 is further separated into five pieces with one second for each piece in order to study various parts of A3. We also study the first $l \in 0.4, 0.6, 0.8, 1, 1.5$ s of B2. These subsegments are denoted as A21,A22,...,A25 and B21,B22,...,B25. Based on the event markers of the EEG data, we define 12 conditions for session A and 21 conditions for session B. The following table lists all of the conditions.

In testing, for each comparison group, we divided the corresponding data samples into 5 non-overlapping subsets. Each time we picked one subset out and trained the PSVM classifier by the data samples of another set. The samples of the left-out subset were considered as unknown samples to test the performance of the trained classifiers. Repeating this procedure again for another set, the averaged prediction accuracy over the 5-fold runs was used to indicate the degree of separability of the EEG signals of musicians and non-musicians.

To achieve reliable feature selection, we employed an advanced feature selection technique, called minimum redundancy maximum relevance (mRMR) [24], which allows us to select a subset of superior features at a low computational cost in a high dimensional space.

The basic idea of mRMR is to select the most relevant features with respect to class labels while minimizing redundancy amongst the selected features. The mRMR algorithm uses mutual information as a distance measure to compute feature-to-feature and feature-to-class-label non-linear similarities.

## 3    Experimental Results

Before going into the classification results, Fig. 2 shows percentage of hit rate, correct rejection rate and the corresponding standard deviation. We noted that musicians had higher hit rate on picture than non-musicians. Also, musicians performed better in working memory task but they performed worse in long term memory task than non-musicians.

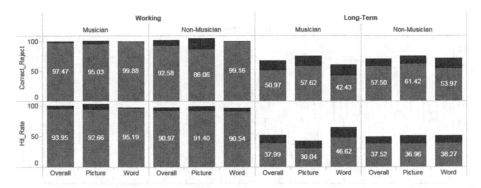

**Fig. 2.** This is a boxplot of AUC of all models using only one sub-feature at a time among various epochs aggregated by condition. For each box, there are 68 sub-features, 8 to 10 epochs and so there are roughly 700 results. Obviously, working memory (condition 1 to 12) have better classification results than long term memory.

Table 4 is a summary of classification accuracy on various conditions. On response period (B2) of long-term memory data as well as maintain period (A3) and response period (A4) of working memory, we obtained high classification accuracy. We also observed that miss events obtained high classification accuracy in general.

**Table 4.** Summary of classification accuracy on various conditions and epochs in working and long-term memory tasks.

|  | Study period (working memory) | | | | | Test period (long-term memory) | | |
|---|---|---|---|---|---|---|---|---|
|  | A1 | A2 | A3 | A4 | A5 | B1 | B2 | B3 |
| Conditions | Pre-stim | Stim1 | Maintain | Response | Post-stim | Pre-stim | Response | Post-stim |
| All samples | 83.78 | 70.27 | 83.78 | 83.78 | 72.97 | 66.67 | 75 | 69.44 |
| Pictures | 75.68 | 70.27 | 72.97 | 72.97 | 67.57 | 78.78 | 75 | 72.22 |
| Words | 81.08 | 72.97 | 86.49 | 78.38 | 64.86 | 88.89 | 69.44 | 62.86 |
| All hit | 64.86 | 72.97 | 81.08 | 78.37 | 72.97 | 87.5 | 91.67 | 64.29 |
| All - miss | 64.86 | 70.27 | 83.78 | 83.78 | 72.97 | 82.61 | 83.33 | 90.63 |
| All corr. rej | 89.19 | 67.57 | 78.35 | 83.78 | 67.57 | 52.17 | 88.89 | 80.65 |
| Picture hit | 78.38 | 78.38 | 67.57 | 70.27 | 70.27 | 63.64 | 75 | 73.53 |
| Picture - miss | 78.38 | 83.78 | 72.97 | 72.97 | 78.38 | 73.68 | 75 | 72.41 |
| Picture - corr. rej | 62.16 | 70.27 | 72.97 | 64.86 | 59.46 | 79.95 | 72.22 | 80.65 |
| Word hit | 59.46 | 64.86 | 75.68 | 67.57 | 67.57 | 55 | 86.11 | 68.75 |
| Word - miss | 59.46 | 78.38 | 64.86 | 70.27 | 78.38 | 73.68 | 77.78 | 80 |
| Word corr. rej | 72.97 | 70.27 | 83.78 | 67.57 | 64.86 | 84.21 | 69.44 | 75.86 |

Figure 3 shows that conditions 1 to 12 (Group A) have higher area under the curve (AUC). It is obvious that EEG of musicians and non-musicians have the most difference during short term memory task.

Figure 4 are the topographies of band power of musicians (left) and non-musicians (right). We note that musicians have larger range of bandpower values than non-musicians. Also, musicians tend to be active on multiple locations while

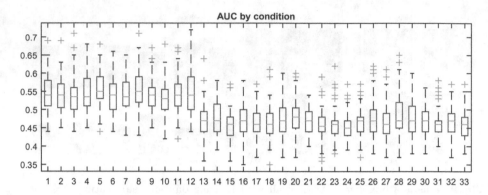

**Fig. 3.** This is a boxplot of AUC of all models using only one sub-feature at a time among various epochs aggregated by condition. For each box, there are 68 sub-features, 8 to 10 epochs and so there are roughly 700 results. Obviously, working memory (condition 1 to 12) have better classification results than long term memory.

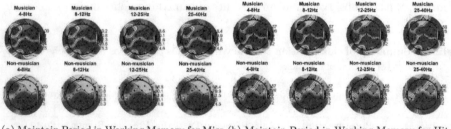

(a) Maintain Period in Working Memory for Miss conditions  (b) Maintain Period in Working Memory for Hit conditions

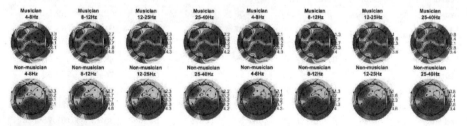

(c) Response Period in Long Term memory for Miss conditions  (d) Response Period in Long-Term memory for All Hit

**Fig. 4.** Comparison for averaged four EEG band power between musicians and non-musicians in response and maintain period. In all conditions, musicians demonstrate higher level of activity in frontal area. Their values are about 50 % higher than non-musicians. Musicians are also more active in several more areas (right area, central area and left middle area) while non-musicians mainly only use their frontal area. This pattern is more obvious in long term memory.

non-musicians tend to be active only on the front lobe. In this study, we also investigated the effect of ICA artifact removal and found that the effect was significant. It improves the classification accuracy by 10 % in general.

## 4   Conclusion and Future Work

In this study, we made a comprehensive EEG data mining study to investigate and compare cognitive memory processing for musicians and non-musicians. We presented a computational EEG pattern analysis and classification framework, which integrated the most recent advances in automated spatiotemporal artifact removal, a broad selection of most popular EEG feature extraction techniques, an information-theory-based feature selection, and a PSVM classification model. The experimental results show that the EEG patterns of the active memory encoding process at the maintain period indeed demonstrated significant differences between musicians and non-musicians. Our study found that musicians overall demonstrated better and more accurate memory performance in both short-term and long-term memory tasks. In particular, the EEG brainwave differences of musicians were more significant on the short-term memory tasks compared to the non-musician group. From the four common EEG band power study, we noted that the musicians were significant more active in frontal areas in alpha, beta, and low gamma bands than non-musicians. This may indicate that the long-time music training can sharpen brain pathways in memory processing with a more active brain activity during memory tasks. More analysis on EEG spatiotemporal patterns and memory brain network will be investigated in future works. The integrated computational framework developed in this study also provides a powerful tool to perform EEG signal processing and pattern analysis, and can be useful in many other applications that involve pattern recognition or abnormality detection in multivariate EEG signals.

## References

1. Lin, Y.-P., Wang, C.-H., Jung, T.-P., Wu, T.-L., Jeng, S.-K., Duann, J.-R., Chen, J.-H.: EEG-based emotion recognition in music listening. IEEE Trans. Biomed. Eng. **57**(7), 1798–1806 (2010)
2. Murugappan, M., Nagarajan, R., Yaacob, S.: Comparison of different wavelet features from EEG signals for classifying human emotions. In: IEEE Symposium on Industrial Electronics and Applications ISIEA 2009, vol. 2, pp. 836–841. IEEE (2009)
3. Lin, Y.-P., Wang, C.-H., Wu, T.-L., Jeng, S.-K., Chen, J.-H.: Support vector machine for EEG signal classification during listening to emotional music. In: 2008 IEEE 10th Workshop on Multimedia Signal Processing, pp. 127–130. IEEE (2008)
4. Croft, R., Barry, R.: Removal of ocular artifact from the EEG: a review. Clin. Neurophysiol. **30**, 5–19 (2000)
5. Mognon, A., Jovicich, J., Bruzzone, L., Buiatti, M.: Adjust: an automatic EEG artifact detector based on the joint use of spatial and temporal features. Psychophysiology **48**(2), 229–240 (2011)
6. Wang, S., Lin, C., Wu, C., Chaovalitwongse, W.: Early detection of numerical typing errors using data mining techniques. IEEE Trans. Syst. Man Cybern. Part A: Syst. Hum. **41**(6), 1199–1212 (2011)

7. Grimes, D., Tan, D., Hudson, S., Shenoy, P., Rao, R.: Feasibility and pragmatics of classifying working memory load with an electroencephalograph. In: Proceedings of the SIGCHI Conference on Human Factors in Computing Systems, vol. 08, pp. 835–844 (2008)

8. Olsen, D., Lesser, R., Harris, J., Webber, R., Cristion, J.: Automatic detection of seizures using electroencephalographic signals, U.S. Patent 5311876

9. Esteller, R., Echauz, J., Cheng, T., Litt, B., Pless, B.: An efficient feature for seizure onset detection. In: Proceedings of the 23rd International Conference of IEEE Engineering Medicine Biology Society, vol. 2, pp. 1707–1710 (2001)

10. Kaiser, J.: On a simple algorithm to calculate the energy of a signal. In: Proceedings of 1990 International Conference of Acoustis, Speech, Signal Processing, vol. 1, pp. 381–384 (1990)

11. Agarwal, R., Gotman, J.: Adaptive segmentation of electroencephalographic data using a nonlinear energy operator. In: Proceedings of 1999 IEEE International Symposium on Circuits and Systems, vol. 4, pp. 199–202 (1999)

12. Addison, N.: The illustrated wavelet transform handbook: introductory theory and applications in science, engineering, medicine, and finance, Taylor and Francis

13. Yuvaraj, R., Murugappan, M., Ibrahim, N.M., Omar, M.I., Sundaraj, K., Mohamad, K., Palaniappan, R., Mesquita, E., Satiyan, M.: On the analysis of EEG power, frequency and asymmetry in Parkinsons disease during emotion processing. Behav. Brain Func. **10**(1), 12 (2014)

14. Rosso, O., Martin, M., Figliola, A., Keller, K., Plastino, A.: EEG analysis using wavelet-based information tools. J. Neurosci. Methods **153**(2), 163–182 (2006)

15. Subasi, A.: EEG signal classification using wavelet feature extraction and a mixture of expert model. Expert Syst. Appl. **32**(4), 1084–1093 (2007)

16. Rosso, O., Blanco, S., Yordanova, J., Kolev, V., Figliola, A., Schourmann, M., Basar, E.: Wavelet entropy: a new tool for analysis of short duration brain electrical signals. J. Neurosci. Methods **105**(1), 65–75 (2001)

17. Blankertz, B., Curio, G., Muller, K.: Classifying single trial EEG: towards brain computer interfacing. Adv. Neural Inf. Process. Syst. **14**(2), 157–164 (2002)

18. Lal, T., Hinterberger, T., Widman, G., Schroer, M., Hill, J., Rosenstiel, W., Elger, C., Schokopf, B., Birbaumer, N.: Methods towards invasive human brain computer interfacess. In: Advances in Neural Information Processing Systems, vol. 17, pp. 737–744. MIT Press (2005)

19. Rakotomamonjy, A., Guigue, V., Mallet, G., Alvarado, V.: Ensemble of SVMs for improving brain computer interface P300 speller performances. In: Duch, W., Kacprzyk, J., Oja, E., Zadrożny, S. (eds.) ICANN 2005. LNCS, vol. 3696, pp. 45–50. Springer, Heidelberg (2005). doi:10.1007/11550822_8

20. Kaper, M., Meinicke, P., Grossekathoefer, U., Lingner, T., Ritter, H.: BCI competition 2003-data set IIb: support vector machines for the P300 speller paradigm. IEEE Trans. Biomed. Eng. **51**(6), 1073–1076 (2004)

21. Garrett, D., Peterson, D., Anderson, C., Thaut, M.: Comparison of linear, nonlinear, and feature selection methods for EEG signal classification. IEEE Trans. Neural Syst.Rehabil. Eng. **11**(2), 141–144 (2003)

22. Mangasarian, O., Wild, E.: Proximal support vector machine classifiers. In: Proceedings of Knowledge Discovery and Data Mining, pp. 77–86 (2001)

23. Stone, M.: Cross-validatory choice and assessment of statistical predictions. J. Roy. Stat. Soc.: Ser. B (Statistical Methodological) **36**(2), 111–147 (1974)

24. Peng, H., Long, F., Ding, C.: Feature selection based on mutual information criteria of max-dependency, max-relevance, and min-redundancy. IEEE Trans. Pattern Anal. Mach. Intell. **27**(8), 1226–1238 (2005)

# Thought Chart: Tracking Dynamic EEG Brain Connectivity with Unsupervised Manifold Learning

Mengqi Xing[1], Olusola Ajilore[2], Ouri E. Wolfson[3],
Christopher Abbott[4], Annmarie MacNamara[2], Reza Tadayonnejad[2],
Angus Forbes[3], K. Luan Phan[2], Heide Klumpp[2], and Alex Leow[1,2(✉)]

[1] Department of Bioengineering,
University of Illinois at Chicago, Chicago, IL, USA
mxing3@uic.edu
[2] Department of Psychiatry, University of Illinois at Chicago, Chicago, IL, USA
{oajilore, amacnamara, rtadayon,
klphan, hklumpp, aleow}@psych.uic.edu
[3] Department of Computer Science,
University of Illinois at Chicago, Chicago, IL, USA
{owolfson, aforbes}@uic.edu
[4] Department of Psychiatry, University of New Mexico, Albuquerque, USA
cabbott@salud.unm.edu

**Abstract.** Assuming that the topological space containing all possible brain states forms a very high-dimensional manifold, this paper proposes an unsupervised manifold learning framework to reconstruct and visualize this manifold using EEG brain connectivity data acquired from a group of healthy volunteers.

Once this manifold is constructed, the temporal sequence of an individual's EEG activities can then be represented as a trajectory or *thought chart* in this space. Our framework first applied *graph dissimilarity space embedding* to the temporal EEG connectomes of 20 healthy volunteers, both at rest and during an emotion regulation task (ERT), followed by local neighborhood reconstruction then nonlinear dimensionality reduction (NDR) in order to reconstruct and embed the learned manifold in a lower-dimensional Euclidean space. We showed that resting and ERT *thought charts* represent distinct trajectories, and that the manifold resembles dynamical systems on the torus. Additionally, new trajectories can be inserted on-line via out-of-sample embedding, thus providing a novel data-driven framework for classifying brain states, with potential applications in neurofeedback via real-time *thought chart* visualization.

**Keywords:** *Thought chart* · Graph dissimilarity embedding · Nonlinear dimensionality reduction · EEG connectome · Emotion regulation

## 1 Introduction

Inspired by the Nash embedding theorems [1, 2], which showed that any compact Riemannian *n*-manifold can be $C^1$ isometrically embedded in a Euclidean space of dimension $2n + 1$, and by *Theorema Egregium,* which showed that the *Gauss curvature*

© Springer International Publishing AG 2016
G.A. Ascoli et al. (Eds.): BIH 2016, LNAI 9919, pp. 149–157, 2016.
DOI: 10.1007/978-3-319-47103-7_15

of a 2-manifold embedded in 3D depends only on the *first fundamental form* and is thus invariant when it is bent without stretched or torn (i.e., complete isometric mappings preserve the Gauss curvature), the goal of this study is to understand the manifold properties or the *intrinsic geometry* of the mind's topological space. We develop this framework around the conjecture that, at least with non-invasive functional brain imaging, this manifold is smooth and differentiable (i.e., local neighborhoods are homeomorphic to a Euclidean space with the same number of dimensions). Our conjecture ultimately relies on the intuition that at least on a macroscopic spatiotemporal scale brain dynamics are continuous, or simply put do not abruptly "jump" from one state to the next. To test this hypothesis, we utilized resting-state and task EEG data from healthy participants performing an emotional regulation task. We hypothesized that the reconstructed manifold will reflect different properties of the brain's state at rest and during the performance of the task. Additionally, by sampling the space, we can extract specific aspects of the manifold that reflect task performance.

## 2    Methods

### 2.1    Subject Recruitment and Data Acquisition

EEG data were collected from 20 psychiatrically healthy participants (age: $27.2 \pm 9.3$) using the Biosemi system (Biosemi, Amsterdam, Netherlands) with an elastic cap with 34 scalp channels. Each participant underwent one recording session of an eight minute eye-open resting state and one separate session of Emotion Regulation Task (ERT). During ERT, participants were requested to look at pictures displayed on the screen, and listen to a corresponding auditory guide. Two types of pictures will be on display for seven seconds in random orders: emotionally neutral pictures (landscape, everyday objects, etc.) and negative pictures (car crash, nature disasters, etc.). The auditory guide will come after the picture on display for one second, instructing the participant to "*look*": viewing the neutral pictures; to "*maintain*": viewing the negative pictures as they normally would; or to "*reappraise*": viewing the negative pictures while attempting to reduce their emotion response by reinterpreting the meaning of pictures [3, 4]. EEG data were preprocessed using *Brain Vision Analyzer* (Brain Products, Gilching Germany), by first segmenting task trials into 7 s segments with a window size of 0.05 s (the first and last 5 time points were discarded, resulting in 130 time points per task; resting state data was similarly preprocessed). Frequencies-of-interest were set from 1 Hz to 50 Hz in increments of 1 Hz. The final output of each subject was averaged over trials within the same task (Fig. 1).

### 2.2    Weighted Phase Lag Index Based EEG Connectome

As functional communications between two brain regions result in synchronized or *phase-coupled* EEG readouts, in this study we used *weighted phase lag index* (WPLI) computed [5] between the times series of two channels to form EEG connectomes (each of which a symmetric 34 by 34 matrix). Mathematically, WPLI is defined as:

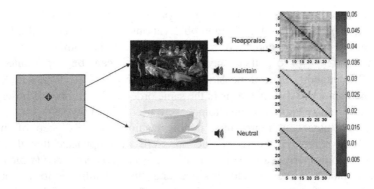

**Fig. 1.** An illustration of a typical ERT session. A fixation point is on display before each trial, then followed by either a neutral or negative picture on the screen. An audio instruction will ask test subjects to *maintain*, *reappraise* or stay *neutral*.

$$WPLI_{xy} = \frac{n^{-1} \sum_{t=1}^{n} |imag(S_{xyt})| sgn(imag(S_{xyt}))}{n^{-1} \sum_{t=1}^{n} |imag(S_{xyt})|} \tag{1}$$

Where *imag(Sxyt)* indicate the cross-spectral density at time t in the complex plane *xy*, and *sgn* is the *sign* function (−1, +1 or 0) [5]. The connectivity matrices were generated with the *MATLAB* toolbox *Fieldtrip* (Donders Centre for Cognitive Neuroimaging, Nijmegen, Netherlands). The final output time-dependent EEG connectome for an individual task of each subject is arranged as 34 * 34 * 50 * 130 (channel * channel * frequency * time). Given several lines of evidence suggesting the role of theta EEG (4–7 Hz) in emotion regulation [6, 7] and our recent graph analyses further demonstrating distinct theta wave changes during ERT, in this study we primarily focused on the manifold informed by theta wave EEG connectomes.

## 2.3 Learning the Manifold with Graph Dissimilarity Space Embedding and Nonlinear Dimensionality Reduction (NDR)

In order to learn the intrinsic geometry of a high-dimensional manifold, one needs a sufficiently large amount of data points. Thus, we treat the EEG connectomes from *all* subjects at *all* time points as sampling possible states of the manifold that is shared among all subjects. Then, graph *dissimilarity space embedding* is used to represent each connectome as a point in a very high-dimensional space (number of dimensions equal to the number of *prototype* graphs as described below). This is then followed by (1) *manifold learning* via local neighborhood reconstruction and (2) *manifold embedding* into a lower dimensional Euclidean space using *nonlinear dimensionality reduction* (NDR). Once this is achieved, *thought chart* of any given individual can be constructed by tracing the trajectory of the time-dependent connectome of that subject for any given task.

Next, we describe the graph *dissimilarity space embedding* procedure [8, 9]. Let $G = \{G_1, ..., G_n\}$ be $n$ "prototype" graph observations $G_i \in \mathbb{G}$ (the set of all possible graphs under consideration) and $d$ a distance metric that can be computed between two graphs $d : \mathbb{G} \times \mathbb{G} \rightarrow [0, \infty)$, then any graph $X \in \mathbb{G}$ can be represented using $\varphi_n^G : \mathbb{G} \rightarrow \mathbb{R}^n$, defined as the n-dimensional vector $\varphi_n^G(X) = [d(X, G_1), ... d(X, G_n)]$. Note here the number of dimensions is in the same order as the number of observations in the dataset (in this study all connectomes were used as prototypes).

Once connectomes are represented in this fashion, the next step of manifold learning is local neighborhood reconstruction. Here we emphasize that this step is crucial in order to properly learn the manifold's *intrinsic geometry*, as $d$ (which is used to define coordinates in the embedding space, and thus not intrinsic to the manifold) will not properly inform geodesics (the shortest paths on the manifold, which is an intrinsic property) except in local neighborhoods. While such a construction calls for a "good" choice of the distance function $d$, we posit that given a sufficiently large amount of data points the learned manifold will converge to the true manifold with any reasonably chosen $d$. Given two connectome matrices $X$ and $Y$ a natural choice, which we adopted here, is the *Euclidean* distance: $d(X, Y) = \sqrt{\sum_{ij} (X_{ij} - Y_{ij})^2}$ and $\varphi_n^G(X) - \varphi_n^G(Y) = \sqrt{\sum_i (d(X, G_i) - d(Y, G_i))^2}$.

Once local neighborhood is learned, the next step is to reduce the manifold that is currently in a very-high dimensional space (recall this dimension is the number of *prototype* graphs used, here in the order of $10^4$) and further embed it in a more manageable lower-dimensional space. Using the prototypical isometric embedding procedure *isomap* as an example, this step thus entails the computation of geodesics based on neighborhood information followed by (quasi-) isometric embedding of the geodesics.

Here, let us pause for a moment and point out the resemblance between *dissimilarity space embedding* and Frechet's classical isometric embedding argument, showing that any n-point $(x_1, ..., x_n)$ metric space can be isometrically embedded in $l_\infty^{n-1}$ [10, 11] by simply placing any point $x \in \{x_1, ..., x_n\}$ at the coordinates: $d(x, x_1), d(x, x_2), ... d(x, x_{n-1})$ where $d$ is the metric (interestingly, this result was later improved to $l_\infty^{n-2}$).

## 2.4    Out-of-Sample Embedding

Once this manifold is constructed, a series of dynamic connectomes acquired from a new subject can then be embedded on-line if we exploit *out-of-sample* extensions for NDR techniques [12]. Again using *isomap* as an example (in this case the procedure is called *landmark isomap* [13]) where pairwise geodesics need to be approximated using neighborhood information followed by *eigendecomposition* of the resulting squared distance matrix, this is particularly relevant as this step turns out to be the bottleneck of the algorithm. Using *out-of-sample* embedding will thus allow us to precompute and store the dimensionally-reduced manifold representation and the corresponding embedding, with which we can then perform online computation given new observations.

In brief, in the case of *isomap* the second step relies on applying the classic *multidimensional scaling* (MDS) to the centered squared geodesic distance matrix $\Delta_c = \frac{-1}{2} H_n \Delta_n H_n$, whose eigendecomposition provides the basis for lower dimensional embedding. Mathematically, it can be shown that the $n$ column vectors denoting coordinates for the $n$ landmark points in a lower $k$-dimensional space is simply given by truncating the following matrix at the $k$-th row:

$$L = \begin{pmatrix} \sqrt{\lambda_1} v_1^T \\ \vdots \\ \sqrt{\lambda_n} v_n^T \end{pmatrix} \tag{2}$$

Here the eigenvalues $\lambda_i$ are arranged from high to low, while $\Delta_n$ is the squared geodesic matrix of the landmark points and the centering matrix $H_n = I - \frac{1}{n} 11^T$.

Then the *out-of-sample* embedding of any new observation can be obtained by first forming the column vector $\delta = (\delta_1, \delta_2, \ldots \delta_n)^T$ that stores this new point's squared geodesic distances to all pre-embedded observations in the training dataset, followed by forming the "interpolated" embedded coordinates: $\frac{-1}{2} L_k^{\#} (\delta - \overline{\delta_n})$.

Here $\overline{\delta_n}$ is the mean of the n column vectors in $\Delta_n$ and $L_k^{\#}$ the pseudoinverse of truncated at the k-th row:

$$L_k^{\#} = \begin{pmatrix} v_1^T / \sqrt{\lambda_1} \\ \vdots \\ v_k^T / \sqrt{\lambda_k} \end{pmatrix} \tag{3}$$

# 3   Results

After averaging across theta frequencies (4–7 Hz) and combining both resting and ERT theta connectomes for all time points, 20 healthy subjects thus contributed a total of 10400 connectomes (130 * 20 * 4). Using the classic *isomap* (local neighborhood of each connectome operationally defined as its 30 nearest neighbors; the number of dimensions reduced from 10400 to 3), the reconstructed theta-EEG manifold exhibited a *principal* dimension that is shared by all 4 states (x-axis in Fig. 2; also see a front view of the manifold in Fig. 4) with a secondary small-amplitude rotation around it. Visually, this manifold thus resembles the shape of a snake by spiraling around its main axis. Moreover, the amplitude of the rotation follows an ordered transition: (from low- to high- amplitude) *resting* (red), *neutral* (green), *maintain* (purple) and *reappraise* (blue), corresponding to increasing cognitive load of the tasks. Insets of Fig. 2 further show the corresponding embedding using *locally linear embedding* (LLE [14]), which exhibits a similar rotation-along-main-axis shape (LLE is another prototype NDR technique that is however *non-isometric*), and the embedding generated using simple *PCA* (a linear technique) that does not recover the complex shape seen in either *isomap* or *LLE*.

Using out-of-sample embedding, the mean group *though chart* for *neutral, maintain* and *reappraise* (computed by averaging, for each time point, theta EEG

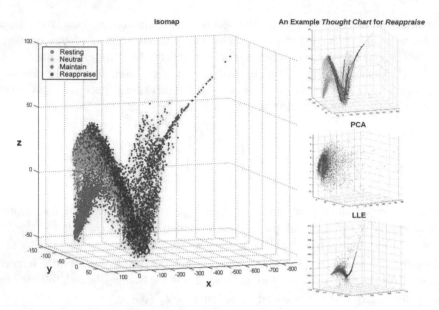

**Fig. 2.** An example *thought chart* during *reappraise* learned from the temporal EEG connectomes of 20 healthy subjects, both at rest and during ERT, using NDR methods of Isomap and LLE, as well as standard PCA. Visually, NDR methods yielded a rotation around the manifold's principal dimension (x-axis), with the amplitude of rotation following an ordered transition from *resting, neutral, maintain* to *reappraise.*

connectomes across all subjects for that task) can also be embedded and visualized (note while mathematically doable, it is inappropriate to compute mean resting *thought chart* as resting state is not stimuli-evoked). Interestingly, there exists a similar ordered antero-posterior transition from *neutral, maintain* to *reappraise*, indicating that the posterior section of the manifold (more negative along the x-axis) represents states that require higher cognitive demands (Fig. 3).

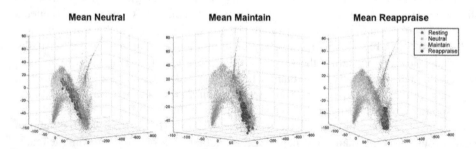

**Fig. 3.** Out-of-sample embedding of the mean group *thought chart* for *neutral, maintain,* and *reappraise* (note that we cannot time-average the resting-state *thought chart* across subjects). Similar to Fig. 2 there is an ordered antero-posterior transition from *neutral, maintain,* to *reappraise.*

To further understand theta-EEG connectome dynamics, we additionally studied the four distinct sub-regions of the manifold (i.e. segments of the "snake"): the *head* (primarily *resting*), the *mid body* (primarily *neutral*), the *posterior body* (a mixture of *neutral, maintain* and *reappraise*) and the *tail* (primarily *maintain* and *reappraise;* Fig. 4). Sampling these segments reveals marked connectome differences. Analysis of the top 10 edge strengths in the *head* region (Fig. 4a) demonstrated increased theta coupling in fronto-parieto-occipital leads while the *body (neutral*-predominant, Fig. 4b; *maintain/reappraise* dominant, Fig. 4c) is characterized with predominantly increased theta coupling between occipital leads. Last, the *tail* (*maintain/reappraise* only, Fig. 4d) revealed increased theta coupling between frontal and parietal leads. Thus, the manifold comprises subspaces representing resting, visual processing (common feature of *neutral, maintain* and *reappraise*) and cognitive control (distinct feature of *maintain* and *reappraise*). Edge strength analyses of the manifold-sampled EEG connectomes demonstrated increased patterns of theta coupling that are highly consistent with previous reports of frequency-band coupling associated with the resting-state [15], visual processing [16], and cognitive control [17].

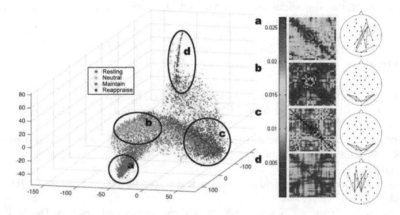

**Fig. 4.** Mean 34 * 34 theta EEG connectomes of four distinct segments of the *Neurospace*: the *head* (a), the *mid* and *posterior body* (b, c) and the *tail* (d) (left). For each mean connectome, its ten strongest edges were visualized on the layout of the electrodes (right).

## 4  Discussion and Conclusion

In this study we proposed a novel unsupervised manifold learning framework to construct a state space, in the form of a manifold embedded in 3D that quasi-isometrically visualizes EEG connectome dynamics. Moreover, in this space one can visualize time-dependent brain activities as a trajectory or *thought chart*. We applied this approach to a group of healthy controls, both at rest and during tasks, and showed that the reconstructed manifold exhibits a complex and highly structured geometry, with distinct sub-regions corresponding to different mental states. Our results suggested that the manifold has a principal dimension that is primarily linear, and a rotation around this principal dimension whose amplitude increases with cognitive demands.

In this context, this manifold resembles dynamical systems on the *torus* [18] (the surface of a doughnut), in that trajectories are generated by the product of two circles: the large torus circle corresponding to the principal dimension while the small or *minor* circle corresponding to the secondary rotation around it (and that cognitive demands change the ratio between the radii of the two circles).

Limitations of our approach merit further discussion. First, as a quasi-isometric technique *isomap* aims to preserve the pairwise geodesics on the manifold, i.e., approximating global isometry when the embedding is constrained to a given dimension. By contrast other classes of local NDR methods such as LLE unfold the manifold by preserving local linear reconstruction relationship (i.e., local parameterization) of each point within its neighborhood. Moreover, as the *Theorema Egregium* only guaranteed the invariance of Gauss curvature for complete isometric embeddings of 2-manifolds, it is unclear if the manifold constructed using one NDR technique is necessarily more "correct". Nevertheless, both *LLE* and *isomap* recover a principal dimension and a rotation around it, while simple linear techniques such as PCA did not. We thus posit that the highly structured complex geometry recovered using our framework may indeed inform the hidden properties of brain dynamics and the underlying neurophysiological mechanisms that generate them.

# References

1. Nash, J.: C1 isometric imbeddings. Ann. Math. **60**(3), 383–396 (1954)
2. Nash, J.: The imbedding problem for Riemannian mainfolds. Ann. Math. **63**(1), 44–64 (1956)
3. Parvaz, M.A., et al.: Event-related induced frontal alpha as a marker of lateral prefrontal cortex activation during cognitive reappraisal. Cogn. Affect. Behav. Neurosci. **4**(12), 730–741 (2012)
4. Gross, J.J.: The emerging field of emotion regulation: an integrative review. Rev. Gen. Psychol. **2**, 281–292 (1998)
5. Cohen, M.X.: Analyzing Neural Time Series Data: Theory and Practice. The MIT Press, Lodon (2013)
6. Knyazev, G.G., et al.: Anxiety and oscillatory responses to emotional facial expressions. Brain Res. **1227**, 88–174 (2008)
7. Balconia, M., Grippab, E., Vanutellia, M.E.: What hemodynamic (fNIRS), electrophysiological (EEG) and autonomic integrated measures can tell us about emotional processing. Brain Cogn. **95**, 67–77 (2015)
8. Bunke, H., Riesen, K.: Graph classification based on dissimilarity space embedding. In: da Vitoria Lobo, N., Kasparis, T., Roli, F., Kwok, J.T., Georgiopoulos, M., Anagnostopoulos, G.C., Loog, M. (eds.) SSPR & SPR 2008. LNCS, vol. 5342, pp. 996–1007. Springer, Heidelberg (2008)
9. Duin, R.P., Loog, M., Pękalska, E., Tax, D.M.: Feature-based dissimilarity space classification. In: Çataltepe, Z., Aksoy, S., Ünay, D. (eds.) ICPR 2010. LNCS, vol. 6388, pp. 46–55. Springer, Heidelberg (2010)
10. Benyamini, Y., Lindenstrauss, J.: Geometric Nonlinear Functional Analysis, vol. 1. American Mathematical Society Colloquium, Providence (2000)
11. Matousek, J.: Lectures on Discrete Geometry. Springer, New York (2012)

12. Bengio, Y., et al.: Out-of-sample extensions for LLE, Isomap, MDS, Eigenmaps, and spectral clustering. Adv. Neural Inf. Process. Syst. **16**, 177–184 (2003)
13. Silva, V., Tenenbaum J.B.: Sparse multidimensional scaling using landmark points. Technical report, Stanford Mathematics (2004)
14. Roweis, S., Saul, J.: Nonlinear dimensionality reduction by locally linear embedding. Science **290**(5500), 2323–2327 (2000)
15. Albrecht, M.A., et al.: The effects of dexamphetamine on the resting-state electroencephalogram and functional connectivity. Hum. Brain Mapp. **37**, 570–589 (2016)
16. Keil, A., et al.: Tagging cortical networks in emotion: a topographical analysis. Hum. Brain Mapp. **33**, 2920–2931 (2013)
17. Griesmayr, B., et al.: EEG theta phase coupling during executive control of visual working memory investigated in individuals with schizophrenia and in healthy controls. Cogn. Affect. Behav. Neurosci. **14**, 1340–1356 (2014)
18. Tozzi, A., Peters, J.F.: Towards a fourth spatial dimension of brain activity. Cogn. Neurodyn. **10**, 1–13 (2016)

# Brain Big Data Analytics, Curation and Management

# User Interests Analysis and Its Application on the Linked Brain Data Platform

Yi Zeng[1,2(✉)], Dongsheng Wang[1,2], and Hongyin Zhu[1,2]

[1] Institute of Automation, Chinese Academy of Sciences, Beijing, China
yi.zeng@ia.ac.cn
[2] Center for Excellence in Brain Science and Intelligence Technology,
Chinese Academy of Sciences, Shanghai, China

**Abstract.** User-centric academic resource service platforms are essential for scientific researchers, since hundreds of new literatures and data sets are produced every single day, and no one can keep him/herself most up-to-date and handle these resources to find, read and understand the most relevant ones completely manually. In this paper, we introduce some user interests analysis methods and apply them to build personalized recommendation services as a user-centric sub system for the Linked Brain Data (LBD) platform, which is an integrated data and knowledge platform for users, especially Neuroscientists and Artificial Intelligence researchers, to explore and better understand the brain and support their research. For interests analysis, we obtain user related data from relatively static data sources (e.g. user profiles maintained by uses), and more dynamic resources (e.g. publications and online social network contents generated by users, which are with chronological information). For recommendation service, we automatically recommend extracted knowledge in the brain association graph and related articles based on the understanding of research interests of the LBD platform users. Through use case studies, we illustrate the importance and potential value of user-centric services for brain and neuroscience related research.

**Keywords:** Linked Brain Data · Linked data · User interests analysis · Neuroinformatics · Brain knowledge base

## 1 Introduction

A great volume of scientific data and knowledge are produced every day, and many of them are publicly available on the Web to push forward the advancement of science. This phenomenon is especially true for neuroscience and brain research. On the one hand, how to integrate and synthesis the data and knowledge from various sources need to be investigated [1], on the other hand, how to help researchers to deal with the information overload and assist them to find the data and knowledge which are most relevant to their research is essential [2]. In our previous work, we proposed a framework for analyzing user interests and discussed potential applications in various

---

Yi Zeng and Dongsheng Wang contributed equally to the work and serve as co-first authors.

G.A. Ascoli et al. (Eds.): BIH 2016, LNAI 9919, pp. 161–172, 2016.
DOI: 10.1007/978-3-319-47103-7_16

domains [2, 3]. In this paper, we introduce and adapt the efforts to the Linked Brain Data platform to provide user centric services for Brain and Neuroscience researchers.

Linked Brain Data (LBD)[1] is a platform where worldwide data and knowledge are integrated, linked and analyzed for comprehensive understanding of the brain. It contains brain data from multiple scales, multiple species, and multiple sources and a reorganized by using a formal ontology. CAS Brain knowledge base, the core of LBD, is a large scale brain knowledge base based on automatic knowledge extraction and integration. The current knowledge sources include but not limited to PubMed, Allen Reference Atlas, Neuroscience Information Framework (NIF), NeuroLex, Neuromorpho.org project, and Wikipedia, etc. Although the data and knowledge in LBD has been digested in some way, user centric services are still essential so that it can assist the end users more efficiently.

For providing such academic services, user profiling is an important step. Resources that can be used to build the user profile are distributed in various sources and ways. User accession log is the most direct information for acquiring user interests. In addition, publications which are with chronological information are essential resource for obtaining users' research interests. On the LBD platform, users can also provide their profile information by filling in relevant tables. However, some users are not willing to do the manual work, especially keep the content up-to-date. In this case, for those how provide author names and affiliations, we use the PubMed data to collect all relevant articles for the users and analyze their research interests.

In this paper, we introduce two types of analysis methods based on (1) relatively static data sources such as profile information manually input by users, and the one based on (2) dynamic data sources such as publications and other user records associated with concrete temporal information. For the recommendation services based on user interests analysis, we do not recommend articles directly, instead, we associate knowledge triples in the association graph with user interests, and recommend relevant knowledge triples as well as related publications. In addition, the most recently updated contents in the association graph will be recommended.

In the case study, we first demonstrate the ranking results of interest terms with two different computation methods. Then we rank term combination based on the interests ranking results and output the contents in the association graph which are extracted from research articles. On one hand, the article recommendation is driven by term combinations, and on the other hand, the most related and most recently updated association graph can be recommended to users. Based on this study, user interests analysis is enabled on the Linked Brain Data platform to interact with the end users and provide them with user centric content services.

## 2  Related Works

This paper is about user analysis and application on the LBD platform, which was named as "Linked Neuron Data (LND)" in our previous works (The name was changed since the extension and coverage for the scope of the platform) [1]. LBD contains

---

[1] Linked Brain Data: http://www.linked-brain-data.org/.

millions of triples obtained from structured knowledge sources from various research organizations and through knowledge extractions and organizations based on unstructured sources (e.g. PubMed abstracts, books). All the integrated and extracted knowledge are expressed in RDF/OWL with hierarchical organizations. Links among different data sources are built up with the entity linking algorithm proposed in [4].

Since LBD is a fundamental platform that provides service for Brain and Neuroscience researchers. The user interests analysis and related user centric services are essential for the future of this platform. In our previous work [1], we propose a method to track the evolution process of user interests. A person may be interested in a topic for a period of time but may gradually lose this interest if it does not show up for a long time in user logs. Thus, interests can be assigned with different weights according to their appearance, and the weights may decay. In this paper, we adopt the method to analyze the research interests of Brain and Neuroscience researchers and provide user centric services based on our LDB platform.

User interests analysis is an essential topic. In [5], the authors analyze the browsing behavior to judge the interest degree and relationships. In [6], the authors track user's interest degree based on historical-domain ontology. User's access frequency, access breadth and the properties of concepts in the domain ontology are considered for the calculation of user interests.

## 3 User Interests Analysis

In this section we will discuss user interest analysis method in detail. In Sect. 3.1, we discuss what kinds of data sources from users we can collect and utilize, and introduce the method of linking users to PubMed articles. In Sect. 3.2, we depict two interest analysis methods and related algorithms. Finally, we demonstrate the association graph based recommendation mechanism in Sect. 3.3.

### 3.1 Data Sources Collection and User Mapping to PubMed

In order to recommend proper content to users, we need to accurately analyze the users' interests. We first list possible data sources where we can acquire from the users to analyze their interests, and they are shown in Table 1.

For registered users, they are asked to fill in their basic profile information in the registration form which can be considered as a static data source. In addition, the knowledge base and association graph on LBD is considered as static data sources since they contain neuroscience lexicons and hierarchical relationships among them. As for dynamic resources, publication information in PubMed is essential. It contains more

**Table 1.** Data sources that can be used to acquire user interests.

| Relatively static resources | Dynamic resources |
| --- | --- |
| Manually input user profiles | Publications |
| Knowledge base (including the association graph) | Social network data, click stream data and query logs |

than 20 million articles in the last 200 years. If a user has publications on PubMed, it is possible to map the user to PubMed publications and extract all relevant articles with publication time to build the user interests list. Users' social network data, click stream data, and query logs can reflect their interests chronologically. Therefore, static and dynamic resources are complementary to each other since they provide understandings of users from different perspectives. Hence, they are all very important for analyzing and modeling user interests.

ORCID[2] is an identifier that distinguishes every researcher by giving a persistent digital number. Researcher's ORCID identifier is unique and will not change when authors change their affiliations. In addition, the identifier distinguishes researchers who are with the same name. On the LBD platform, it is recommended for users to provide their ORCIDs, and if it is given, we can map them to PubMed in a direct way.

For people who do not provide their own ORCID, as a first try, we use direct name mapping algorithms to map the user to PubMed articles. One of our previous works for entity linking and disambiguation introduced in [4] has illustrated satisfactory results and is adopted by the LBD platform. In this way, we can extract and synthesis all the articles of the user from PubMed.

### 3.2    Interests Analysis and Value Assignment

LBD is a domain specific platform, so the interest terms or topics can be based on particular domain lexicons. The lexicons we utilize here are primarily on Brain and Neuroscience, and they are mainly integrated from NeuroLex and Allen Reference Atlas, Wikipedia, etc. The number of domain lexicons is listed in Table 2. It contains various cognitive functions, brain diseases and brain building blocks at multiple scales, which ranges from brain regions to neurotransmitters.

**Table 2.** The number of domain lexicons related to Brain and Neuroscience

| Lexicon | Brain diseases | Brain regions | Neurons | Neurotransmitters | Cognitive functions | Protein | Gene |
|---------|----------------|---------------|---------|-------------------|---------------------|---------|------|
| Number  | 422            | 2,999         | 774     | 363               | 108                 | 358     | 38,329 |

Given the lexicon of terms, we can extract users' interests from their interests related data sources. Based on our previous work [2], here we adopt two methods to do statistics and assign weight values for the extracted interest terms.

For the first one, we named it as the cumulative interest analysis method which mainly captures the frequency of the appeared interests in a certain time slot [2].

$$CI(t(i), n) = \sum_{j=1}^{n} y_{t(i),j} \tag{1}$$

---

[2] ORCID: Universal identifier for scientific researchers: http://orcid.org/.

As shown in Formula 1, Cumulative Interest(CI in short) is expressed as $CI(t(i),n)$, which is used for calculating the appearance times of a specific interest $t(i)$ within a certain time slot composed of $n$ time intervals. $N$ denotes the number of time intervals and $j$ indicates one specific time interval. $y_{t(i),j}$ indicates the number of appearance times for topic $t(i)$.

For the other, we named it as the Retained Interest (RI in short) analysis method, which emphasize on the dynamic characteristics of user interests [2]. This method is primarily inspired by research on human memory [7].

$$RI(t(i), n) = \sum\nolimits_{j=1}^{n} y_{t(i),j} \times AT_{t(i)}^{-b} \tag{2}$$

As shown in Formula 2, $T_{t(i)}$ is the duration of the topic $t(i)$ that a user is interested in. For every time interval $j$, the interest $t(i)$ appears $y_{t(i),j}$ times, and $y_{t(i),j} \times AT_{t(i)}^{-b}$ is the total retention of an interest contributed by the specific time interval. b is the decay factor. We use the parameters A = 0.855 and b = 1.295 which is validated to be practical for describing research interests in [2].

### 3.3 Association Graph Based Recommendation

Traditional recommendation is based on pure term matching techniques, which returns a ranked list of articles which contains specific keywords. However, there may be thousands of articles that share the same combination of keywords, which may need several pages to display, and thus may not provide a more comprehensive recommendation results. In the Linked Brain Data platform, we extract associations among various concepts in Neuroscience, and the research articles are organized under these extracted associations. Therefore, we recommend research articles through firstly linking interests terms to knowledge triples in the Association graph, then the PubMed articles which are organized by these association knowledge triples are presented. We firstly rank the keywords according to their weights, then we retrieve the term combinations that appeared in articles and are extracted for building the association graph. When a user is interested in one combination, he/she can click it and refer to the relevant articles.

The interactions between LBD and the end users are also reflected in the association graph, allowing the users to manually check whether the combination of the terms is related. Moreover, the construction process for the association graph is a real-time mining process from PubMed, which can be utilized to recommend the most recently updated association records to the users. Section 4 will provide a case study.

In short, we can summarize the recommendation architecture as shown in Fig 1. User information is extracted, and he/she is mapped with the ORCID or by mapping and disambiguation algorithm to PubMed. Then, a set of synthesized text is achieved and the interest term extraction and evaluation process could be conducted with two different analysis methods. After that, the value of research Interest pairs are calculated for each combination and ranked. Irrelevant combination terms are filtered out according to association graph which are linked to recommendation articles. Finally

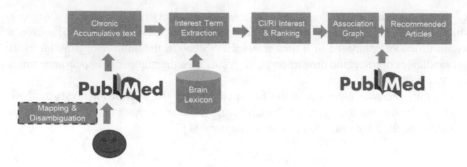

**Fig. 1.** The architecture of the LBD service recommendation based on user interests analysis.

PubMed article data were used again to support searching the relevant articles that are grouped by the association graph, the knowledge triples that are related to user interests and the relevant articles are recommended to users together.

## 4    A Case Study

In this section, we first bring up an overall evaluation of user satisfaction when using different recommendation methods, followed by demonstrating some interest analysis and recommendation results, and the difference of them when using different interest calculation methods. As the demonstrating case in Sects. 4.1 and 4.2, we use the data related to Henry Markram as an example.

### 4.1    CI Driven Recommendation Based on Association Graph

We firstly investigate cumulative interests based on Formula 1 and get the Top-11 *CI* interests. The result is shown in Table 3.

**Table 3.**  Top-11 interest terms ranked by interest values from CI perspective.

| Interest terms | CI |
|---|---|
| Neocortex | 38.0 |
| Interneuron | 17.0 |
| Receptors | 11.0 |
| Depression | 8.0 |
| Glutamate | 8.0 |
| Neurotransmitter | 7.0 |
| Aspartate | 7.0 |
| CA1 | 6.0 |
| Acetylcholine | 5.0 |
| Ion channels | 5.0 |
| P1 | 5.0 |

Subsequently, the Top-15 recommendations of knowledge triples in the association graph which are linked to PubMed articles are shown in Table 4.

**Table 4.** Top-15 knowledge triples in the association graph which are related to Henry Markram's cumulative interests

| Term1 | Term2 | Cumulative interest | Article number |
|---|---|---|---|
| Interneuron | Neocortex | 55 | 312 |
| Receptors | Neocortex | 49 | 173 |
| Glutamate | Neocortex | 46 | 183 |
| Depression | Neocortex | 46 | 120 |
| Aspartate | Neocortex | 45 | 84 |
| Neurotransmitter | Neocortex | 45 | 52 |
| CA1 | Neocortex | 44 | 82 |
| P1 | Neocortex | 43 | 23 |
| Ion_channels | Neocortex | 43 | 1 |
| Acetylcholine | Neocortex | 43 | 130 |
| Receptors | Interneuron | 28 | 145 |
| Depression | Interneuron | 25 | 192 |
| Glutamate | Interneuron | 25 | 535 |
| Aspartate | Interneuron | 24 | 103 |
| Neurotransmitter | Interneuron | 24 | 192 |

As shown in Table 4, two terms are correlated and their cumulative interest values are added together in the third column. In addition, the number of articles that are related to this combination is demonstrated in the fourth column. The first combination, for example, means Interneuron and Neocortex are correlated, which may be the combination that Henry Markram is most interested in, and for this combination, there are currently 312 articles in PubMed which he can refers to.

In order to validate the overall recommendation method, we conduct a survey on 18 neuroscience related researchers and students from Chinese Academy of Sciences (CAS). They are required to input their interests keywords and the system would return two lists of results based on two methods: originally keyword searching and CI driven recommendation. When they are asked how many results are they interested, 33.3 % of the results from original keyword search are preferred, and 65.0 % of the results from CI driven recommendations are preferred.

### 4.2   RI Driven Recommendation Based on Association Graph

We secondly investigate on the retained interest value based on Formula 2. The Top 11 interest terms are listed in Table 5.

Thus, we can list the two ranking results together in Table 6 to see whether they have some overlaps and whether the orders changed much.

**Table 5.** Top-11 interest terms ranked by *RI* interest value

| Interest | Retained interest |
|----------|-------------------|
| Neocortex | 2.581149 |
| TRPA1 | 1.203443 |
| Receptors | 1.039845 |
| Interneuron | 0.972932 |
| Insulin receptor | 0.855 |
| Insulin | 0.855 |
| P1 | 0.744833 |
| Ion channels | 0.423197 |
| GEM | 0.398128 |
| Glutamate | 0.37202 |
| TRPM8 | 0.348443 |

As shown in Table 6, many of the interests terms changed, only with "Neocortex" as the top one stay still. Many interests terms seem not as important as in the CI list when the time factor is involved. For example, the user showed fewer interests to "Glutamate" in the RI list compared to the CI list. Here a picture is generated to show the relationships among some shared interest terms from the two perspectives.

**Table 6.** Comparison between the two rank lists from the *CI* and *RI* perspectives.

| Sequence | CI | RI |
|----------|-----|-----|
| 1 | **Neocortex** | **Neocortex** |
| 2 | **Interneuron** | TRPA1 |
| 3 | **Receptors** | **Receptors** |
| 4 | Depression | **Interneuron** |
| 5 | **Glutamate** | Insulin receptor |
| 6 | Neurotransmitter | Insulin |
| 7 | Aspartate | **P1** |
| 8 | CA1 | **Ion channels** |
| 9 | **Acetylcholine** | GEM |
| 10 | **Ion channels** | **Glutamate** |
| 11 | **P1** | TRPM8 |

The *RI* values which locate in the bottom of Fig. 2, is ranked in a decreasing order and we can observe the CI sequence respectively. We can find that the overall trends are consistent but some ranking sequence of terms is changed. Take "Glutamate" as an example, from the cumulative interests perspective, it appears in Henry Markram's publications quite often, but most of them are from his previous publications years ago. Thus, it is ranked relatively lower in the RI ranking list.

Following the same way, we get Top-10 recommendations of association correlations from the perspectives of retained interests, as shown in Table 7.

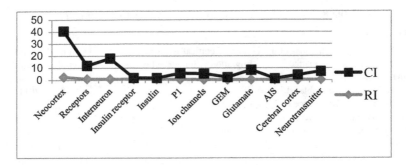

**Fig. 2.** The interest values with two different method, CI and RI, respectively.

**Table 7.** Top-10 knowledge triples in the association graph which are related to Henry Markram's retained interests

| Term1 | Term2 | RI value | Article number |
|---|---|---|---|
| Receptors | Neocortex | 3.6209946454949744 | 173 |
| Interneuron | Neocortex | 3.5540812104404536 | 312 |
| Insulin_receptor | Neocortex | 3.4361491902134427 | 1 |
| Insulin | Neocortex | 3.4361491902134427 | 2 |
| P1 | Neocortex | 3.325981717207573 | 23 |
| Ion_channels | Neocortex | 3.0043461558424096 | 1 |
| Glutamate | Neocortex | 2.97927724288924 | 183 |
| TRPM8 | Receptors | 2.929592612315565 | 28 |
| TRPA1 | Interneuron | 2.1763754423291335 | 1 |
| Receptors | Interneuron | 2.0127774755085426 | 145 |

If Henry Markram wants to check the articles related to the second associative relation (Interneuron Related To Neocortex), then he can click and open the articles (312 citations) as shown in the following:

As illustrated in Table 8, the first line gives the specific sentence in which the combination of interest terms appeared. The second column is the title of the paper, followed by the third column for the rest of the citation information. The link is available for users to click into the publication source on the LBD page.

As discussed in Table 1, social networks are also essential resources to extract researcher's most up-to-date interests, since they may share some articles or leave comments related to their field of research. Various social network data may support acquisition of these kinds of data. Here we investigate the contents users shared on LOOP[3], a social network for Neuroscience researchers. The results for user interests analysis from the perspectives of CI and RI based on LOOP short messages are provided in Table 9.

---

[3] The Loop academic social network: http://loop.frontiersin.org/.

**Table 8.** Recommended articles linked with association graph

| Related sentence | Title | Reference |
|---|---|---|
| In particular, we suggest that loss of a repellant signal from the medial **neocortex**, which is greatly decreased in size in hem-ablated mice, allows the early advance of **interneurons** and that reduction of another secreted molecule from C-R cells, the chemokine SDF-1/CXCL12, permits early radial migration into the CP | Timing of cortical interneuron migration is influenced by the cortical hem | Caronia-Brwon G, et al., Cerebral Cortex, 21 (4), 748-55, 2011 |
| The population of pyramidal cells significantly outnumbers the inhibitory **interneurons** in the **neocortex**, while at the same time the diversity of interneuron types is much more pronounced | A cortical attractor network with Martinotti cells driven by facilitating synapses | Krishnamurthy P, et al., PLoS ONE 7(4): e30752, 2012 |
| Modulation and function of the autaptic connections of layer V fast spiking **interneurons** in the rat **neocortex** | Modulation and function of the autaptic connections of layer V fast spiking interneurons in the rat neocortex | Connelly WM. et al. Journal of physiology, 588, 2047-63, 2010 |
| These principles suggest that inhibitory synapses could shape the impact of different **interneurons** according to their specific spatiotemporal patterns of activity and that GABAergic interneuron and synapse diversity may enable combinatorial inhibitory effects in the **neocortex** | Organizing principles for a diversity of GABAergic interneurons and synapses in the neocortex | Gupta A. et al. Science,287, 273-8, 2000 |

......

**Table 9.** Henry Markram's Top-15 research interests from CI and RI perspectives based on social network data from LOOP

| Interest terms | CI value | Interest term | RI value |
|---|---|---|---|
| Brain | 11 | Health | 0.245306884 |
| Neuroscience | 5 | Brain | 0.233092804 |
| Health | 3 | Bioinformatics | 0.20610764 |
| Brain disease | 1 | DNA | 0.20610764 |
| Cell | 1 | Gene | 0.20610764 |
| Gene | 1 | Neuroscience | 0.205444044 |
| Alzheimer's disease | 1 | Disorders | 0.083996317 |
| Membrane | 1 | Membrane | 0.083996317 |
| Disorders | 1 | Clinical data | 0.015614524 |
| DNA | 1 | Dementia | 0.015614524 |
| Bioinformatics | 1 | Alzheimer's disease | 0.015614524 |
| Dementia | 1 | Brain disease | 0.015614524 |
| Clinical data | 1 | Neocortical Structure | 0.014741055 |
| Neocortex | 1 | Neocortex | 0.014741055 |
| Neocortical structure | 1 | Cell | 0.013950589 |

Compared to the results based on publications (as shown in Table 6), the extracted research interests from LOOP is comparatively broader, while research interests from publications are relatively more concrete and specific. In addition, the list of Top-N research interests from different resources complement with each other, and they collectively provide a more comprehensive view for understanding of researcher's interests.

## 5   Conclusion and Future Work

Analyzing the users and providing them with customized service are significant for LBD. We first introduce the interest analysis method based on (1) static material such as user profile and existing knowledge base, and the one based on (2) dynamic materials such as publications and user records with the consideration of interest evolving with time. Through a case study, we illustrate its application and recommendation results with different ranking methods. The case study demonstrates that user interest analysis can enable LBD to interact with the users dynamically with association graph and to recommend relative articles the author is most likely concerned with.

In the future, we will consider the hierarchical relationship between terms when analyzing user interests [8]. For example, CA1 and hippocampus are two terms that are calculated separately for their weights, while CA1 is actually part of Hippocampus. Hence, the appearing times of CA1 can be added to Hippocampus. We will consider this situation in our future works to have more accurate interests analysis.

**Acknowledgement.** This study was funded by the Strategic Priority Research Program of the Chinese Academy of Sciences (XDB02060007), and Beijing Municipal Commission of Science and Technology (Z151100000915070, Z161100000216124).

## References

1. Zeng, Y., Wang, D.S., Zhang, T.L, Xu, B.: Linked neuron data (lnd): a platform for integrating and semantically linking neuroscience data and knowledge. In: Frontiers of Neuroinformatics. Conference Abstract: The 7th Neuroinformatics Congress (2014)
2. Zeng, Y., Zhou, E.Z., Wang, Y., Ren, X., Qin, Y.L., Huang, Z.S., Zhong, N.: Research interests: their dynamics, structures and applications in unifying search and reasoning. J. Intell. Inf. Syst. **37**(1), 65–88 (2011)
3. Zeng, Y., Hao, H.W., Zhong, N., Ren, X., Wang, Y.: Ranking and combining social network data for web personalization. In: Proceedings of the International Workshop on Data-driven User Behavioral Modelling and Mining from Social Media, Co-located with the 21st ACM International Conference on Information and Knowledge Management, pp. 15–18 (2012)
4. Zeng, Y., Wang, D.S., Zhang, T.L., Wang, H., Hao, H.W.: Linking entities in short texts based on a Chinese semantic knowledge base. Commun. Comput. Inf. Sci. **400**, 266–276 (2013)

5. Li, J.T., Ye, G., Tang, Z.J.: User interest degree calculating based on analysis users' browsing behaviors. Comput. Eng. Des. **33**(3), 968–972 (2012)
6. Ye, J.M., Chen, J.R., Zhang, X., Wang, L.: Interest degree calculation based on modified SPBN model. Int. J. Adv. Comput. Technol. **4**(19), 115–121 (2012)
7. Anderson, J.R., Schooler, L.J.: Reflections of the environment in memory. Psychol. Sci. **2**(6), 396–408 (1991)
8. Ma, Y., Zeng, Y., Ren, X., Zhong, N.: User interests modeling based on multi-source personal information fusion and semantic reasoning. In: Callaghan, V., Ghorbani, A.A., Hu, B., Zhong, N. (eds.) AMT 2011. LNCS, vol. 6890, pp. 195–205. Springer, Heidelberg (2011)

# Content-Based fMRI Brain Maps Retrieval

Alba G. Seco de Herrera$^{(\boxtimes)}$, L. Rodney Long, and Sameer Antani

Lister Hill National Center for Biomedical Communications,
National Library of Medicine, Bethesda, USA
{albagarcia,l.long,sameer.antani}@nih.gov
https://lhncbc.nlm.nih.gov

**Abstract.** The statistical analysis of functional magnetic resonance
imaging (fMRI) is used to extract functional data of cerebral activation
during a given experimental task. It allows for assessing changes in cerebral function related to cerebral activities. This methodology has been
widely used and a few initiatives aim to develop shared data resources.
Searching these data resources for a specific research goal remains a
challenging problem. In particular, work is needed to create a global
content–based (CB) fMRI retrieval capability.

This work presents a CB fMRI retrieval approach based on the brain
activation maps extracted using Probabilistic Independent Component
Analysis (PICA). We obtained promising results on data from a variety
of experiments which highlight the potential of the system as a tool that
provides support for finding hidden similarities between brain activation
maps.

**Keywords:** fMRI retrieval · PICA · Brain activation map

## 1 Introduction

Functional Magnetic Resonance Imaging (fMRI) is a powerful tool used in the
study of brain function. It can non-invasively detect signal changes in areas of the
brain where neuronal activity is varying [19]. Following each stimulus the scanner
generates a time-series of 3-D volumetric data, where each voxel represents the
time course of the Blood Oxygen Level Dependent (BOLD) response at that
voxel. Subsequent statistical processing generates additional 3-D brain maps, in
which each voxel represents the probability that a statistically significant change
in BOLD response occurred between a stimulus and corresponding control [16].
In order to obtain the statistical brain maps, the General Linear Model (GLM)
has been extensively used [15]. However, Probabilistic Independent Component
Analysis (PICA), a variant of the traditional Independent Component Analysis
(ICA) is becoming more popular for fMRI data analysis [1]. In this work PICA
components are used as the retrieval unit.

Data sharing is becoming increasingly common, but despite encouragement
and facilitation by some research efforts most neuroimaging data acquired today
is still not shared due to political, financial, social, and technical barriers [10].

© Springer International Publishing AG 2016
G.A. Ascoli et al. (Eds.): BIH 2016, LNAI 9919, pp. 173–180, 2016.
DOI: 10.1007/978-3-319-47103-7_17

Some efforts have been made to develop fMRI repositories. However, a global content-based (CB) fMRI retrieval capability is still lacking. Such a capability would allow a researcher to retrieve studies relevant to a specified study or interest.

Most of the work carried out addresses the problem of the classification of brain images. Some researchers try to detect activation volumes in the same brain image sequence [13,14], while others try to distinguish experiments with different cognitive tasks [9]. In these studies, machine learning (ML) methods (k-nearest neighbors  [14], Bayesian [14], Support Vector Machines (SVM) [13,14] and Fishers Discriminant Analysis [9] are applied to the time series of voxels [13, 14], or results from additional processing, such as t-maps [9] generated by the General Linear Model (GLM). All ML methods characterize the distribution of some set of features for labeled training datasets, and use these characteristics to classify other datasets.

Some work has been done on CB fMRI retrieval [3,5,20]. Laconte [13] assumes a priori knowledge exists in the temporal characteristics of the data. Bai [2] applied several similarity measures to retrieve the brain maps calculated using PICA. Shapiro et al. [16] retrieve fMRI signals based on prior matching of the raw signal data to eight signal templates. In 2013, Tungaraza et al. [18] proposed a method for retrieving similar fMRI statistical images given a query fMRI statistical image. The method thresholds the voxels within those images and extracts spatially distinct regions from the voxels that remain. Each region is defined by a feature vector containing several geometrical values. The similarity between two images is obtained by the summed minimum distance (SMD) of their constituent feature vectors.

A new method for CB fMRI brain maps retrieval is proposed in this work.

The remainder of the paper is organized as follows. Section 2 presents the techniques proposed in this paper as well as the database used to evaluate them. The experiments that we carried out are presented in Sect. 3. Finally, a discussion and the conclusions are given in Sect. 4.

## 2   Methods

This section describes the techniques developed to create a CB fMRI retrieval system. A description of the dataset and framework used to evaluate the proposed system is also given.

### 2.1   Dataset

In this paper the data and evaluation scenario provided by Bai et al. [4] are used. The data used is obtained from 359 subjects during 8 experiments. However, the number of subjects per experiment is not uniformly distributed. From each subject 10 PICA components are used, as provided by Bai et al. [4]. PICA components were calculated using FLS[1] library Each PICA component is a complete brain map (with dimension $91 \times 109 \times 91$) where each voxel has an associated statistical $z$-value which indicates the level of activation. Table 1 shows the distribution of the number of subjects participating in each experiment. The experiments consist of fMRI brain activity comparisons during various tasks. Brain activity of each subject was recorded for each separate experiment (i.e. for each task). A variety of tasks are covered in the various experiments, such as watching films, using moral dilemmas as probes or doing basic memory exercises.

**Table 1.** Number of subject per experiment.

| Experiment | N. subjects |
|---|---|
| Oddball-visual | 4 |
| Oddball-auditory | 4 |
| Event perception–House Active | 27 |
| Event perception–Study Active | 25 |
| Morality | 248 |
| Study-Recall | 27 |
| Recall-Only | 9 |
| Romantic | 15 |
| Total | 359 |

## 2.2 Techniques

This section describes the basic techniques that we used in in this study. Figure 1 puts together all the basic components in our retrieval system.

We used brain map extracted with PICA as the retrieval unit. Bai et al. [4] used a whole-brain voxel–wise strategy as a brain map descriptor. That method is computationally expensive, sensitive to noise and difficult to interpret [8]. Instead, we present two alternative descriptors: a map layout descriptor (MLD) and a whole–brain ROIs–wise descriptor.

*MLD* is similar to the Color Layout Descriptor [12] commonly used in 2D CB image retrieval (CBIR). It is designed to capture the spatial distribution of intensity in a volume. The feature extraction process consists of a grid based representative intensity selection.

*Whole–Brain Region of Interest (ROI)–Wise* – combines voxels into functionality distinct ROIs. The human brain atlas provided by Craddock et al. [8] (see Fig. 2) is used in this paper because it is functionally homogeneous, spatially

---

[1] http://fsl.fmrib.ox.ac.uk/fsl/f.

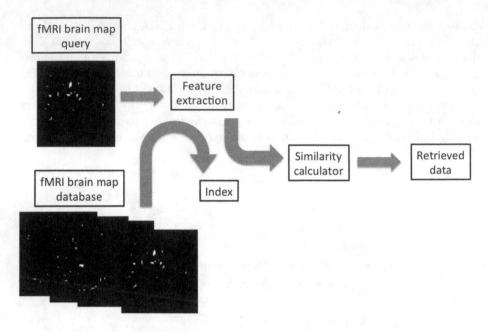

**Fig. 1.** Outline of the basic elements of the retrieval system.

contiguous, and it represent the functional connectivity (FC) patterns of the brain. The feature extraction process comprises the following process. For each brain map $B_i, i = 1, \ldots, n$, there is a set of MNI coordinates[2] $C = \{c_1, \ldots, c_m\}$, where $m$ is the number of voxels in each brain map, (if they are not MNI coordinates they are converted to MNI). Each coordinate contains the $z$-values from the PICA component. The histogram $\mathbf{h} \in \mathbb{B}^{200}$ is defined as:

$$\mathbf{h_k} = \begin{cases} 1 \text{ if } \exists c_j \subset R_k \\ 0 \text{ otherwise} \end{cases} \quad (1)$$

where $R_k$ is the k-th Craddock ROI, $\forall k, k = 1, \ldots 200$. If the MNI coordinates $c_j$ lie outside the brain but they are within 5 voxels of Craddock ROI $R_k$, then $\mathbf{h_k} = \mathbf{1}$.

These descriptors allow the extraction of the main features of the fMRI brain activation maps.

In this work, two measures are tested for the similarity comparison for each of the descriptors: histogram intersection (HI) [17] and Euclidean distance. For each subject only the nearest PICA component is considered. CombSum is the fusion strategy applied to combine results of each of the descriptors of the same fMRI brain activation map. See [11] for more details on the chosen fusion strategies.

---

[2] The Montreal Neurological Institute (MNI) defined a standard brain, which is representative of the population, by using a large series of MRI scans on normal controls.

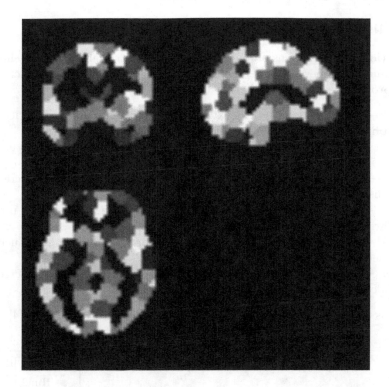

**Fig. 2.** Atlas provided by Craddock et al. consisting on 200 ROIs.

## 2.3 Evaluation

The main objective of this work is to evaluate the effectiveness of the techniques discussed in Sect. 2 for fMRI brain activation map retrieval based on PICA components. Therefore, the evaluation scenario used in this work is reused from Bai et al. [4] for comparison. The scenario considers a retrieved brain map relevant to a query if they both belong to the same experiment. This assumption is actually too strict and not totally accurate because there can be hidden similarities among different experiments. Despite the limitations of the evaluation framework, it provides a basic scenario to compare the proposed approaches with the state-of-the-art.

Each brain map in the dataset (see Sect. 2.1) is used as a query. Every brain map belonging to the same subject as the query is excluded. The area under the ROC curve is calculated for every experiment. Results are compared with the best run proposed by Bai et al. [4].

## 3    Experimental Results

This section details the runs produced for fMRI CB retrieval using the techniques and evaluation framework presented in Sect. 2. The characteristics of each of the 6 runs proposed are presented below:

- *Run1* – the MLD descriptor is extracted and HI is used for similarity comparison;
- *Run2* – the whole–brain ROIs–wise descriptor is extracted and HI is used for similarity comparison;
- *Run3* – the MLD and whole–brain ROIs–wise descriptors are extracted and HI is used for similarity comparison.
- *Run4* – the MLD descriptor is extracted and Euclidean distance is used for similarity comparison;
- *Run5* – the whole–brain ROIs–wise descriptor is extracted and Euclidean distance is used for similarity comparison;
- *Run6* – the MLD and whole–brain ROIs–wise descriptors are extracted and Euclidean distance is used for similarity comparison.

This runs are also compared with the best run proposed by Bai et al. [4].

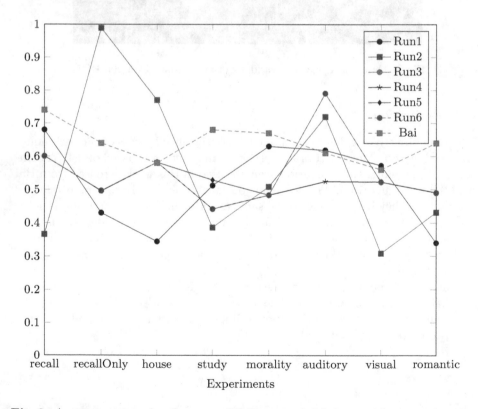

**Fig. 3.** Average area under the curve ROC per each of the experiments using the various runs and compared with the baseline proposed by Bai et al.

Table 2. Average area under the curve ROC.

| | Recall | RecallOnly | House | Study | Morality | Auditory | Visual | Romantic |
|---|---|---|---|---|---|---|---|---|
| *Run1* | 0.68 | 0.43 | 0.34 | 0.51 | 0.63 | 0.62 | 0.57 | 0.34 |
| *Run2* | 0.37 | 0.99 | 0.77 | 0.39 | 0.51 | 0.72 | 0.31 | 0.43 |
| *Run3* | 0.6 | 0.5 | 0.58 | 0.44 | 0.48 | 0.79 | 0.52 | 0.49 |
| *Run4* | 0.6 | 0.5 | 0.58 | 0.44 | 0.48 | 0.52 | 0.52 | 0.49 |
| *Run5* | 0.6 | 0.5 | 0.58 | 0.53 | 0.48 | 0.79 | 0.52 | 0.49 |
| *Run6* | 0.6 | 0.5 | 0.58 | 0.44 | 0.48 | 0.79 | 0.52 | 0.49 |
| Bai | 0.74 | 0.64 | 0.58 | 0.68 | 0.67 | 0.61 | 0.56 | 0.64 |

Figure 3 shows the average area under the ROC curve for each experiment. A more detailed view of the results can be found in Table 2. Results show that there is a big difference between experiments probably due to the uneven distribution of subjects between experiments. However, the use of the proposed descriptors achieved results comparable with the previous work of Bai et al. [4].

## 4 Conclusions

This article describes the methods and results applied to a novel method for fMRI brain activation map retrieval process. This is an area of research which has not been extensively explored. We propose two new descriptors to represent fMRI brain activation maps and simplify the retrieval of relevant cases.

Experimental data provided by Bai et al. [4] is used for the evaluation of the techniques. We note that it is difficult to assess when a fMRI brain activation map is relevant for a given query and plan to explore additional methods, such as the combination of human judgments with statistical methods [6,7]. Despite this limitation, the framework provides a basic approach to compare alternative feature descriptors and similarity measures with the limited state-of-the-art available in this field.

The results are promising but there is a big difference between experiments. Future work will expand the experimental data set and incorporate better fusion of several descriptors to help the retrieval. Further investigation on applications of CB fMRI brain activation retrieval will also be carried out.

**Acknowledgments.** This research was supported by the Intramural Research Program of the National Institutes of Health (NIH), National Library of Medicine (NLM), and Lister Hill National Center for Biomedical Communications (LIINCBC). Thanks to Dr. Bing Bai and Prof. Paul Kantor for providing us the fMRI experimental data.

## References

1. Ao, J.: An optimized statistical analysis of fMRI data using independent component analysis. Ph.D. thesis, Texas Tech University (2010)

2. Bai, B.: Feature extraction and matching in content-based retrieval of functional magnetic resonance images. Ph.D. thesis, The State University of New Jersey (2007)
3. Bai, B., Kantor, P., Cornea, N., Silver, D.: IR principles for content-based indexing and retrieval of functional brain images. In: Proceedings of 15th ACM International Conference on Information and Knowledge Management, pp. 828–829. ACM (2006)
4. Bai, B., Kantor, P., Shokoufandeh, A., Silver, D.: fMRI brain image retrieval based on ICA components. In: Conference on Current Trends in Computer Sciencel, pp. 10–17. IEEE (2007)
5. Bai, B., Kantor, P.B., Cornea, N.D., Silver, D.: Toward content-based indexing and retrieval of functional brain images. In: RIAO (2007)
6. van den Broek, E.L., Kisters, P.M., Vuurpijl, L.G.: The utilization of human color categorization for conten-based image retrieval. In: Proceedings of SPIE, Human Vision and Electronic Imaging IX, pp. 351–362 (2004)
7. van den Broek, E.L., Kisters, P.M., Vuurpijl, L.G.: Content-based Image retrieval benchmarking: utilizing color categories and color distributions. J. Imaging Sci. Technol. **49**, 293–301 (2005)
8. Craddock, R.C., James, G.A., Holtzheimer, P.E., Hu, X.P., Mayberg, H.S.: A whole brain fMRI atlas generated via spatially constrained spectral clustering. Hum. Brain Mapp. **33**(8), 1914–1928 (2012)
9. Ford, J., Farid, H., Makedon, F., Flashman, L.A., McAllister, T.W., Megalooikonomou, V., Saykin, A.J.: Patient classification of fMRI activation maps. In: Ellis, R.E., Peters, T.M. (eds.) MICCAI 2003. LNCS, vol. 2879, pp. 58–65. Springer, Heidelberg (2003). doi:10.1007/978-3-540-39903-2_8
10. Haselgrove, C., Poline, J.B., Kennedy, D.N.: A simple tool for neuroimaging data sharing. Front. Neuroinformatics **8**, 82 (2014)
11. García Seco de Herrera, A., Schaer, R., Markonis, D., Müller, H.: Comparing fusion techniques for the ImageCLEF 2013 medical case retrieval task. Comput. Med. Imaging Graph. **39**, 46–54 (2015)
12. Kasutani, E., Yamada, A.: The MPEG-7 color layout descriptor: a compact image feature description for high-speed image/video segment retrieval. In: Proceedings of International Conference on Image Processing, ICIP 2001, pp. 674–677 (2001)
13. LaConte, S., Strother, S., Cherkassky, V., Anderson, J., Hu, X.: Support vector machines for temporal classification of block design fMRI data. NeuroImage **26**(2), 317–329 (2005)
14. Mitchell, T.M., Hutchinson, R., Niculescu, R.S., Pereira, F., Wang, X., Just, M., Newman, S.: Learning to decode cognitive states from brain images. Mach. Learn. **57**(1–2), 145–175 (2004)
15. Poline, J.B., Brett, M.: The general linear model and fMRI: does love last forever? Neuroimage **62**(2), 871–880 (2012)
16. Shapiro, L.G., Atmosukarto, I., Cho, H., Lin, H.J., Ruiz-Correa, S., Yuen, J.: Similarity-based retrieval for biomedical applications. In: Perner, P. (ed.) Case-Based Reasoning on Images and Signals. SCI, vol. 73, pp. 355–387. Springer, Berlin (2008)
17. Swain, M.J., Ballard, D.H.: Color indexing. Int. J. Comput. Vis. **7**(1), 11–32 (1991)
18. Tungaraza, R., Guan, J., Shapiro, L., Brinkley, J., Ojemann, J., Franklin, J.: A similarity retrieval tool for functional magnetic resonance imaging statistical maps. Int. J. Biomed. Data Min. **2**, 1–12 (2013)
19. Woolrich, M.W., Beckmann, C.F., Nichols, T.E., Smith, S.M.: Statistical analysis of fMRI data. In: Filippi, M. (ed.) fMRI Techniques and Protocols. Neuromethods, vol. 41, pp. 179–236. Springer, Berlin (2009)
20. Zhang, J., Megalooikonomou, V.: An effective and efficient technique for searching for similar brain activation patterns. In: 2007 4th IEEE International Symposium on Biomedical Imaging: From Nano to Macro, ISBI 2007, pp. 428–431. IEEE (2007)

# A Domain-Driven Literature Retrieval Method for Systematic Brain Informatics

Wenjin Sheng[1,2,4](✉), Hongxia Xu[1,2,4], Jianzhuo Yan[1,2,4], Jianhui Chen[3,4,5], Bin Shi[1,4], Dongsheng Wang[3,4,6], Hongzhi Kuai[1,2,4], and Ningning Wang[3,4]

[1] Beijing Advanced Innovation Center for Future Internet Technology,
Beijing University of Technology, Beijing 100124, China
{932767262,kuaihongzhi}@emails.bjut.edu.cn,
{xhxccl,yanjianzhuo}@bjut.edu.cn, shiyuquan@163.com
[2] College of Electronic Information and Control Engineering,
Beijing University of Technology, Beijing 100024, China
[3] International WIC Institute, Beijing University of Technology,
Beijing 100024, China
{chenjianhui,dswang}@bjut.edu.cn, wangningning@emails.bjut.edu.cn
[4] Beijing Key Laboratory of MRI and Brain Informatics, Beijing, China
[5] Beijing International Collaboration Base on Brain Informatics and Wisdom
Services, Beijing, China
[6] School of Computer Science and Engineering, Institute of Intelligent Transport
System, Jiangsu University of Science of Technology, Zhenjiang 212003, China

**Abstract.** Systematic brain informatics (BI) research depends on a large amount of prior knowledge and scientific literatures are a kind of important knowledge source. However, the increasing number of scientific literatures has led to information overload. For researchers, it is difficult to find appropriate literatures. Developing literature retrieval technologies and systems becomes an important issue during systematic BI researches. However, most of existing literature retrieval technologies optimize query conditions only based on user interests and cannot effectively reflect domain interests. This paper proposes a domain-driven literature retrieval method which adopts the spread activation model to combine the dynamic and static domain models for ranking query results. The proposed method has been applied to the PubMed dataset. The experiment results show the efficiency of our method for retrieving literatures about brain informatics.

## 1 Introduction

Brain informatics (BI) [1] is an emerging interdisciplinary and multidisciplinary research field that combining cognitive neuroscience with advanced information processing technologies [2]. Aiming at complex thinking-centric researches, BI adopts a systematic methodology which depends on a large amount of prior knowledge obtained from existing similar experimental and analytical researches. Scientific literatures are a kind of important prior knowledge sources. Therefore,

G.A. Ascoli et al. (Eds.): BIH 2016, LNAI 9919, pp. 181–189, 2016.
DOI: 10.1007/978-3-319-47103-7_18

it is important for BI researchers to find related literatures from scientific literature databases and obtain necessary prior knowledge about experiments and analyses. In recent years, the number of literatures has been increased rapidly. According to the statistical data of literatures released by the public biomedical literature dataset PubMed, from 2012 to 2014, researchers had published about 3314256 literatures, while the number in 2014 was 4.2 % higher than in 2013. And it is predictable that the growth trend won't change in the short term. On the one hand, users can fully enjoy the convenience that all needed information can be obtained from massive literatures. On the other hand, it is difficult for users to obtain the information they really need quickly and accurately from such massive literatures. For example, when we want to retrieve literatures about "depression" from PubMed, 347316 results can be obtained. It will be time-consuming to find the needed literatures from these results.

Information retrieval [3] is a process to organize information in a certain way and find information users need. Knowledge Retrieval [7] emphasizes the search object is knowledge, specially the semantics-based content structure and it is a special case of information retrieval. In recent years, it mainly focuses on ontology based application. Literature retrieval is an important branch of information retrieval. It provides an effectively approach to find the needed literatures from massive query results, for quickly searching previous experience and achievements and timely grasping the latest developing trend in BI related field. In this paper, we propose a domain-driven literature retrieval method for brain informatics. It combines dynamic domain interests with static domain interests by using the spread activation model.

The rest of this paper is organized as follows. Section 2 discusses background and related work. Section 3 illustrates the details of the proposed method. Experiments are presented in Sect. 4. Finally, Sect. 5 gives conclusion and future work.

## 2    Background and Related Work

### 2.1    The Data-Brain

Brain informatics attempts at a long-tem, comprehensive perspective to understand the principles, models and mechanisms of human information processing systems [2]. Aiming to complex brain science problems, BI adopts a systematic methodology, including four core issues: a systematic investigation of human thinking centric mechanisms, systematic design of cognitive experiments, systematic human brain data management and systematic human brain data analysis and simulation. Such a systematic methodology proposes a standardization idea to solve complex problems.

In order to support systematic BI studies, BI needs a Data-Brain to integrate key data, information, and knowledge for various data requests of systematic BI studies. The Data-Brain is a domain-driven conceptual model of brain data, which represents multi-aspect relationships among multiple human brain data sources, with respect to all major aspects and capabilities of human information processing system (HIPS), for systematic investigation and understanding of human intelligence. It is divided into four dimensions, including the function dimension, experiment dimension, data dimension and analysis dimension, which corresponds to four aspects of systematic methodology. By using the domain-driven modeling method [4], the Data-Brain models static domain interests of BI researches. This paper focuses on Brain informatics. Hence, we use the Data-Brain as the static domain model.

## 2.2   Literature Retrieval

Literature retrieval is the process of acquiring literatures according to the need of studies and work. Many literature retrieval methods have been developed. For examples, Jimenez-Castellanos et al. [5] developed a method to enhance scientific literature searches from various sources, by including patient information in the retrieval process. Sondhi et al. [6] worked on finding relevant full-text articles from literatures in response to a medical case query submitted by a healthcare professional. However, most of these methods adopt user interests to optimize query conditions. The limitation of users' knowledge and experience makes it difficult to excavate domain interests by using these literature retrieval methods.

Ontology is an explicit specification of conceptualization and it is a body of knowledge describing some domain, typically common sense knowledge domain. It defines concepts and relations from different levels of formal models for machine understanding and reasoning. As domain ontology can capture useful prior knowledge in a domain, it is a good method to construct static domain interests by utilizing domain ontology in literature retrieval. Traditional literature retrieval methods focus on optimizing query conditions to improve the recall rate. For instance, Ontoseek [8] formulated queries based on ontologies to improve the precision of literature retrieval. Guha et al. [9] employed ontologies to improve traditional web search by augmenting the search results with the related concepts in the ontology. Different from these researches, OntoSearch [13] proposed a method to optimize query results based on the spread activation theory. However, only classification information in domain terminology ontology was used. In this paper, we adopt the Data-Brain as domain research ontology to optimize query results based on the spread activation theory. Besides classification information, other types of relationship information are also be used.

## 3   A Domain-Driven Literature Retrieval Method

As shown in Fig. 1, our method consists of three parts: modeling literatures, modeling domain interests, and calculating the similarity between domain interests and literatures. The details will be discussed as follows.

### 3.1   Modeling Literatures

In this process we use vector space model (VSM) [10] to index every literature. VSM is a general mean for modeling textual objects and has been

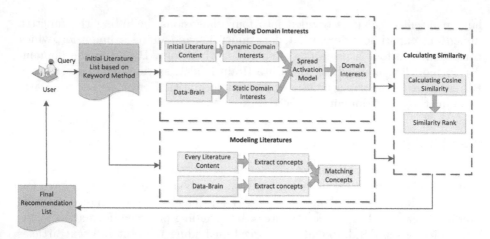

**Fig. 1.** The framework of domain-driven literature retrieval method.

used in many previous researches. For the literature $d_j$, it can be modeled as $d_j = (c_{1,j}, c_{2,j}, \cdots, c_{n,j})$, in which n is the number of non-repetitive concepts of domain ontology, $c_{i,j}$ represents the weight of concept $c_i$ of the Data-Brain in the literature $d_j$. Different from the OntoSearch based method, we use the traditional tf/idf measure [11] to calculate $c_{i,j}$, i.e., $c_{i,j} = freq_{i,j} \times log\frac{N}{n_i}$, where $freq_{i,j}$ is the frequency of $c_i$ in $d_j$, N represents the total number of literatures in the dataset, and $n_i$ represents the number of literatures including $c_i$.

## 3.2   Modeling Domain Interests

Domain interests can be divided into two types: static domain interests and dynamic domain interests. Static domain interests represent long-term and commonly acknowledged research foci in the domain. They can be represents by domain ontologies, such as the Data-Brain. Dynamic domain interests represent current research foci in the domain. We can get dynamic domain interests based on the user's query. Combining dynamic domain interests with static domain interests, it is possible to get better retrieval results. The spread activation model [12] can be used to confirm this idea. The spread activation theory was firstly used in the field of artificial intelligence, in recent years it was often used in concept searching. Given some initial concepts and constraints, it will find concepts closely related to the initial concepts in domain ontology. Because the spread activation theory is an effective way of knowledge reasoning, we use spread activation theory on the Data-Brain, which is also a kind of semantic network, in this paper.

In the semantic network, concepts are represented as nodes and connected by relationships. The information processing of semantic network abides by the spread activation theory that the activation value of each node spreads to neighbor nodes. The whole spread activation process can be described by using the following formula [13]:

$$O = [\varepsilon - (1 - \alpha)\omega^T]^{-1} I_q \tag{1}$$

where $I_q = [I_{1,q}, I_{2,q}, \cdots, I_{n,q}]^T$ is the initial input of the network, $\omega$ is the relation matrix of the network and each element of $\omega_{ij}$ represents the link between concept $c_i$ and concept $c_j$, $\varepsilon$ is an identity matrix of order n, $\alpha$ is the decay factor, $O = [O_1, O_2, \cdots, O_n]^T$ is the output matrix of the spread activation process in which $O_i$ represents the activation value of concept $c_i$. In the process of spread activation the energy will decay, so we use the attenuation factor to represent the decay process. Referring to [14], $\alpha$ is set as 0.2.

In order to apply the spread activation theory to literature retrieval, we firstly get an initial concept list. By using the spread activation theory in the Data-Brain, domain interests can be extended. The input of the spread activation process is the mapping of initial literature contents in the Data-Brain and represents dynamic domain interests. Different from the OntoSearch retrieval method, we extract concepts from initial literature contents and then match them with concepts in Data-Brain for forming dynamic domain interests. $I_q$ is a $n \times 1$ matrix composed by the initial concept list. $I_{i,q}$ represents the initial activation value of concept $c_i$ and is calculated by the following formula:

$$I_{i,q} = \begin{cases} \frac{freq(c_i)}{\sum_{c_j} freq(c_j)} & c_i, c_j \in LC_{initial} \cap DB_{BI} \\ 0 & c_i \notin LC_{initial} \cap DB_{BI} \end{cases} \tag{2}$$

where $freq(c_i)$ represents the frequency of concept $c_i$ in the literatures acquired by the keyword based query method. $LC_{initial}$ represents the initial literature content, $DB_{BI}$ represents the Data-Brain. The elements of initial concept list are the concepts in Data-Brain. The sum of all elements in the input matrix is 1.

Once acquiring the input matrix, the nodes in the Data-Brain will be activated in different degrees and finally reach a steady state. In the literature retrieval algorithm, $\omega$ represents the relation matrix of Data-Brain in which $\omega_{ij}$ represents the proportion of relationship $r_{ij}$ in the Data-Brain and can be calculated by the following formula:

$$\omega_{i,j} = \begin{cases} \frac{freqr_{i,j}}{\sum_j freqr_{i,j}} & rel \in subClassOf \\ \frac{0.8 freqr_{i,j}}{\sum_j freqr_{i,j}} & rel \in domain \\ \frac{0.6 freqr_{i,j}}{\sum_j freqr_{i,j}} & rel \in others \end{cases} \tag{3}$$

Different from the OntoSearch retrieval method, we consider relationship types in the process of spread activation. For different relationship types, we set different weights In this study, we set weight 1, 0.8, 0.6 to the relationship subClassOf, domain, and the others respectively. The values of weight were acquired from the experiments which got the best retrieval results. When the spread activation process is over, we can acquire the output matrix O corresponding to domain interests which combining dynamic domain interests with static domain interests.

### 3.3   Outputting Retrieval Literatures

After the above steps, we can get the literature vector $d_j$ and the output vector O. Based on these two vectors, the cosine similarity method can be used to calculate their correlation. The formula is as follows:

$$Sim(d_j, O) = \frac{\sum_{i=1}^{n} d_{i,j} * O_i}{\sqrt{\sum_{i=1}^{n}(d_{i,j})^2} * \sqrt{\sum_{i=1}^{n}(O_i)^2}} \tag{4}$$

The similarity varies from 0 to 1. 0 is completely dissimilar and 1 represents exactly similar. Ranking literatures based on the similarity values, a recommendation list of literatures will be obtained.

## 4   Experiments and Evaluation

### 4.1   Experimental Data

PubMed maintained by the National Library of Medicine is a database of biomedical research articles containing over 21 million citations. The PubMed dataset provides publication information, title, abstract, keywords, authors and so on. Our literature retrieval method is oriented to BI researches. The main purpose is to provide the retrieval service for BI researchers. Hence, we choose experiment data related to brain informatics. The core of PubMed dataset is biomedical, so we choose PubMed as our experiment data source. We extract the literatures which were published from 2005 to 2007 in three top neuroscience journals, including Trends in neurosciences, Nature neuroscience and Neuron. We use the Data-Brain prototype stated in [4].

### 4.2   Experiment Process

Most previous studies invite domain experts to decide the accuracy. However, such a method lacks persuasion. Hence, besides experts' assessments, we assess the retrieval accuracy by judging whether the literatures are relevant to brain area. We compare retrieval results with the keyword based method and the OntoSearch based method.

**The First Step is to Observe the PubMed Dataset.** In this process, the PubMed dataset is divided into five aspects, including brain, symptom, diagnosis, gene and the others. We input the query "depression", and then the retrieved literature list was obtained. For the keyword based method, this list is just final results. For the OntoSearch based method and our method, new lists will be obtained by using this list as the input. Observing each one in top 20 literatures and judging which aspect it belongs to, we can get the result shown in Table 1.

**Table 1.** The result based on the query "depression"

|                            | Brain | Symptom | Diagnosis | Gene | Others |
|----------------------------|-------|---------|-----------|------|--------|
| Keyword based method       | 9     | 2       | 6         | 3    | 0      |
| OntoSearch based method    | 15    | 0       | 5         | 0    |        |
| The improved method        | 16    | 0       | 4         | 0    | 0      |

**The Second Step is to Calculate the Average Precision.** In order to verify the accuracy of our method, ten queries were input. The keywords include "attention", "cognitive", "computation", "depression", "emotion", "induction", "learning", "fMRI", "EEG", "memory". Different from the first step, we only need to judge whether the literature is relevant to brain area. Table 2 gives the results of the three methods based on top1, top7, top14, and top20 retrieved literatures.

**Table 2.** The average precision of three methods

|                            | 1    | 7     | 14    | 20    |
|----------------------------|------|-------|-------|-------|
| Keyword based method       | 0.60 | 0.557 | 0.536 | 0.515 |
| OntoSearch based method    | 0.90 | 0.871 | 0.779 | 0.745 |
| The improved method        | 0.90 | 0.886 | 0.80  | 0.775 |

**The Third Step is to Calculate the 11-point Average Precision.** As shown in Fig. 2, we present the 11-point average precision scores of three methods in retrieving literatures based on "attention".

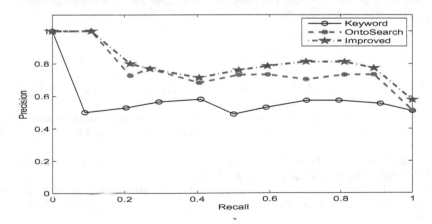

**Fig. 2.** A comparison of three methods measure based on a query on "attention"

## 4.3 Evaluation Results and Discussion

Table 1 shows that our method can provide more brain related results in top 20 literatures than the keyword based method and the OntoSearch based method. Table 2 is the average precision of three methods based on the top1, top7, top14, and top20 retrieved literatures. Experimental results show that our method has the higher average precision than the keyword based method and the OntoSearch based method.

Figure 2 is the comparison of experiment results between three methods. This figure shows that there is a big gap between three method's precisions when the recall is low. This means our method outperforms both the keyword based method and the OntoSearch based method significantly when the recall value is low.

## 5 Conclusion and Future Work

In this paper we put forward a literature retrieval method for supporting systematic BI researches. We use Data-Brain as static domain ontology and use the spread activation model on query results to combine static domain ontology with dynamic domain interests. Furthermore, we consider relationship types in the process of spread activation. The experimental results show that our method can improve the precision of retrieved literatures. Our method makes it possible for researchers to retrieve literatures relevant to BI more easily and effectively. In the future, we need to consider the indirect relationship between concepts and solve the problem of data sparseness for improving the effectiveness and speed of literature retrieval.

**Acknowledgments.** The work is supported by National Key Basic Research Program of China (2014CB744605), National Natural Science Foundation of China (61272345), Research Supported by the CAS/SAFEA International Partnership Program for Creative Research Teams, the Japan Society for the Promotion of Science Grants-in-Aid for Scientific Research (25330270).

## References

1. Zhong, N., Bradshaw, J.M., Liu, J.M., Taylor, J.G.: Brain informatics. IEEE Intell. Syst. **26**, 16–20 (2011)
2. Zhong, N., Chen, J.H.: Constructing a new-style conceptual model of brain data for systematic brain informatics. IEEE Trans. Knowl. Data Eng. **24**(12), 2127–2142 (2012)
3. Baeza-Yates, R.A., Berthier, A.: Ribeiro-Neto. Modern Information Retrieval. ACM Press/Addison-Wesley, Boston (1999)
4. Zhong, N., Chen, J.: Constructing a new-style conceptual model of brain data for systematic brain informatics. IEEE Trans. Knowl. Data Eng. **24**(12), 2127–2142 (2012)

5. Jimenez-Castellanos, A., et al.: Biomedical literature retrieval based on patient information. In: Fred, A., Filipe, J., Gamboa, H. (eds.) BIOSTEC 2011. CCIS, vol. 273, pp. 312–323. Springer, Heidelberg (2013)
6. Sondhi, P., Sun, J., Zhai, C.X., Sorrentino, R., Kohn, M.S.: Leveraging medical thesauri and physician feedback for improving medical literature retrieval for case queries. J. Am. Med. Inform. Assoc. **19**(5), 851–8 (2012)
7. Park, M., Lee, K.-W., Lee, H.-S., Jiayi, P., Yu, J.: Ontology-based construction knowledge retrieval system. KSCE J. Civil Eng. **17**(7), 1654–1663 (2013)
8. Guarino, N., Masolo, C., Vetere, G.: Ontoseek: content-based access to the web. IEEE Intell. Syst. **14**(3), 70–80 (1999)
9. Guha, R., McCool, R., Miller, E.: Semanticsearch. In: WWW 2003, pp. 700–709 (2003)
10. Crouch, C.J., Crouch, D.B., Nareddy, K.: Connectionist model for information retrieval based on the vector space model. Int. J. Expert Syst. **7**, 139–163 (1994)
11. Rijsbergen, C.J.V.: Information Retrieval, 2nd edn. Butterworths, London (1979)
12. Anderson, R.J.: A spreading activation theory of memory. J. Verbal Learn. Verbal Behav. **22**, 261–295 (1983)
13. Jiang, X., Tan, A.H.: OntoSearch: A full-text search engine for the semantic web. In: National Conference on Artificial Intelligence, Innovative Applications of Artificial Intelligence Conference, pp. 1325–1330 (2006)
14. Sheng, K.: Design and Implementation Strategy Based on Semantic Network User Ontology Model. University of Electronic Science and Technology of China, Chengdu (2014)

# A Provenance Driven Approach for Systematic EEG Data Analysis

Xian Li[1,2(✉)], Jianzhuo Yan[1,2], Jianhui Chen[3,5], Yongchuan Yu[1,2],
and Ning Zhong[1,3,4,5,6]

[1] Beijing Advanced Innovation Center for Future Internet Technology,
Beijing University of Technology, Beijing 100124, China
lixian1992@emails.bjut.edu.cn, {yanjianzhuo,yuyongchuan}@bjut.edu.cn,
zhong@maebashi-it.ac.jp
[2] College of Electronic Information and Control Engineering,
Beijing University of Technology, Beijing 100024, China
[3] International WIC Institute, Beijing University of Technology,
Beijing 100024, China
chenjianhui@bjut.edu.cn
[4] Beijing Key Laboratory of MRI and Brain Informatics, Beijing, China
[5] Beijing International Collaboration Base on Brain Informatics and Wisdom
Services, Beijing, China
[6] Department of Life Science and Informatics, Maebashi Institute of Technology,
Maebashi 371-0816, Japan

**Abstract.** As an important issue of Brain Informatics (BI) methodology, systematic brain data analysis has gained significant attractions in BI community. However, the existing expert-driven multi-aspect data analysis and distributed analytical platforms excessively depend on individual capabilities and cannot be widely adopted in systematic human brain study. In this paper, we propose a provenance driven approach for systematic brain data analysis, which is implemented by using the Data-Brain, BI provenances and the Global Learning Scheme for BI. Furthermore, a systematic EEG data analysis for emotion recognition which is a key issue of affective computing is described to demonstrate significance and usefulness of the proposed approach. Such a provenance driven approach reduces the dependency of individual capabilities and provides a practical way for realizing the systematic human brain data analysis of BI methodology.

## 1 Introduction

Brain Informatics (BI) [10] is an emerging interdisciplinary and multidisciplinary research field that focuses on studying the mechanisms underlying the human information processing systems (HIPS) for deep understanding of human intelligence eventually. BI emphasizes on a systematic approach generalized as a BI methodology [2], in which systematic brain data analysis is a key issue. Systematic brain data analysis can be regarded as the domain-driven data mining involving a large amount of domain knowledge [3], whose core issue is to integrate

© Springer International Publishing AG 2016
G.A. Ascoli et al. (Eds.): BIH 2016, LNAI 9919, pp. 190–200, 2016.
DOI: 10.1007/978-3-319-47103-7_19

various brain data and analytical methods. This is a very challenging task for beginners or non-domain researchers without a priori knowledge. Hence, it is necessary that the construction of analysis process planning guides the researchers to achieve systematic brain data analysis step by step using the generated analysis workflows. Although some of existing open source softwares (eg.,WEKA) can realize the analysis of brain data for specific mining problems, they only provide analysis methods and no workflow descriptions and analysis planning processes. Furthermore, the results based process optimization should be realized during the analytical process planning.

This paper proposes a provenance driven approach to support the implementation and popularization of systematic EEG data analysis. The rest of this paper is organized as follows. Section 2 discusses the background and related work. Section 3 illustrates the details of the proposed method. Further more, an experiment about emotion recognition is provided in Sect. 4 to describe how to implement a provenance driven approach for systematic EEG data analysis. Section 5 gives concluding remarks and future work. The final section is our sincere acknowledgements.

## 2   Background and Related Work

Provenances are a kind of metadata that describing the origin and subsequent processing of a data set [12]. In systematic BI study, it will produce various original data, derived data, data features and other result data. For effectively managing, sharing and utilizing these data, BI provenances, which are the metadata describing the origin and subsequent processing of various human brain data in systematic BI studies, were defined based on the Data-Brain [11].

Provenance based researches have gained increasing interests in recent years. Many brain databases have been constructed to effectively store and share multiple levels of brain data based on their own provenances. At present, the research based on neuroimaging provenance is one of the most important provenance based researches, which mainly focuses on the description of the analysis process to support the distributed analysis platform such as LONI pipeline[1]. However, it is difficult that most of the ordinary investigators should hold all of domain knowledge because a holistic multi-aspect brain data analysis will integrate various data and analysis methods. Recent studies [2,5] have addressed the aforementioned problems by developing new approaches which integrates a large number of analytical softwares or algorithms for systematic brain data analysis. However, there are still some deficiencies, in which they don't realize the descriptions of analysis results and the optimization of analysis process based on results which is important to construct more efficient workflows.

---

[1] http://pipeline.loni.ucla.edu.

# 3    Method

## 3.1    Systematic EEG Based Emotion Recognition

Emotion is described as a response to an important event that is generated by internal and external events. EEG based emotion recognition as a core issue of affective computing (AC) has been studied by various domains, including human-computer interaction (HCI), cognitive psychology, etc. In this study, the EEG based systematic emotion recognition mainly includes the following steps:

- Data preprocessing. This step includes down sampling, common average referencing, bandpass filtering, artifact elimination, etc.
- Feature extraction. In this step, features are extracted by sliding a 4-s window with a 2-s overlapping. The linear features and nonlinear features are performed to extract EEG features.
- Feature selection. EEG features are selected by using a statistical analysis software SPSS[2] to find emotion-related features.
- Classification and constructing rules. It includes emotion classification using C4.5 algorithm in WEKA [9] and constructing rules based on decision trees.

The C4.5 algorithm as one type of decision tree is used in our research to perform emotion classification and rule construction, because it merely selects the features which are relevant to differentiate each emotional state and is searched sequentially for an appropriate "IF-THEN" statement to be used as a classification rule. The all EEG features are participated in generating rules and the result is achieved using the J48 classifier (a Java implementation of C4.5 algorithm) in WEKA.

## 3.2    Data-Brain Based BI Provenances

The Data-Brain is a conceptual model of brain data, with multi-view and multi-dimension framework to model the four issues of systematic BI methodology by its own four dimensions, namely function dimension, data dimension, experiment dimension, and analysis dimension [4]. It also provides a conceptual model for the construction of BI provenances [11]. Our previous studies have proposed a BI methodology based ontological modeling process for constructing the Data-Brain and a Data-Brain based approach for constructing BI provenances. The Data-Brain based BI provenances forms a knowledge graph about the whole life cycle of brain data.

In this study, the Data-Brain based BI provenances were constructed for describing systematic EEG data analysis, in which all of EEG data were obtained by emotion eliciting experiments. By the BI methodology based ontological modeling approach, a group of key concepts of the Data-Brain can be identified from data and information related to experimental materials, equipment parameters,

---

[2] http://www.ibm.com/analytics/us/en/technology/spss/.

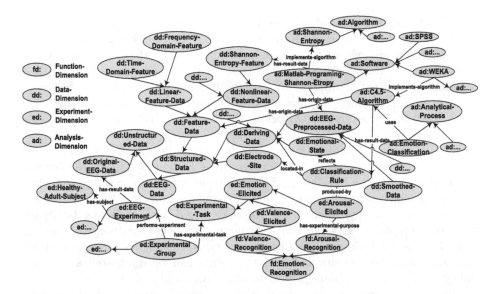

**Fig. 1.** A segment of Data-Brain for modeling the systematic EEG data analysis

participants' information and so on. Figure 1 provides a segment of the Data-Brain, which includes some key concepts and relations for modeling the systematic EEG data analysis. For example, the EEG recording experiment mentioned above is generalized as an "Experimental-Group" which includes a group of "EEG-Experiment" involved with a group of "Healthy-Adult-Subject" and a set of "Original-EEG-Data". Based on the Data-Brain, some key concepts and relations can be identified from the basic information of the EEG analysis process including a group of electrodes, a set of feature data, various software and algorithms, etc. For example, the WEKA based analysis is generalized as an analytical process "Emotion-Classification". It is performed by a "C4.5-Algorithm" whose input data is a group of feature data sets by the concept "EEG-Feature-Data" and relation "has-origin-data". Its results are a group of "Classification-Rule" in which each classification rule is produced by "Arousal-Elicited" and reflects a specific "Emotional-State". Furthermore, the corresponding BI analysis provenances can also be constructed by extracting related information from experimental records or literatures and creating instances of the above concepts.

## 3.3 Global Learning Scheme for BI

As stated earlier, the key issue of the multi-aspect brain data analysis is how to find and integrate the needed data and analytical methods according to different analytical purposes. In order to offset the disadvantages of the existing expert-driven multi-aspect brain data analysis, the Global Learning Scheme for BI (GLS-BI) [5] was designed to perform a Data-Brain driven mining process planning for multi-aspect brain data analysis.

In the GLS-BI, semantic web service technologies are used to wrap physical or virtual data and analysis resources in BI community as various data and analysis agents, whose descriptions are annotated by the Data-Brain based BI provenances. Each data agent is corresponding to one dataset which has the same experimental proposal in BI experimental studies, and each analysis agent is corresponding to a or a group of data operations in BI data analytical studies. For example, we define the $ds_1 = (EEG\text{-}Arousal, Arousal\text{-}Elicited, Arousal\text{-}Recognition, Biosemi\text{-}ActiveTwo, Original\text{-}EEG\text{-}Data)$ to describe a data agent which wraps a dataset getting from a emotion-elicited experiment. And the $as_1 = (Preprocessing, Filtering\text{-}EEG\text{-}Waveforms, EEGLAB, Original\text{-}EEG\text{-}Data, EEG\text{-}Preprocessed\text{-}Data)$ describes an analysis angent which wraps a group of preprocessing operations of EEG waveforms performed by using the open source software EEGLAB[3], including bandpass filtering, eliminating EOG and EMG artifacts, etc. These agents are connected by the Internet and form an open agent society. According to different analysis purposes, these data agents and analysis agents can be integrated as various mining workflows by the multi-aspect mining process planning.

The whole planning process mainly includes three steps: purpose definition, Data-Brain driven agent discovery and workflow extraction. In purpose definition, investigators need to define the analysis purpose based on the Data-Brain. As stated in our previous studies, the whole process of multi-aspect brain data analysis can be generalized as "aiming at an objective function to investigate its information processing course by extracting and analyzing various spatiotemporal features on related data sets". Hence, the purpose definition can be implemented by selecting a specific function concept from the function dimension of Data-Brain and a group of data feature concepts from the data dimension of Data-Brain. For example, the analytical purpose of EEG based arousal recognition can be formally defined as follows.

$$ap1 = (CF1, DF1)$$

where $CF1 = $ "$Arousal\text{-}Recognition$" is a function concept in the function dimension, which means that the current analysis aims at systematic EEG data analysis of arousal recognition. $DF1 = \{$"$Topography\text{-}from\text{-}EEG\text{-}Data$", "$Feature\text{-}Data$", "$Classification\text{-}Result\text{-}of\text{-}Arousal$"$\}$ is a set of data concepts from the data dimension of Data-Brain, which means that investigators attempt to obtain these three kinds of data features from the data dimension of Data-Brain during EEG analysis.

Data-Brain based provenance driven data selection is performed to find the needed data agents according to the objective function $CF1$. Based on the above descriptions, the discovery algorithm of analysis agents is shown in Algorithm 1. Its input parameters are the set of data agent descriptions $Data\text{-}agents$ and the set of data feature concepts $Features$, which is selected in the *purpose definition* step. In this algorithm, finding and organizing analysis agents depend on the subsumption relations between the data concepts which are associated

---

[3] http://sccn.ucsd.edu/eeglab/.

with the *Input* and *Output* of analysis agent descriptions. Taking into account that in the process of EEG based emotion recognition, not all of EEG features are involved in the construction of classification rules. Hence, we can realize the automatic updating of the analysis process based on the classification results by judging whether the EEG features are present in the classification rules *CRS*. Finally, the output is a topology graph, denoted by *TG*, which can be used for workflow extraction. Various mining workflows are extracted from the topology graph *TG* through workflow extraction. Each workflow is just a simple path from an original node (data agent) to a target node (analysis agent) in the directed graph *TG* and can be extracted by the depth-first traversal.

---

**Algorithm 1.** The algorithm of analysis agent discovery for EEG systematic analysis

---

**Input:** *Data-agents* and *Features*
**Output:** a topology graph *TG*.
1. Initialize an empty Topology Graph, *TG*;
2. Initialize an empty analysis request type set, *SRTS*;
3. Initialize an empty classification rule set, *CRS*;
4. For each $ds_i$ in *Data-agents* do
5.     add $ds_i$ as an original node into *TG*;
6.     add $ds_i.Type$ into *SRTS*;
7. End For
8. While($SRTS\langle\rangle empty$) do
9.     Initialize *New-SRTS*=empty;
10.     Initialize *New-AS*=empty;
11.         For each available analysis agent $as_i$ do
12.             For each $ss_i$ in *SRTS* do
13.                 If ($degreeOfMatch(ss_i, as_i.Input)$==*exact* or *plugIn*) then
14.                     IF $as_i.Output$ in *CRS* then
15.                         add $as_i$ as node and relevant edge $e_i$ into *TG*;
16.                         If($e_i$ is a new edge in *TG*) then
17.                             add $as_i$ into *New-AS*;
18.                             add $as_i.Output$ into *New-SRTS*;
19.                         End If
20.                     End If
21.                 End If
22.             End For
23.         End For
24.     Initialize $SRTS = New\text{-}SRTS$;
25.     For each $nss_i$ in *New-SRTS* do
26.         If ($\exists df_i \in Features, degreeOfMatch(df_i, nss_i) == exact$) then
27.             make $as_i$ corresponding to $nss_i$ as a target node;
28.             delete $nss_i$ from *SRTS*;
29.         End If
30.     End For
31. End While

---

# 4   Experiment and Results

The proposed provenance driven approach of brain data analysis can be realized based on the Data-Brain based BI provenances and the GLS-BI. In this section, a case study will be introduced for the above EEG based systematic emotion recognition to demonstrate such an provenance driven approach. Firstly, a dynamic planning process will be performed to obtain candidate workflows. Secondly, the obtained workflows will be performed by calling the WEKA, SPSS, EEGLAB and other Matlab[4] programs. Finally, the analytical results will be integrated into BI provenances to obtain optimized analytical processes by performing the planning again.

## 4.1   Data and Analyses

In this study, one public dataset DEAP [7] which adopts arousal-valence space [16] to quantify emotion has been used to demonstrate the performance characteristics of the proposed provenance driven analysis approach for emotion recognition. The dateset contains EEG and peripheral physiological signals from 32 subjects by using the Biosemi ActiveTwo system[5], in which EEG was recorded at a sampling rate of 512 Hz using 32 active AgCl electrodes placed according to the international 10–20 system. A full experimental description of the dataset has given in the literature [7]. The corresponding data agents and analysis agents were created by using data and analysis provenances, respectively. The creation of data provenances mainly includes: describing experimental group, describing experimental task, describing measuring instrument, etc. And the creation of analysis provenances mainly includes: describing analytical process, describing analytical inputs, describing analytical tools, describing analytical results, etc. Based on these data and data/analysis provenances, two data agents and a group of analysis agents were constructed in the GLS-BI. For simplifying descriptions of workflows, each analysis agent is corresponding to not an atomic data operation but a group of data operations whose results can be used for multiple analytical methods.

## 4.2   The Process Planning of Systematic EEG Based Emotion Recognition

A systematic EEG data analysis for emotion recognition can be presented as "aiming at the objective function *Emotion-Recognition* to investigate its information processing course by extracting, analysis and classifying various spatiotemporal features on related dataset". This purpose can be defined as an objective function "*Arousal-Recognition*" and three types of data features, namely, "*Topography-from-EEG-Data*", "*Feature-Data*" and "*Classification-Result-of-Arousal*" were chosen. Each workflow represents a

---

[4] http://www.mathworks.com.
[5] http://www.biosemi.com.

possible mining process which aims at the experimental data corresponding to the "*Arousal-Recognition*". Figure 2(a) shows the corresponding workflow of EEG systematic analysis which represents a mining process for emotion recognition.

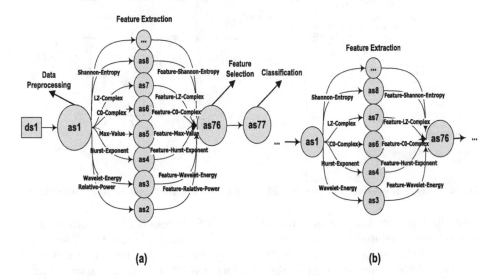

**Fig. 2.** (a) A mining workflow of EEG systematic analysis for emotion recognition; (b) An improved workflow for EEG analysis after optimization based on classification rules

In this figure, the data agent *ds*1 represents the EEG data set obtained by the "*Arousal-Elicited*" task. The analysis agent *as*1 which represents a series of EEG data preprocessing methods integrated into EEGLAB includes bandpass filtering, EOG and EMG removal, etc. Subsequently a group of feature extraction methods which were wrapped into a group of analysis agents to extract EEG feature, including linear features (e.g., standard deviation, relative power, etc.) and nonlinear dynamics features (e.g., LZ-complex, sample entropy, etc.). A statistical analysis software SPSS which is wrapped into the analysis agent *as*76 are used to perform feature selection. The agent *as*77 represents the software WEKA which integrates a series of machine learning algorithm including various classification algorithms.

### 4.3   Workflow Performance and Optimization

Figure 3 shows a segment of decision trees based on C4.5 algorithm and classification result when arousal recognition is performed by using four famous machine learn algorithms, namely C4.5, SVM, MLP and k-NN. According to the classification result, the classification rules reach an average classification rate of 75.52 % on arousal using C4.5 with 10-fold cross validation which is highest among these four classification algorithms. From the classification rules as

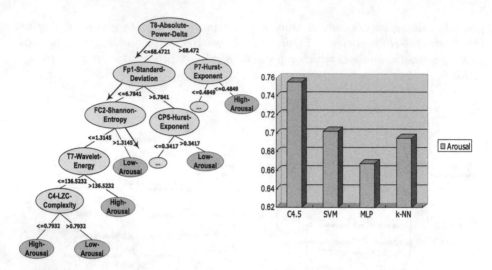

**Fig. 3.** A segment of decision tree by C4.5 and classification result of four algorithms

shown in Fig. 3 we can see that not all of EEG features obtained from various analysis agents related to various feature extraction methods are useful for emotion recognition because some features are not involved in the construction of the classification rule set. Hence, the obtained workflow includes many redundant and useless nodes which will lead to enormous amount of computation and time consumption. In order to address this problem and realize the optimization of workflows, the obtained classification rules are represented by using semantic Web technologies, such as the Jena rule and integrated into the Data-Brain provenances. For example, a rule shown by the arrow in Fig. 3 can be represented as follows:

String rule =
"[Rule 1: (?EEG_feature1 rdf:type base: Absolute-Power-Delta)
(?EEG_feature1 base:hasValue ?value1)lessThanOrEqual(?value1, 68.4721)
(?EEG_feature1 base:onElectrode ?electrode1)
(?electrode1 rdfs:label "T8")
(?EEG_feature2 rdf:type base: Standar-Deviation)
(?EEG_feature2 base:hasValue ?value2)lessThanOrEqual(?value2, 6.7841)
(?EEG_feature2 base:onElectrode ?electrode2)
(?electrode2 rdfs:label "FP1")
(?EEG_feature3 rdf:type base: Shannon-Entropy)
(?EEG_feature3 base:hasValue ?value3)greaterThan(?value3, 1.3145)
(?EEG_feature3 base:onElectrode ?electrode3)
(?electrode3 rdfs:label "FC2")
(?arousal rdf:type base:Emotion)
(?arousal base:has Symbol "1")
(?user base:hasEmotion ?emotion)]".

The Jena rules which are composed of all of paths from the root node to leaf node can be created to infer the subjects' emotional state with the "IF-THEN" structure according to the concepts and properties defined in Data-Brain based BI provenances. Based on this new knowledge, the adaptive adjustment strategy stated in Algorithm 1 in Sect. 3 can be activated. By performing the process planning again, a new improved workflow which has deleted those redundant and useless nodes according to classification rules is shown in Fig. 2(b).

The above scenario illustrates a case study on the provenance driven systematic human brain data analysis. During such a provenance driven data mining process, the Data-Brain, BI provenances and the GLS-BI guided a systematic analysis process to integrate various data and analyses for EEG based systematic emotion recognition step by step.

## 5 Conclusions and Future Work

Our proposed approach has the following contributions. Firstly, a dynamic planning method is proposed based on the BI provenances and GLS-BI to generate candidate workflows for guiding the systematic brain data analysis. Secondly, knowledge about both analytical processes and analytical results is integrated into BI provenances to realize a self-learning mechanism for the continuous optimization of process planning. The investigators who lack enough domain and data related knowledge can also easily apply multiple analytical methods to systematically analyze various brain data.

Our studies only obtained some preliminary results, the future work mainly includes wrapping more data and analytical methods into the GLS-BI, performing the further analysis based on public brain databases and embedding the GLS-BI into a mature distributed computing environment (e.g., LONI pipeline).

**Acknowledgments.** This work is supported by National Key Basic Research Program of China (2014CB744605), National Natural Science Foundation of China (61272345), Research Supported by the CAS/SAFEA International Partnership Program for Creative Research Teams, the Japan Society for the Promotion of Science Grants-in-Aid for Scientific Research (25330270).

## References

1. Zhong, N., Liu, J., Yao, Y., Wu, J., Lu, S., Qin, Y., Li, K., Wah, B.: Web intelligence meets brain informatics. In: Zhong, N., Liu, J., Yao, Y., Wu, J., Lu, S., Li, K. (eds.) WImBI 2006. LNCS (LNAI), vol. 4845, pp. 1–31. Springer, Heidelberg (2006). doi:10.1007/978-3-540-77028-2_1
2. Motomura, S., Zhong, N.. Multi-aspect data analysis for investigating human computation mechanism. Cogn. Syst. Res. **11**(1), 3–15 (2010)
3. Cao, L.B., Zhang, C.Q.: The evolution of KDD: towards domain-driven data mining. Int. J. Pattern Recogn. Artif. Intell. **21**(4), 677–692 (2007)
4. Chen, J.H., Zhong, N.: Data-brain modeling based on brain informatics methodology. In: IEEE and WIC and ACM International Conference on Web Intelligence, WI 2008, 9–12 December 2008, Sydney, pp. 41–47 (2008)

5. Zhong, N., Chen, J.H.: Data-brain driven multi-aspect mining process planning. In: 2010 International Joint Conference on Neural Networks (IJCNN), pp. 1–4 (2010)
6. Brazdil, P.: Metalearning: applications to data mining. Cognitive Technologies (2009)
7. Koelstra, S., Muhl, C., Soleymani, M., et al.: DEAP: a database for emotion analysis using physiological signals. IEEE Trans. Affect. Comput. 3(1), 18–31 (2011)
8. Klyne, G., Carroll, J.J., et al.: Resource description framework (RDF): concepts and abstract syntax. In: World Wide Web Consortium Recommendation (2004)
9. Garner, S.R., et al.: WEKA: the waikato environment for knowledge analysis. In: Proceedings of the NewZealand Computer Science Research Students Conference, pp. 57–64. Citeseer (1995)
10. Zhong, N., Bradshaw, J.M., Liu, J.M., Taylor, J.G.: Brain informatics. IEEE Intell. Syst., pp. 26–20 (2011)
11. Zhong, N., Chen, J.H.: Constructing a new-style conceptual model of brain data for systematic brain informatics. IEEE Trans. Knowl. Data Eng. 24(12), 2127–2142 (2012)
12. Simmhan, Y.L., Plale, B., Gannon, D.: A survey of data provenance in e-Science. Sigmod Rec. 3(34), 31–36 (2005)
13. Buneman, P., Khanna, S., Wang-Chiew, T.: Why and where: a characterization of data provenance. In: Bussche, J., Vianu, V. (eds.) ICDT 2001. LNCS, vol. 1973, pp. 316–330. Springer, Heidelberg (2001). doi:10.1007/3-540-44503-X_20
14. Chen, J.H., Zhong, N., Huang, R.: Towards systematic human brain data management using a data-brain based GLS-BI system. In: Yao, Y., Sun, R., Poggio, T., Liu, J., Zhong, N., Huang, J. (eds.) BI 2010. LNCS (LNAI), vol. 6334, pp. 365–376. Springer, Heidelberg (2010). doi:10.1007/978-3-642-15314-3_35
15. Noy, N.F., Musen, M.A.: Specifying ontology views by traversal. In: McIlraith, S.A., Plexousakis, D., Harmelen, F. (eds.) ISWC 2004. LNCS, vol. 3298, pp. 713–725. Springer, Heidelberg (2004). doi:10.1007/978-3-540-30475-3_49
16. Russell, J.A.: A circumplex model of affect. J. Pers. Soc. Psychol. 6(39), 1161–1178 (1980)

# Concept Recognition of Depression Drugs in Biomedical Literatures Using the Domain Relevance Measure

Jianhui Chen[1,2,3,4,5]($\boxtimes$), Zhongcheng Zhao[1], Ningning Wang[2,3], and Shaofu Lin[1]

[1] Beijing Advanced Innovation Center for Future Internet Technology, Beijing University of Technology, Beijing 100024, China
{chenjianhui,linshaofu}@bjut.edu.cn, zhaozhongch@163.com
[2] College of Electronic Information and Control Engineering, Beijing University of Technology, Beijing 100024, China
[3] International WIC Institute, Beijing University of Technology, Beijing, China
[4] Beijing International Collaboration Base on Brain Informatics and Wisdom Services, Beijing, China
[5] Beijing Key Laboratory of MRI and Brain Informatics, Beijing, China

**Abstract.** Concepts of depression drugs are a kind of important domain knowledge and need to be integrated into the Data-Brain, which is a multi-dimension knowledge framework, for supporting systematic brain informatics studies on the depression. Though some open biomedical knowledge sources have already provided depression drug ontologies, it is still necessary to realize automatic concept recognition of depression drugs from biomedical literatures because of the quick development of depression-related studies and the constant appearance of new depression drugs. However, various nomenclatures and a large number of abbreviations make it difficult to extract depression drug concepts precisely only using existing methods. This paper proposes a new method of concept recognition based on the domain relevance measure, in which new independence assumptions and the domain bias function are defined. The experimental results show that both the precision and recall of concept recognition can been improved obviously comparing with existing methods.

## 1 Introduction

The study of brain and mental disorders is an important viewpoint of brain informatics (BI) [1,2] and can be regarded as the "control group" for understanding human information processing mechanism in depth. At present, depression studies of BI are being performed based on the systematic BI methodology [3], to reveal the pathology of depression for developing new diagnosis and treatment technologies [4]. Such systematic studies need a Data-Brain [3] which is a conceptual brain data model and can be used to integrate the valuable data, information and knowledge in the whole research process of BI for various data requests

© Springer International Publishing AG 2016
G.A. Ascoli et al. (Eds.): BIH 2016, LNAI 9919, pp. 201–210, 2016.
DOI: 10.1007/978-3-319-47103-7_20

coming from different aspects of systematic BI studies. By using the BI methodology based ontological modeling approach [3], a multi-dimension framework of Data-Brain can be constructed. Furthermore, text-based ontology learning technologies should be developed to extract new knowledge, especially domain concepts, for enriching the Data-Brain quickly.

Concepts of depression drugs are a kind of important domain concepts for constructing the Data-Brain and developing intelligent auxiliary diagnosis and treatment technologies of depression. Some open biomedical knowledge sources, such as SNOMED Clinical Terms (SNOMED CT) [5], have already provided depression drug ontologies. However, it is still necessary to develop automatic technologies for recognizing concepts of depression drugs from biomedical literatures because of the quick development of depression-related studies and the constant appearance of new depression drugs. Furthermore, owing to various nomenclatures and a large number of abbreviations, the concept recognition of depression drugs cannot be effectively realized only using the existing text-based concept recognition technologies. Thus, this paper proposes a method of concept recognition based on the domain relevance measure (DRM) [6]. New independence assumptions and the domain relevance function are defined.

The rest of this paper is organized as follows. Section 2 discusses background and related work. Section 3 proposes a direct assumption based domain relevance measure for concept recognition of depression drugs. Experiments are presented in Sect. 4. Finally, Sect. 5 gives concluding remarks.

## 2   Background and Related Work

An ontology is a specification of a conceptualization [7] and concepts are its core contents. Recognizing concepts from texts, especially scientific literatures, is a key issue of ontology learning. Related methods can be divided into three types: dictionary-based, rule-based, and statistics and machine learning-based. Dictionary-based methods are faced with the problems of name collision and limited dictionary scope. Rule-based methods require much time to construct recognition rules. Hence, statistics and machine learning-based methods become research focuses.

The DRM is a kind of important statistics-based method for concept recognition. It is to calculate the domain relevance of candidate concepts based on the target domain corpus and the contrasting corpus, for recognizing domain concepts. Compared with machine learning-based methods, such as conditional random fields, support vector machine, neural networks [8–11], the DRM don't need a large number of train data and is fit for recognizing domain-specific concepts, such as depression drug names, gene names. Roberto Navigli et al. [6] proposed the DR-DC method which bound the domain relevance and domain consensus to calculate the weight of candidate concepts for recognizing domain concepts. Xing Jiang et al. [12] proposed the CRCTOL method which used the log-likelihood ratio to measure the domain relevance of candidate concepts based on the target domain corpus and the contrasting corpus. However, the independence assumptions of above methods are mainly based on the probability of occurrence of the candidate concept, which are decided by word frequencies of both the candidate concept and other concepts in texts. Hence, these methods have poor robustness properties and their results are greatly affected by the quality of texts.

Aiming the above deficiency, this paper proposes a new DRM-based method for concept recognition, called the direct assumption-based domain relevance measure (DA-DRM), in which new independence assumptions and the domain bias function are defined. The detail will be introduced in the following section.

## 3   The Direct Assumption Based Domain Relevance Measure for Concept Recognition of Depression Drugs

Figure 1 gives the technological framework of DA-DRM. As shown in this figure, the whole process of concept recognition includes two phases: generating candidate concepts and recognizing depression drug concepts.

### 3.1   Generating Candidate Concepts

The first phase is to extract candidate concepts from text sets by text analysis. Domain concepts are nouns or noun phrase with adjectives, adverbs and other modifiers [13]. Text analysis is just to perform part-of-speech (POS) tagging, syntactic parsing and lemmatization for constructing the parse tree of texts, and then choose candidate domain concepts based on the above rule of domain concepts.

Furthermore, three preprocessing operations are performed on candidate concepts. Firstly, adjectives, articles and other stop words are removed from obtained candidate concepts. Secondly, long candidate concepts are divided into the shorter concepts, such as dividing "amitriptyline treatment" into "amitriptyline". Lastly, the final candidate concept set is obtained by removing duplicate concepts.

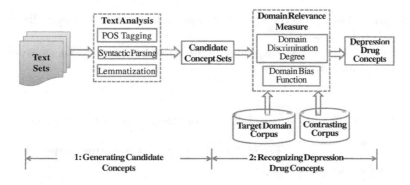

**Fig. 1.** The technological framework of DA-DRM.

## 3.2    Recognizing Depression Drug Concepts

The second phase is to calculate the domain relevance based on the target domain corpus and the contrasting corpus for recognizing depression drug concepts from candidate concepts. The target domain corpus consists of texts related to depression drugs and the contrasting corpus consists of texts not related to depression drugs. Thus, depression drug concepts can be recognized by choosing the candidate concepts which have the higher domain relevance with the target domain corpus. In this study, the domain relevance measure is performed by using the domain discrimination degree and the domain bias function.

**The Domain Discrimination Degree.** Referring to existing studies [6,12], the DA-DRM method adopts the log-likelihood ratio of independence assumptions to calculate the domain discrimination degree of candidate concepts between the target domain corpus and the contrasting corpus. Most of existing methods, such as CRCTOL [12], adopt the independence assumption "Suppose the probabilities of $t$'s occurrence in $A$ and $\bar{A}$ are $p_1$ and $p_2$, respectively". $A$ is the target domain corpus and $\bar{A}$ is the contrasting corpus. $p_1 = \frac{a}{a+c}$ where $a$ is the frequency of candidate concept $t$ in $A$ and $c$ is the frequency of other candidate concepts in $A$. $p_2 = \frac{b}{b+d}$ where $b$ is the frequency of candidate concept $t$ in $\bar{A}$ and $d$ is the frequency of other candidate concepts in $\bar{A}$. As stated above, such an independence assumption is decided by word frequencies of both the candidate concept and other concepts in texts, and has poor robustness properties. Thus, this paper defines the following new independence assumptions to calculate the domain discrimination degree of candidate concepts based on distribution proportions of word frequency.

Suppose the contingency table of word frequencies of a candidate concept $t$ is given in Table 1. Then, $p_1 = \frac{m}{m+n}$ is the distribution proportion of word frequency of $t$ in the target domain corpus $A$ and $p_2 = \frac{n}{m+n}$ is the distribution proportion of word frequency of $t$ in the contrasting corpus $\bar{A}$. In order to calculate the domain discrimination degree of $t$, two assumptions are given as follows:

- Assumption $Ass_1$: $t$ has the same distribution proportion $p$ of word frequency in $A$ and $\bar{A}$, i.e., $p = p_1 = p_2 = 50\%$.
- Assumption $Ass_2$: $t$ has the different distribution proportions of word frequency in $A$ and $\bar{A}$, i.e., $p_1 \neq p_2$.

**Table 1.** The contingency table of word frequencies of $t$ in $A$ and $\bar{A}$.

|  | Target domain corpus $A$ | Contrasting corpus $\bar{A}$ |
|---|---|---|
| Word frequency of $t$ | m | n |

The log-likelihood ratio can be used to measure the difference of possibility between two assumptions. Using the binomial distribution hypothesis, the log-likelihood ratio of above two assumptions can be calculated as follows (base 2):

$$\lambda_{TF}(t) = Log\frac{L(Ass_1)}{L(Ass_2)} = Log\frac{b(n; m+n, p)b(m; m+n, p)}{b(m; m+n, p_1)b(n; m+n, p_2)}$$

$$= Log\frac{p^m(1-p)^n p^n(1-p)^m}{p_1^m(1-p_1)^n p_2^n(1-p_2)^m}$$

$$= Log\frac{0.5^m(1-0.5)^n 0.5^n(1-0.5)^m}{(\frac{m}{m+n})^m(1-\frac{m}{m+n})^n(\frac{n}{m+n})^n(1-\frac{n}{m+n})^m}$$

The bigger value of $\lambda_{TF}(t)$ means the bigger possibility of $Ass_2$.

In the above formula, the domain discrimination degree of $t$ is calculated based on its word frequencies in $A$ and $\bar{A}$. The bigger occurrence number of $t$ in a corpus means that $t$ is more similar to the corpus. Referring to the DR-DC algorithm [6], the document frequency can also be used to calculate the domain discrimination degree. The more documents contain $t$ in a corpus means that $t$ is more similar to the corpus. Hence, the corresponding log-likelihood ratio can be calculated as follows (base 2):

$$\lambda_{DF}(t) = Log\frac{L(Ass_1')}{L(Ass_2')} = Log\frac{0.5^{m'}(1-0.5)^{n'} 0.5^{n'}(1-0.5)^{m'}}{(\frac{m'}{m'+n'})^{m'}(1-\frac{m'}{m'+n'})^{n'}(\frac{n'}{m'+n'})^{n'}(1-\frac{n}{m'+n'})^{m'}}$$

where $m'$ is the document frequency of $t$ in $A$, $n'$ is the document frequency of $t$ in $\bar{A}$, $p_1' = \frac{m'}{m'+n'}$ is the distribution proportion of document frequency of $t$ in $A$ and $p_2' = \frac{n'}{m'+n'}$ is the distribution proportion of document frequency of $t$ in $\bar{A}$.

Based on two types of log-likelihood ratios, the domain discrimination degree of $t$ can be calculated as follows:

$$DD_t = \beta \times \lambda_{TF}(t) + (1-\beta) \times \lambda_{DF}(t), 0 < \beta < 1;$$

The bigger value of $DD_t$ means that $t$ has higher discrimination degree between $A$ and $\bar{A}$.

**The Domain Bias Function.** The domain discrimination degree $DD_t$ is used to calculate the difference of domain relevance of $t$ between $A$ and $\bar{A}$. However, it cannot measure whether $t$ is more related to $A$ or $\bar{A}$. In order to recognize domain concepts, which are more related to $A$, the domain bias function is needed.

Candidate concepts include many noun phrases. According to the "head-modifier" principle stated in [14], main meanings of terms are represented by their head words. Hence, the independent variable of the domain bias function can adopt the domain ratio of head word $Drh = \frac{n_h}{m_h}, m_h > 0, n_h \geq 0$, in which $m_h$ and $n_h$ represent word frequencies of $t$ in $A$ and $\bar{A}$ respectively. Furthermore, in order to recognize domain concepts, the domain bias function should have the following characteristics:

- When $Drh \to 1$, word frequencies of $t$ in $A$ and $\bar{A}$ are similar. The relevance of $t$ to $A$ is very small and the value of the domain bias function is close to 0.
- When $Drh \to 0$, the word frequency of $t$ in $A$ is far bigger than in $\bar{A}$. The relevance of $t$ to $A$ is very big and the value of the domain bias function is close to 1.
- When $Drh$ increases between 0 and 1, The relevance of $t$ to $A$, i.e., the value of the domain bias function, decreases nonlinearly.

Based on the above characteristics, the domain bias function can be defined as follows:

$$CF(t) = e^{-\gamma * Drh * ln2}$$

in which $\gamma > 0$ is a regulating factor. Figure 2 describes the change of value of $CF(t)$.

**The Domain Relevance Measure.** Based on the domain discrimination degree and the domain bias function, the domain relevance measure (DRM) of $t$ can be calculated as follows:

$$DRM_t = DD_t * CF(t).$$

The bigger value of $DRM_t$ means that $t$ has the higher relevance to the target domain corpus. By defining a threshold, depression drug concepts can be recognized from candidate concepts.

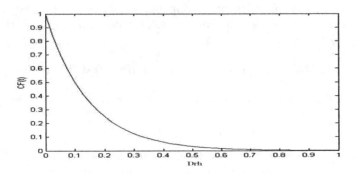

**Fig. 2.** The domain bias function.

## 4    Experiments

In this section, we assess the performance of our proposed method. All experiments were performed based on abstracts in PubMed and NSF (National Science Foundation, United States).

## 4.1    Data Sets

**The Target Domain Corpus.** Five thousands of depression related literature abstracts in PubMed were used to construct the target domain corpus. Each abstract includes a or several depression drug concepts of SNOMED CT which is the world's largest clinical terminology and provides broad coverage of clinical medicine, including findings, diseases, and procedures for use in electronic medical records [15].

**The Contrasting Corpus.** Four thousands of research abstracts in NSF and one thousand of literature abstracts in PubMed were used to construct the contrasting corpus. Abstracts in NSF involve with multiple research domains, including physics, mathematics, computer science, geology, biology, etc. Abstracts in PubMed are related to depression but don't include depression drug concepts.

**The Test Dataset.** The test dataset was constructed based on literature abstracts in PubMed. Five psychiatry related journals were selected as source journals, including "ActapsychiatricaScandinavica", "The Journal of clinical psychiatry", "Neuropharmacology", "European", and "Psychopharmacology". 500 literature abstracts were randomly extracted from these source journals, with the earliest publications dating to 2005, and the latest to 2007. Based on SNOMED CT, 34 depression drug concepts in these abstracts were recognized and annotated.

## 4.2    Experimental Results

Defining 0.001 as the threshold of DRM, 49 concepts can be extracted from the test dataset. Table 2 gives results of concept recognition. Values of DRM in this table were obtained by performing the normalization $DRM_i/DRM_{max}$, in which $DRM_{max}$ is the maximum value of $DRM$. There are 27 right concepts in Table 2. Thus, the accuracy rate is $P = 27/49 = 55.1\%$ and the recall rate is $R = 27/34 = 79.41\%$.

As shown in Table 2, three new concepts, i.e., venlafaxine XR, risperidone and buspirone, were recognized. Though they are not included in depression drug terms of SNOMED CT, proofs from the search engine can prove that they are depression related drug concepts. There are also three abbreviations, i.e., SSRI, IMI and DMI. Taking these new concepts and abbreviations into account, the accuracy rate is $P = 27 + 6/49 = 67.35\%$ and the recall rate is $R = 27/34 = 79.41\%$. Figure 3 gives a comparison between our proposed method and other previous studies. As shown in this figure, the proposed method greatly improves the accuracy rate and the recall rate compared with some existing similar methods.

**Table 2.** The extracted concept list.

| ID | Concept | DRM | Memo | ID | Concept | DRM | Memo |
|----|---------|-----|------|----|---------|-----|------|
| 1 | Fluoxetine | 1 | Right | 26 | ATYP | 0.163753 | Error |
| 2 | Citalopram | 0.97034 | Right | 27 | Escitalopram | 0.128901 | Right |
| 3 | Venlafaxine | 0.785515 | Right | 28 | ESS | 0.117978 | Error |
| 4 | Imipramine | 0.719399 | Right | 29 | Milnacipran | 0.114392 | Right |
| 5 | Paroxetine | 0.532477 | Right | 30 | SSRI | 0.11334 | Abbreviation |
| 6 | Amitriptyline | 0.427257 | Right | 31 | DDR | 0.11168 | Error |
| 7 | Sertraline | 0.419555 | Right | 32 | IMI | 0.107353 | Abbreviation |
| 8 | Reuptake | 0.387391 | Error | 33 | Maprotiline | 0.106194 | Right |
| 9 | Desipramine | 0.378649 | Right | 34 | MADRS | 0.084576 | Error |
| 10 | Olanzapine | 0.333844 | Right | 35 | Manic-depressive | 0.073185 | Error |
| 11 | Bupropion | 0.314916 | Right | 36 | Tryptophan | 0.071311 | Right |
| 12 | ADM | 0.281015 | Error | 37 | Multicenter | 0.069071 | Error |
| 13 | Mirtazapine | 0.272987 | Right | 38 | Amoxapine | 0.068702 | Right |
| 14 | Lithium | 0.259998 | Right | 39 | Cytochrome P450 | 0.062056 | Error |
| 15 | Fluvoxamine | 0.256762 | Right | 40 | Venlafaxine XR | 0.061323 | New concept |
| 16 | Clomipramine | 0.250431 | Right | 41 | Risperidone | 0.058759 | New concept |
| 17 | Manic | 0.249679 | Error | 42 | Phenelzine | 0.057994 | Right |
| 18 | Nefazodone | 0.232453 | Right | 43 | CBT | 0.052052 | Error |
| 19 | SRIs | 0.227553 | Error | 44 | tranylcypromine | 0.049944 | Right |
| 20 | Monoamines | 0.222114 | Error | 45 | Mania | 0.049059 | Error |
| 21 | Mianserin | 0.213747 | Right | 46 | CGI-S | 0.048643 | Error |
| 22 | Reboxetine | 0.203953 | Right | 47 | DMI | 0.048615 | Abbreviation |
| 23 | Trazodone | 0.189291 | Right | 48 | ESM | 0.048372 | Error |
| 24 | Nortriptyline | 0.179066 | Right | 49 | Buspirone | 0.047489 | New concept |
| 25 | Duloxetine | 0.175063 | Right | | | | |

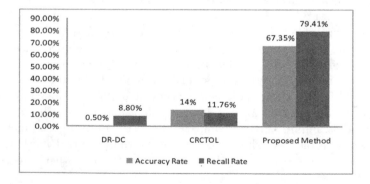

**Fig. 3.** A comparison between the proposed method and some previous studies.

# 5   Conclusions

Recognizing depression drug concepts from literatures is an important task for supporting systematic depression studies of BI. This paper proposes a new method of concept recognition based on the domain relevance measure. Compared with previous similar studies, such as CRCTOL, the proposed method provides the following advantages:

– defining new independence assumptions to decrease the influence of other concepts in texts and improve the robustness of method,
– adding the domain bias function to recognize domain concepts, which are more related to the target domain corpus.

The experimental results show that the proposed method not only has the higher accuracy rate and recall rate but also can recognize new concepts and abbreviation of depression drugs. Thus, it has the high practicability though term ontologies of depression drugs have been existed.

**Acknowledgments.** The work is supported by National Basic Research Program of China (2014CB744600), International Science & Technology Cooperation Program of China (2013DFA32180), National Natural Science Foundation of China (61272345), Research Supported by the CAS/SAFEA International Partnership Program for Creative Research Teams, Open Foundation of Key Laboratory of Multimedia and Intelligent Software (Beijing University of Technology), Beijing, the Japan Society for the Promotion of Science Grants-in-Aid for Scientific Research (25330270), and Support Center for Advanced Telecommunications Technology Research, Foundation (SCAT), Japan.

# References

1. Zhong, N.: Impending brain informatics research from web intelligence perspective. Int. J. Inf. Technol. Decis. Mak. **5**(4), 713–727 (2006)
2. Zhong, N., Liu, J., Yao, Y., Wu, J., Lu, S., Qin, Y., Li, K., Wah, B.W.: Conversational informatics where web intelligence meets brain informatics. In: Zhong, N., Liu, J., Yao, Y., Wu, J., Lu, S., Li, K. (eds.) WImBI 2006. LNCS, vol. 4845, pp. 1–31. Springer, Heidelberg (2006)
3. Zhong, N., Chen, J.H.: Constructing a new-style conceptual model of brain data for systematic brain informatics. IEEE Trans. Knowl. Data Eng. **24**(12), 2127–2142 (2012)
4. Li, M., Zhong, N., Lu, S.F., Wang, G., Feng, L., Hu, B.: Cognitive behavioral performance of untreated depressed patients with mild depressive symptoms. PLoS One, 05 January 2016. doi:10.1371/journal.pone.014635
5. Elkin, P.L., Brown, S.H., Husser, C.S., Bauer, B.A., Wahner-Roedler, D., Rosenbloom, S.T., Speroff, T.: Evaluation of the content coverage of SNOMED CT: ability of SNOMED clinical terms to represent clinical problem lists. In: Mayo Clinic Proceedings, vol. 81, no. 6, pp. 741–748 (2006)
6. Navigli, R., Velardi, P.: Learning domain ontologies from document warehouses and dedicated web sites. Comput. Linguist. **30**(2), 151–179 (2004)

 7. Gruber, T.: Towards principles for the design of ontologies used for knowledge sharing. Int. J. Hum.-Comput. Stud. **43**(5/6), 907–928 (1995)
 8. Hourali, M., Montazer, G.A.: A new approach for automating the ontology learning process using fuzzy theory and ART neural network. J. Convergence Inf. Technol. **6**(10), 24–32 (2011)
 9. Hai, D., Khadeer, H.F.: SOT: a semi-supervised ontology learning-based focused crawler. Concurrency Comput. Pract. Exp. **25**(12), 1755–1770 (2013)
10. Yang, L., Zhou, Y.H.: Exploring feature sets for two-phase biomedical named entity recognition using semi-CRFs. Knowl. Inf. Syst. **40**(2), 439–453 (2014)
11. Tang, B.Z., Feng, Y.D., Wang, X.L., Wu, Y.H., Zhang, Y.Y., Jiang, M., Wang, J.Q., Xu, H.: A comparison of conditional random fields and structured support vector machines for chemical entity recognition in biomedical literature. J. Cheminform. **7**(Suppl 1), S8 (2015)
12. Jiang, X., Tan, A.H.: CRCTOL: a semantic-based domain ontology learning system. J. Am. Soc. Inf. Sci. Technol. **61**(1), 150–168 (2010)
13. Ruiz-Martinez, J.M., Valencia-Garcia, R.: Ontology learning from biomedical natural language documents using UMLS. Expert Syst. Appl. **38**, 12365–12378 (2011)
14. Hippisley, A., Cheng, D., Ahmad, K.: The head-modifier principle and multilingual term extraction. Nat. Lang. Eng. **11**(02), 129–157 (2005)
15. Zhang, G.Q., Zhu, W., Sun, M.M., Tao, S.Q., Bodenreider, O., Cui, L.: MaPLE: a MapReduce pipeline for lattice-based evaluation and its application to SNOMED CT. In: Proceedings of the 2014 IEEE International Conference on Big Data (IEEE Big Data 2014), pp. 754–759 (2014)

# Brain Knowledge Graph Analysis
# Based on Complex Network Theory

Hongyin Zhu[1], Yi Zeng[1,2]([⊠]), Dongsheng Wang[1], and Bo Xu[1,2]

[1] Institute of Automation, Chinese Academy of Sciences, Beijing, China
{zhuhongyin2014,yi.zeng}@ia.ac.cn
[2] Center for Excellence in Brain Science and Intelligence Technology,
Chinese Academy of Sciences, Shanghai, China

**Abstract.** Domain knowledge about the brain is embedded in the literature over the whole scientific history. Researchers find there are intricate relationships among different cognitive functions, brain regions, brain diseases, neurons, protein, gene, neurotransmitters, etc. In order to integrate, synthesize, and analyze what we have known about the brain, the brain knowledge graph is constructed and released as part of the Linked Brain Data (LBD) project, to reveal the existing and potential relationships of brain related entities. However, there are some incorrect and missing relationships in the extracted relations, and researchers also cannot find the key topics overwhelmed in the massive relations. Some researchers analyze the properties of vertices based on the network topology, but they cannot verify and infer the potential relations. In order to address the above problems, we propose a framework which consists of 3 parts. Firstly, based on complex network theory, we adopt the embeddedness to verify the relations and infer the potential links. Secondly, we use the network topology of existing knowledge to build the self-relations graph. Finally, the structural holes theory from sociology is adopted to discover the key and core vertices in the whole brain knowledge graph and we recommend those topics to users. Compared with logic inference methods, our methods are lightweight and capable of processing large-scale knowledge efficiently. We test the results about relation verification and inference, and the result demonstrates the feasibility of our method.

**Keywords:** Complex network · Brain knowledge graph · Relation inference · Network analysis · Linked Brain Data

## 1 Introduction

There is a long history of the research on the brain from the perspectives of its cognitive functions, its building blocks, and related brain diseases, etc. Brain research is not only useful because it is highly related to answer the question of who we are, the understanding of the brain is also important for the development of Artificial Intelligence. There is massive known and unknown knowledge about the brain, while knowledge engineering can help to extract, organize, and

© Springer International Publishing AG 2016
G.A. Ascoli et al. (Eds.): BIH 2016, LNAI 9919, pp. 211–220, 2016.
DOI: 10.1007/978-3-319-47103-7_21

analyze these domain knowledge. Under this background, The Linked brain data (LBD) project is developed and the platform is released[1]. It's aim is to extract, synthesize, and analyze the data and knowledge about the brain from the World Wide Web [16]. However, it is inevitable that errors and missing relations exists in the LBD knowledge base. Besides, it is also hard to find the key topics which are overwhelmed in the enormous knowledge network.

Our work focuses on the network topology analysis to obtain new knowledge and new understandings based on the existing LBD brain knowledge graph. In [7], clustering coefficient is used to analyze the network topology of extracted information. In [8], graph theory based method is used to generate the document summarization. Their works mainly analyze the properties of vertices or relations according to their degrees. However, they cannot infer the potential links or verify the relations. Our contribution is the relation verification and inference based on the complex network theory.

In this paper, we propose a framework of analyzing brain knowledge graph by complex network theory. Firstly, the embeddedness is adopted to improve the accuracy of extracted relations and infer potential relations. Secondly, as an extension to the existing brain knowledge graph in Linked Brain Data, which focused on category inter-relationship, this paper extract category intra-relationship construction. Namely, the correlation of entities in the same categories (i.e. the category of cognitive functions, brain diseases, brain regions, neurons, proteins, genes, neurotransmitters). Finally, the structural holes theory [2] is adopted to find key topics for users.

## 2    Related Works

From the spatial perspective, domain knowledge on the brain is distributed around the world, such as different universities, laboratories and institutes, different literature sources, different databases. From the temporal perspective, they have been distributed almost in the whole history of Science. Although they are physically distributed, these knowledge on the brain are connected implicitly by nature, and they collectively provide a more comprehensive understanding of the brain. Nevertheless, the brain is still a mystery, and scientists are still on the way to provide a hologram of the brain. Most brain scientists focus on specific directions and scales for the investigation, and it is impractical for a brain scientist to know every scientific conclusion of existing brain research.

Under this background, the Linked Brain Data platform makes an effort to integrate and extract distributed knowledge on the brain and make a 10 million scale brain knowledge base accessible to all academic and industry communities. It integrates multi-source data and knowledge and links them semantically [16]. For the next stage, we not only plan to provide a brain knowledge graph that users could explore, but also want to provide domain knowledge based services (such as research recommendations).

---

[1] Linked Brain Data: http://www.linked-brain-data.org/.

For the relation verification, Liu et al. propose a method to verify "isa" relation based on specific features and rules [9], while the method is relation specific and cannot generalize to other relations. Zhang et al. propose an ontology based method to verify semantic relations, and their work needs a domain ontology and a vector space model [17]. Our paper proposes a model free method to verify the relations merely depending on the topology of the knowledge graph. As for the relation inference, Schoenmackers et al. propose a method to learn the inference rules from Web text [13]. Our method applies the existing topological structure to infer potential relations without rules. Currently, many efforts on recommender system focus on the adaptability to users [11]. Nevertheless, to the best of our knowledge, the work concerning recommending the key topics in the knowledge graph attracts little attention. Catanese et al. adopt the clustering coefficient to analyze the structural properties of Facebook Graph [4]. Here, we adopt clustering coefficient to find key topics in the brain knowledge graph.

## 3   Relation Verification and Inference

Since the domain knowledge is automatically extracted from scientific literatures, uncertainty are inevitable due to the reason that understanding of the brain may be inconsistent and the limitation of current automatic knowledge extraction techniques. The embeddedness [5] is the number of common neighbors of 2 vertices. The high embeddedness means high confidence, stability and consistency, and vice versa [1,6,12]. As for the knowledge graph, the relation confidence can be represented by embeddedness which also represents the strength or probability of a relationship.

The embeddedness of relations is calculated by Algorithm 1. Our first step is to find the corresponding entity pair according to the relation list in the knowledge graph. After getting the specific vectors, we can calculate their summation. If there is a common vertex, the corresponding element is 2 in the summation of the 2 vectors. For example, dementia is correlated with working memory. At the same time, the dementia is also correlated with white matter which is also correlated with working memory. So the white matter is the common vertex of the relation between dementia and working memory. It also means there is a triadic closure.

The higher the embeddedness value is, the stronger the binary relationship is. This method can support the correctness of the existing relations from a specific perspective. In addition, embeddedness can be used to infer currently unknown relations. More common vertices are available, more likely that a binary relation exists between the vertex pair. For example, based on the current brain knowledge graph in LBD, there is no direct relationship between the Zona incerta and the Lysine, but they have 36 common vertices, so the relationship between them may exist with a high probability. Hence, the method can support researchers to validate existing relations and predict unknown relationships.

We propose that we acquire new relations, the embeddedness calculation process is being carried out simultaneously as a supporting factor. We propose

**Algorithm 1.** Binary Relation Embeddedness Calculation Algorithm

---

**Require:** The adjacency matrix of vertices and the relation lists between those vertices
**Ensure:** The embeddedness of every vertices pair
  **procedure** CE($String[][]$ $matrix$,$List$ $relation$)
    **for** $i \leftarrow 0, relation.length - 1$ **do**
      $row[2]$=findRows($relation[i]$)
      **for** $j \leftarrow 1, relation.length - 1$ **do**
        $ele[j] = matrix[row[0]][j] + matrix[row[1]][j]$
      **end for**
      **for** $j \leftarrow 1, relation.length - 1$ **do**
        **if** $ele[j] > 1$ **then**
          $multi$++
        **else if** $ele[j] == 1$ **then**
          $single$++
        **end if**
        $emr = multi/(multi + single)$
      **end for**
    **end for**
  **end procedure**

---

this method as statistical topology inference (STI) which investigate on the probability of relations from a completely different perspective compared to logic inference. It transforms the topological properties of a graph into statistical features to infer the potential relations and support analysis on existing relations.

# 4 Category Intra-relationship Inference and Verification

For the previous version of the brain knowledge graph in Linked Brain Data, links are mainly established between entities in different categories, since for the first stage, we want to obtain relationships among different cognitive functions, brain diseases, and brain building blocks at multiple scales. However, links within the same category are also very important. For example, connections among different type of neurons are essential to understand the structural connectivity mechanism of the brain.

Category intra-relationship for cognitive functions (such as correlated relations of different cognitive functions) are also very important. Sometimes one kind of cognitive function does not play a separate role. Many cognitive functions serve as closely related building blocks to complex cognitive tasks. For example, Moscovitch et al. took the experiments to investigate on the relationship between long-term memory and episode memory in the same patient [10]. Now, by statistical topology inference, we may obtain possible relationships among different cognitive functions even before the experimental studies. Besides, possible correlated relations among brain diseases are also very important. This effort can be used to help doctors and medical researchers find potential relationships among different brain diseases to support their medical diagnosis and treatment.

# 5  Key Topics Discovery and Recommendation

Within the brain knowledge graph, some of the topics (domain terms) are essential from the topology point of view. The topology structure of a vertex can reflect its degree of importance compared to others. Here, we adopt the structural holes theory to find the key topics. Our method can find some topics located at a significant or special position of this knowledge graph.

In Sociology, there are some vertices with low embeddedness which are called structural holes [2,3]. The structural hole has many properties. For example, it is the connection vertex between several communities [2,3]. Based on its structural characteristic, the structural hole, the traffic hub of information, has higher power than other vertices. In the social network, the person, who is in the position of the structural hole, has a lot of interpersonal relations and becomes the key to communicating among several communities [2,3]. As for the knowledge graph, the structural holes are key concepts playing an important role in the connection of different local knowledge networks. In our experimental brain knowledge graph, there are only a few structural holes in the strict sense. In order to extend the result, we make some improvement to increase the number of candidates, and we can also get some vertices which are very similar with structural holes from topology perspective. When we increase the threshold of being a structural hole, the key vertices are more likely to show up.

Given the special position of structural holes in a network, their presence or disappearance will greatly affect the connectivity of the network. For example, it makes human more vulnerable to some extent that structural holes sometimes establish a shortcut for the diseases. It also reminds us of an effective way to eliminate the factors that can cause brain disease. Finding the structural holes would help people to prevent diseases with more explicit targets. If we removed the structural holes, a specific disease would only occur when several other conditions are satisfied together. Because we have already cut off this short path so that this disease only appears when it finds another complete pathway. It means that we can reduce the probability of a specific disease once we cut off the connectivity to structural holes. For example, the left fusiform gyrus correlated with various brain diseases and cognitive functions, as illustrated in Fig. 1(a). However, based on the partial knowledge graph, the semantic memory does not connect to brain diseases directly and it only connects to the left fusiform gyrus directly. If the semantic memory disorder symptom occurs in a patient, we may need to pay attention to the left fusiform gyrus, although it may be with no problem. The correlated vertices have the higher probability to be affected than those uncorrelated ones. If we take care of the left fusiform gyrus, we can predict or prevent the diseases, since based on the partial knowledge graph, semantic memory is not directly related to anorexia nervosa, amblyopia, etc. through the left fusiform gyrus, as shown in Fig. 1(a). It means paying special attention to these key vertices may can decrease the disease incidence, especially when the related vertices are starting lesion in patients.

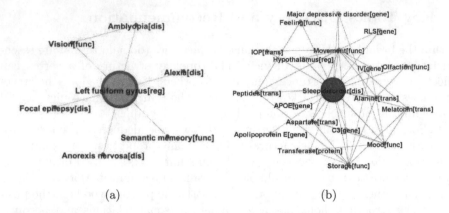

(a)                                                    (b)

**Fig. 1.** (a) An example of structural hole, Left fusiform gyrus, and its related nodes. (b) An example of core vertex, the Sleep disorder, which has more triadic closures and is topologically very different from the structural holes.

The formation of structural holes is decided by the existing knowledge graph, so the relationships in this area may have not been revealed completely by scientists. We adopt the Algorithm 2 to find the structural holes.

There is another kind of important vertices, core vertices, which have more triadic closures around and present a totally different characteristic with the structural holes. Those core vertices can be found by the clustering coefficient [15], as shown in Eq. (1). $c_i$ represents the clustering coefficient of vertex $i$. $t_i$ is the number of edges among the neighbors of vertex $i$, and $k_i$ is the number of its neighbors [14].

$$c_i = \frac{t_i}{C_{k_i}^2} \tag{1}$$

We adopt Algorithm 2 to calculate the clustering coefficient. Those vertices with the higher clustering coefficient are the core of stable communities which influence the whole network stability [15]. For example, the sleep disorder has many triadic closures around, as Fig. 1(b) shows. The sleep disorder has the capacity to form an intensive correlation with the surrounding vertices. This special structure characteristic represents special meaning to the whole structure. The key and core vertices can be recommended to the users.

## 6    Experiments

We take all the none duplicated correlated relations (265,946 relations) and related vertices (16,890) in Linked Brain Data to perform our experiments (The original data are brain related literature titles and abstracts from PubMed, ranging from the year 1874 to 2014). We take the above vertices and relations as seeds to generate 142,627,605 possible relations. In the relations, we found that 597,946

---

**Algorithm 2.** Calculating the clustering coefficient

---
**Require:** The adjacency matrix of vertices
**Ensure:** The structural holes and the clustering coefficient of every vertex
    **procedure** CLUS(*String*[][] *matrix*)
        **for** $row \leftarrow 1, matrix.length - 1$ **do**
            List<Integer> $li$ = findOnes($matrix[row]$)
            **for** $i \leftarrow 0, li.length - 1$ **do**
                initialize *indexList*
                **for** $j \leftarrow i + 1, li.length - 1$ **do**
                    $x = li.get(i)$
                    $y = li.get(j)$
                    $indexList$.add(combinationIndex($x$,$y$))
                **end for**
                clusteringCofficient(*indexList*)
            **end for**
        **end for**
    **end procedure**

---

relations have more than 20 common vertices in their neighbors between different categories and 602,389 relations in the same category, some examples are shown in Table 1. $S$ represents the number of the neighbors which only have one relationship with Entity 1 or Entity 2. The $EM$ represents the number of common vertices of a specific entity pair. The $EMR$ is the embedding ratio. The gene, reg, dis, protein, trans, func and neu represent the gene, brain regions, brain diseases, protein, neurotransmitters, cognitive functions and neurons respectively. When we sort relations by $EMR$ (with a threshold $EMR > 0.5$), there are only 8,250 relations between different categories and 204,345 relations without category limitation. The huge difference indicates that there are extensive relations in the same category and the portion of common vertices of many entity pairs is small.

In the existing relations, 155,729 relations have more than 20 common vertices. The cardinal number of common vertices can be very big, but the embedding ratio of most relations is less than 40 %. It implies that most of the neighbors are correlated with only one entity of the two entities in a specific relation pair. According to the various situation mentioned above, we design some rules to find the relations with both high cardinal number and embedding ratio. These relations are considered as the highly confident ones.

We randomly select 1000 verified relations about brain regions, brain diseases and cognitive functions from the extracted relations, and we manually check the correctness of them. Our experimental results show the verification precision is 95.3 % when we set the EM > 20. This method can filter some of the incorrect relations. As for the inferred relations, they are to some extent generated hypothesis, and we expect and invite Brain Scientists to investigate on these hypothesis

**Table 1.** Example relations and their corresponding parameters

| Entity1 | Entity2 | S | EM | EMR |
|---|---|---|---|---|
| Schizophrenia [dis] | Encoding [func] | 6672 | 1140 | 0.14592 |
| Atherosclerosis [dis] | Encoding [func] | 6534 | 865 | 0.11690 |
| CA2 [reg] | Encoding [func] | 6290 | 1226 | 0.16311 |
| Hippocampus [reg] | Movement [func] | 1798 | 616 | 0.25517 |

and verify them by biological experiments[2]. The above inference function can be considered as a novel way to find the potential links.

**Table 2.** Some examples of the inferred brain region correlations which are not extracted directly

| Entity1 | Entity2 | S | EM | EMR |
|---|---|---|---|---|
| CA2 [reg] | Hippocampus [reg] | 1391 | 737 | 0.34633 |
| Hypothalamus [reg] | CA2 [reg] | 1278 | 558 | 0.30392 |
| Cerebellum [reg] | Hippocampus [reg] | 1091 | 763 | 0.41154 |
| CA2 [reg] | CA1 [reg] | 1179 | 553 | 0.3192 |
| Hypothalamus [reg] | Forebrain [reg] | 810 | 469 | 0.36669 |

In the category intra-relation inference experiment, some examples of the inferred relations about brain regions are shown in Table 2. We randomly select 100 inferred relations between brain regions and manually check the correctness of them. The precision is currently 85 % when we set EM > 20.

**Table 3.** Examples of the key vertices in the brain knowledge graph

| Structural holes | Num |
|---|---|
| NO [protein] | 47 |
| GABA [protein] | 43 |
| Knowledge retrieval [func] | 7 |
| Core of nucleus accumbens [reg] | 7 |
| Barbiturate dependence [dis] | 5 |

**Table 4.** Some examples of the core vertices in the knowledge graph

| VERTICES | R | V | CC |
|---|---|---|---|
| Encoding [func] | 195765 | 7277 | 0.0074 |
| Movement [func] | 96921 | 1630 | 0.0730 |
| Alzheimer [dis] | 91519 | 1582 | 0.0732 |
| Schizophrenia [dis] | 68227 | 1675 | 0.0487 |

As for the topics discovery experiments, some examples of the key vertices are shown in Table 3 where *Num* denotes the number of neighbors of a specific vertex. Most of the key vertices have high value of *Num* and many relations with

---

[2] Inferred relationships can be accessed through Linked Brain Data.

their neighbor vertices. Some examples of the core vertices in the brain knowledge graph is shown in Table 4. $R$ represents the number of relationships with the neighbors of a corresponding vertex. $V$ represents the number of neighbor vertices. $CC$ is the value of the clustering coefficient. Some vertices with low $CC$ value but high $R$ value also can be considered as the core vertices since they also have many triadic closures. Finally, users can get some structurally important vertices and relations overwhelmed in the massive knowledge on the Brain.

# 7    Conclusion and Future Work

Based on complex network theories, we propose a framework to address the problems of relation verification, inference and key topics discovery on brain knowledge graph. Firstly, the verification and inference of relation extraction are investigated based on the embeddedness. We test our verified results based on the annotated data. The experimental results demonstrate the feasibility of our method. Secondly, we investigate on the category intra-relations and use embeddedness for verification. Finally, the discovery function of key and core topics is realized by the structural holes algorithm which is borrowed from sociology.

Our future work will consider extracting the specific types of the correlated relations in the brain knowledge graph. We will also invite brain scientists to verify the potential links that we generated based on the prediction model introduced in this paper.

**Acknowledgments.** This study was funded by the Strategic Priority Research Program of the Chinese Academy of Sciences (XDB02060007), and Beijing Municipal Commission of Science and Technology (Z151100000915070, Z161100000216124).

# References

1. Bearman, P.S., Moody, J.: Suicide and friendships among American adolescents. Am. J. Pub. Health **94**(1), 89–95 (2004)
2. Burt, R.S.: Structural holes and good ideas. Am. J. Sociol. **110**(2), 349–399 (2004)
3. Burt, R.S.: Structural Holes: The Social Structure of Competition. Harvard University Press, Cambridge (2009)
4. Catanese, S., Meo, P.D., Ferrara, E., Fiumara, G., Provetti, A.: Extraction and analysis of facebook friendship relations. In: Abraham, A. (ed.) Computational Social Networks, pp. 291–324. Springer, Berlin (2012)
5. Granovetter, M.: Economic action and social structure: the problem of embeddedness. Am. J. Sociol. **91**, 481–510 (1985)
6. Kossinets, G., Watts, D.J.: Empirical analysis of an evolving social network. Science **311**(5757), 88–90 (2006)
7. Li, X.: Graph-based learning for information systems. Ph.D. thesis, The University of Arizona (2009)
8. Li, Y., Cheng, K.: Single document summarization based on clustering coefficient and transitivity analysis. In: Proceedings of the 10th International Conference on Accomplishments in Electrical and Mechanical Engineering and Information Technology, pp. 26–28 (2011)

9. Liu, L., Zhang, S., Diao, L., Yan, S., Cao, C.: Automatic verification of "ISA" relations based on features. In: Proceedings of the Sixth International Conference on Fuzzy Systems and Knowledge Discovery, vol. 2, pp. 70–74. IEEE Press (2009)

10. Moscovitch, M., Nadel, L., Winocur, G., Gilboa, A., Rosenbaum, R.S.: The cognitive neuroscience of remote episodic, semantic and spatial memory. Curr. Opin. Neurobiol. **16**(2), 179–190 (2006)

11. Nanda, A., Omanwar, R., Deshpande, B.: Implicitly learning a user interest profile for personalization of web search using collaborative filtering. In: Proceedings of the 2014 IEEE/WIC/ACM International Joint Conferences on Web Intelligence (WI) and Intelligent Agent Technologies (IAT), vol. 2, pp. 54–62. IEEE (2014)

12. Rapoport, A.: Spread of information through a population with socio-structural bias: Iii. Suggested experimental procedures. Bull. Math. Biophys. **16**(1), 75–81 (1954)

13. Schoenmackers, S., Etzioni, O., Weld, D.S., Davis, J.: Learning first-order horn clauses from web text. In: Proceedings of the 2010 Conference on Empirical Methods in Natural Language Processing, pp. 1088–1098. Association for Computational Linguistics (2010)

14. Soffer, S.N., Vazquez, A.: Network clustering coefficient without degree-correlation biases. Phys. Rev. E **71**(5), 057101 (2005)

15. Watts, D.J., Strogatz, S.H.: Collective dynamics of 'small-world' networks. Nature **393**(6684), 440–442 (1998)

16. Zeng, Y., Wang, D., Zhang, T., Xu, B.: Linked neuron data (lnd): a platform for integrating and semantically linking neuroscience data and knowledge. In: Frontiers in Neuroinformatics. Conference Abstract: The 7th Neuroinformatics Congress (Neuroinformatics 2014), Leiden, The Netherlands, pp. 1–2 (2014)

17. Zhang, X., Chen, H., Ma, J., Tao, J.: Ontology based semantic relation verification for TCM semantic grid. In: Proceedings of 2009 Fourth ChinaGrid Annual Conference, pp. 185–191. IEEE Press (2009)

# Relation Inference and Type Identification Based on Brain Knowledge Graph

Hongyin Zhu[1], Yi Zeng[1,2(✉)], Dongsheng Wang[1], and Bo Xu[1,2]

[1] Chinese Academy of Sciences, Institute of Automation, Beijing, China
{zhuhongyin2014,yi.zeng}@ia.ac.cn
[2] Chinese Academy of Sciences,
Center for Excellence in Brain Science and Intelligence Technology, Shanghai, China

**Abstract.** Large-scale brain knowledge bases, such as Linked Brain Data, integrate and synthesize domain knowledge on the brain from various data sources. Although it is designed to provide comprehensive understanding of the brain from multiple perspectives and multi-scale, the correctness and specificity of the extracted knowledge is very important. In this paper, we propose a framework of relation inference and relation type identification to solve the upper problem. Firstly, we propose a quadrilateral closure method based on the network topology to verify and infer the binary relations. Secondly, we learn a model based on artificial neural network to predict the potential relations. Finally, we propose a model free method to identify the specific type of relations based on dependency parsing. We test our verified relations on the annotated data, and the result demonstrates a promising performance.

**Keywords:** Complex network · Knowledge graph · Relation inference · Neural network · Dependency parsing

## 1 Introduction

Findings of many brain research can be summarized as relations among cognitive functions, brain diseases, and brain building blocks at multiple scales (brain regions, neurons, proteins, genes, neurotransmitters). Automatic knowledge extraction and synthesis can help to organize knowledge about the brain covering the whole scientific history, and make use of them through various analysis methods [17,20]. Although creating a large scale brain knowledge base is essential, much efforts need to be paid to the correctness of extracted knowledge in the brain knowledge graph since the domain knowledge is used to assist user to understand the brain and support scientific research. As for relation extraction, the target sentences can be located according to the co-occurrence of interested entities [9], but it is hard to determine what kind of relations do the two entities have. In this paper, we propose a framework to address the above problems, and apply them to the brain knowledge graph in Linked Brain Data[1].

---

[1] Linked Brain Data: http://www.linked-brain-data.org.

© Springer International Publishing AG 2016
G.A. Ascoli et al. (Eds.): BIH 2016, LNAI 9919, pp. 221–230, 2016.
DOI: 10.1007/978-3-319-47103-7_22

Firstly, we propose a method based on the quadrilateral closure of the network topology to verify and infer the relations. Secondly, we adopt artificial neural network models to improve the performance of relation prediction. Finally, we propose a method to extract the type of relations between two related entities in a specific sentence. It is a model free method which takes the statistic and syntax feature into consideration, and it can identify the original expression of relations in sentences.

## 2     Related Works

The Linked Brain Data (LBD) platform integrates multi-source data on brain science to support scientists accessing the brain knowledge in a more comprehensive way [20]. By using knowledge extraction, representation, and integration techniques, it provides a multi-scale association graph on the relationships among brain regions, neurons, protein, genes, neurotransmitters, cognitive functions, and various brain diseases. In order to increase the quality of the domain knowledge, all the extracted knowledge need to be verified. Liu et al. [14] proposes a method to verify the "isa" relation, but the proposed method is relation specific. Grigni et al. propose topological inference [8], and the method is designed to infer specific types of relation for geographical databases. Our method merely depends on the network topology structure.

The Brain Association Graph highlights to correlated relations among various domain terms related to the Brain, while many users may prefer to have more specific types for these domain knowledge. So it is necessary to extract relation types from the sentences. However, it is hard to summarize all the possible knowledge manually. Culotta et al. adopt the dependency tree kernel methods [5], and Zeng et al. use the convolutional deep neural network [19] to classify the relation types. However, many labeled training data and tedious work for predefining the relation categories are still needed. We propose a model free method to extract relations without predefined relation categories so that we can retain the original relation expression to the most extent.

## 3     The Indirect Statistical Topology Inference Method

In [21], we adopt the number of common vertices of a vertex pair to assess the probability of their relation. It is based on a sociology theory that two persons are more likely to become friends when they have more common friends [11,16]. Due to the current stage for research on the brain, it is impossible to establish all the knowledge about the brain, and the brain knowledge graph is clearly incomplete. We may miss lots of information merely depending on the common vertices algorithm. In order to solve the data sparsity problem, we propose a method to extend the inference and verification capacity.

In social network research, Easley et al. point out the possibility of two persons become friends even they do not have the same neighborhood friends (and their data show that some of their neighborhood friends are friends to each other) [6]. With this observation as a support, we hypothesize two persons have higher possibility to become friends when their distinct friends from two sides respectively have dense relations with each other. We introduce this idea to the investigation of knowledge graph, and we hypothesize there is a higher probability of the relation between two vertices when their distinct neighbors have dense relations. We propose this method as indirect statistical topology inference (ISTI) which uses the indirectly related network topology and statistical information to infer the missing knowledge.

In [18], the clustering coefficient is adopted to calculate how well connected are the neighbors of a vertex in a graph, as shown in Eq. (1). $k_i$ is the degree of a vertex and $t_i$ is the number of edges among its neighbors [18]. Based on it, we propose a method to calculate clustering coefficient of a relation. As shown in Eq. (2), $k_{ij}$ is the number of vertices connected with the vertex pair ($i$ and $j$) and $t_{ij}$ is the number of edges among its neighbors. After getting the experimental result, we find merely calculating the clustering coefficient of a relation is not adequate for ISTI, because some of the relations only come from the neighbor set of one vertex. For example, the set of friend of person $A$ has very dense relations while the set of friend of B has not, but the clustering coefficient of this vertex pair is high. In order to solve the imbalance of single side relations, we add another factor to calculate the relations spanning two sets. As shown in Fig. 1, the adjacency matrix represents the whole structure of the knowledge graph. The sub matrix represents the relations in the neighbors of a relation, and the span matrix represents the relations spanning two sets. In Eq. (3), $s_{ij}$ is the number of edges spanning two groups of neighbors. For example, as shown in Fig. 2, Schizophrenia and Left planum temporale just have 4 common vertices which is relatively a low value, but the neighbor vertices of the Left planum temperate has 1730 connections with the neighbor vertices of the Schizophrenia. In this case, we feel more confident to ensure the relation between the two vertices.

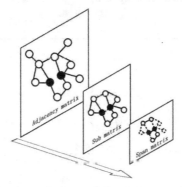

**Fig. 1.** The relations among the adjacency matrix, sub matrix and span matrix of network topology where the black circles represent the central vertex pair

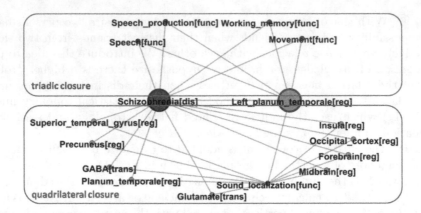

**Fig. 2.** An example of the verified relation between the Left planum temporale and Schizophreria

---

**Algorithm 1.** Calculating the span and sub matrix

---

**Require:** The adjacency matrix of entities and relation list
**Ensure:** The submatrix, spanmatrix and relation clustering coefficient
  **procedure** SPAN($String[][]\ matrix, List\ relation$)
    initialize $subList, spanList1, spanList2$
    **for** $i \leftarrow 0, relation.length - 1$ **do**
      $(x, y) = $ findRows($relation.get(i)$)
      $sublist$.add($x, y$)
      $sublist1 = $ findNeighbors($x$)
      $sublist2 = $ findNeighbors($y$)
      $spanlist1 = $ removeUnspanedEle($sublist, sublist1$)
      $spanlist2 = $ removeUnspanedEle($sublist, sublist2$)
      generateSubMat($matrix, submatrix, sublist$)
      calculatePairClustering($submatrix$)($submatrix$)
      calculateSpan($spanlist1, spanlist2$)
    **end for**
  **end procedure**

---

$$c_i = \frac{t_i}{C_{k_i}^2} \tag{1}$$

$$c_{ij} = \frac{t_{ij}}{C_{k_{ij}}^2} \tag{2}$$

$$c'_{ij} = \frac{s_{ij}}{C_{k_{ij}}^2} \tag{3}$$

If we merely adopted common vertices approach, this relation would be regarded as an unconfident one. As demonstrated in Algorithm 1, we first find the sub matrix which consists of the neighbors of a specific relation, and in terms of the topology structure of the whole group, we can identify those relations spanning two sub groups. After adopting the ISTI, we can find some knowledge missed by the common vertices based inference. In fact, the ISTI is based on the quadrilateral closure where the relations form a quadrilateral relations in the complex network.

## 4    The Neural Network Prediction Model

As mentioned above, we can verify and infer the relations according to the whole graph topology. However, the strengths of the existing relations are various. According to [7,15], we hypothesize the more frequent relations represent the stronger ties. If two vertices, B and C, both have strong ties to A, then B and C have high possibility to have a relation with each other [7]. The relation strength becomes a considerable problem, so we apply the above theory to the knowledge graph. We first adopt the neural network to learn a model of triadic closure in our knowledge graph where the frequency represents the probability of the potential relation to some extent. According to [2], the neural network has strong capacity to fit linear and nonlinear problems. However, the input dimensions are various to different relations, so we add a pre-processing module before putting data to the neural network.

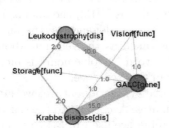

**Fig. 3.** An example of relation inference between the Leukodystrophy and Krabbe disease based on the neural network model

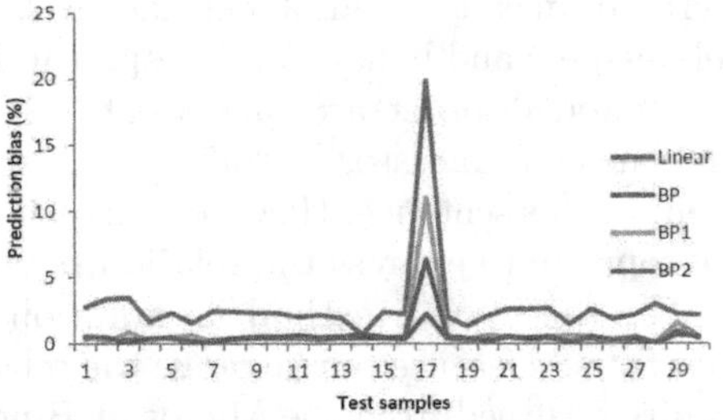

**Fig. 4.** The comparative study of prediction results with different methods

We apply this model to infer the potential relations. For example, the Krabbe disease and Leukodystrophy is not connected directly in this graph. However, according to [12], the Globoid Cell Leukodystrophy (GLD) is also known as Krabbe disease. It means the above two diseases are very closely related. As shown in Fig. 3, these two diseases just have two common vertices, but their connections with the GALC are very strong (the labels on the edges represent the co-occurrence frequency of two vertices).

## 5    Type Identification for Open Relation Extraction

Since the brain knowledge graph contains various domain terms, and the type of relations among them cannot be completely predefined. This is an open relation extraction problem without predefined relation categories [1]. We want to extract relations from the scientific literatures directly without manually predefined relation categories to realize the maximum retention of the original information. We adopt Stanford dependency parser to find the dependency path [4]. Compared with the work in [3], we take the dependency direction into consideration so that we can find the high level ancestor nodes in the dependency tree.

Generally, many entity pairs have more than one common ancestor nodes. We propose three methods to select a representative word. The first method, named as nearest ancestor method, only considers the ranking of common ancestors in the dependency parsing tree, and the lowest ancestor is the candidate to be chosen. For example, in the sentence "Some familial Alzheimer's disease (AD) cases are caused by rare and highly-penetrant mutations in APP, PSEN1, and PSEN2." [10], for a binary relation, the target entities are Alzheimer's disease and APP, and the relation type "caused" is identified correctly. However, sometimes the first method fails. For example, in the sentence "The involvement of adenosine in the pathophysiology of mood disorders was first proposed when increases in endogenous adenosine levels led to behaviour consistent with learned helplessness and behavioural despair in laboratory animals." [13], the adenosine and mood disorder are target entities. According to the dependency parsing, their nearest ancestor is "of", so the word "of" is taken as the relation about them in this sentence. However, instead of "of", the word "involvement" is more appropriate to express the relation between them in this sentence.

For the second method, in addition to the above syntactic feature, we add the statistic feature to rearrange the relation candidates. According to the search results returned from the Microsoft Bing search engine, we use Eq. (4) to calculate a score for the ranking.

$$score = P(o|s, p_r) \times P(s|p_r, o) \tag{4}$$

$$score = \frac{t - r}{t} P(o|s, p_r) \times P(s|p_r, o) \tag{5}$$

As shown in Eqs. (4) and (5), $s$ and $o$ represent the subject and object respectively. $t$ represents the total number of relation candidates. The $r$ represents the initial ranking in the set, and $p_r$ represents the member with the corresponding ranking.

The third method is based on Eq. (5). The ranking information is a penalty term, and the top ranked members have the priority to get a high score. The *score* represents the score of a candidate word. After they are ranked according to the score, the first member, with the highest score, can be considered as the relation. The triple <adenosine, involvement, mood disorder> is what exactly the above example describes. Compared with the first method, this method introduces some statistic features to adjust the ranking of candidates. However, it does not take the syntax structure into consideration, which leads to the lost of syntax features. We find if we use Eq. (5) to increase the weight of closer ancestor node, the result can reflect information from both statistical and syntactical perspectives. Finally, we combine the above three methods to extract the words which represent the relation types among the two vertices in the sentences.

## 6 Experiment

### 6.1 The ISTI Experiment

The experimental data consists of 16,890 vertices and 265,946 relations. We use them as seeds to generate 142,627,605 possible relations. We set 1,000 edges as the threshold to filter out the relations with low credibility. As shown in Table 1, *Relation* represents the number of edges among the neighborhood vertices of an entity pair. *Span* means the relations spanning two groups of neighbors. $E2$ and $E3$ denote the results calculated by Eqs. (2) and (3) respectively.

**Table 1.** Some examples of the entity pairs and their parameters

| Entity1 | Entity2 | Relation | Span | E2 | E3 |
|---------|---------|----------|------|----|----|
| Movement [function] | CA2 [region] | 145727 | 185842 | 0.0485 | 0.0618 |
| Alzheimer [disease] | CA2 [region] | 139024 | 182551 | 0.0482 | 0.0633 |
| Alzheimer [disease] | Storage [function] | 131850 | 181436 | 0.0552 | 0.0759 |

We randomly select 100 verified relations from existing relations about brain regions, brain diseases and cognitive functions, and we manually check the above samples. The method of Eq. (2) has the precision 80 %, and the method of Eq. (3) get the precision 88 %. Using the number of spanning relations can get the best performance, namely, with the precision of 93 %. The reason for Eq. (3) not getting the best result is that the existing relations are not complete in the brain knowledge graph. The ratio of spanning relations cannot work well in a sparse network.

### 6.2 The Neural Network Prediction Experiment

We adopt the multilayer perceptron (MLP) with 3 hidden layers and sigmoid function, and we earn the average deviation 2.01 % without considering the data organization factor. In our experiments, different formats of the input data cause different results with the same method, and we compare 3 kinds of input formats in the pre-processing modules, as shown in Fig. 5. According to the experimental result, dividing the data into the different part is beneficial for the generalization of the neural network model, especially for avoiding the significant deviation. As demonstrated in Fig. 4, $BP1$ and $BP2$ represent the input data follows different

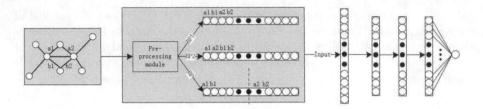

**Fig. 5.** The pre-processing module and the neural network in our method

mixed forms, while $BP$ represents the data divided as follows. We divide the input nodes into two symmetrical groups where the first group is used to receive one edge of every triadic closure with the same common edge. It divides the input area into two parts corresponding to the two edges of each triadic closure. The result shows the average deviation of the neural network is 1.44 %, better than multi-linear regression (3.64 %). We randomly select 30 test samples with the above model, as shown in Fig. 4. According to the results, we found that the performance of the neural network can be changed by changing the organization form of input data. It can improve the performance of prediction that the fixed input nodes are used to receive the fixed attribute data.

### 6.3    The Type Identification Experiment

The extracted predicate candidates are ranked according to the score, the candidate which has the highest score, can be considered as the relation to be chosen. Table 2 shows the results by merely considering the syntactic ranking information. As shown in Table 3, $E4$ represents the results after ranking according to Eq. (4). As illustrated in Table 3, for $E5$, We use Eq. (5) to increase the weight of ancestor nodes in lower levels, and the result can reflect information from both statistical and syntactical perspectives. We randomly select 100 sentences where the portion of the correct relations are 23 %, 25 % and 42 % by the nearest ancestor, Eqs. (4) and (5) respectively.

**Table 2.** The extracted candidates based on the nearest ancestor method

| Subject | Predicate | Candidates | Object |
|---|---|---|---|
| Tyrosine | Affect | Affect; show; expand | Prion disease |
| Adenosine | Of | Of; involvement; proposed | Mood disorder |
| APP | Caused | Caused | Alzheimer |
| Nitric Oxide | Leads | Leads; suggest; | Brain edema |
| Olfactory Nerve | Contain | Contain | Photoreceptor cell |

**Table 3.** The extracted candidates based on Eqs. (4) and (5)

| Subject | E4 | E5 | Object |
|---|---|---|---|
| Tyrosine | Affect; expand; show | Affect; show; expand | Prion disease |
| Adenosine | Involvement; proposed; of | Involvement; of; proposed | Mood disorder |
| APP | Caused | Caused | Alzheimer |
| Nitric Oxide | Suggest; leads | Leads; suggest | Brain edema |
| Olfactory Nerve | Contain | Contain | Photoreceptor cell |

## 7    Conclusion and Future Work

This paper proposes a framework to solve the problems of relation verification, inference and relation type identification. Firstly, we propose a method based on the quadrilateral closure to verify and infer the relations of the brain knowledge graph. Secondly, we adopt the neural network to learn a model to infer relations. Finally, we propose a model free method to extract the relations from natural language sentences without predefined relation types. In order to make the relation type representation more consistent, in the future, we will investigate on unsupervised methods to classify the extracted original relations into automatically generated categories.

**Acknowledgment.** This study was funded by the Strategic Priority Research Program of the Chinese Academy of Sciences (XDB02060007), and Beijing Municipal Commission of Science and Technology (Z151100000915070, Z161100000216124).

## References

1. Banko, M., Cafarella, M.J., Soderland, S., Broadhead, M., Etzioni, O.: Open information extraction from the web. In: Proceedings of the 20th International Joint Conference on Artificial Intelligence, vol. 7, pp. 2670–2676 (2007)
2. Beale, M.H., Hagan, M.T., Demuth, H.B.: Neural Network Toolbox 7 User's Guide. MathWorks Inc., Natick (2010)
3. Bunescu, R.C., Mooney, R.J.: A shortest path dependency kernel for relation extraction. In: Proceedings of the Conference on Human Language Technology and Empirical Methods in Natural Language Processing, pp. 724–731. Association for Computational Linguistics (2005)
4. Chen, D., Manning, C.D.: A fast and accurate dependency parser using neural networks. In: Proceedings of the 2014 Conference on Empirical Methods in Natural Language Processing, pp. 740–750. Association for Computational Linguistics (2014)
5. Culotta, A., Sorensen, J.: Dependency tree kernels for relation extraction. In: Proceedings of the 42nd Annual Meeting on Association for Computational Linguistics, p. 423. Association for Computational Linguistics (2004)
6. Easley, D., Kleinberg, J.: Strong and weak ties. In: Networks, Crowds, and Markets: Reasoning About a Highly Connected World, pp. 47–84. Cambridge University Press (2010)

7. Granovetter, M.S.: The strength of weak ties. Am. J. Sociol. **78**, 1360–1380 (1973)
8. Grigni, M., Papadias, D., Papadimitriou, C.: Topological inference. In: Proceedings of the 14th International Joint Conference on Artificial Intelligence, pp. 901–907 (1995)
9. Hasegawa, T., Sekine, S., Grishman, R.: Discovering relations among named entities from large corpora. In: Proceedings of the 42nd Annual Meeting on Association for Computational Linguistics, p. 415. Association for Computational Linguistics (2004)
10. Jin, S.C., Pastor, P., Cooper, B., Cervantes, S., Benitez, B.A., Razquin, C., Goate, A., Cruchaga, C.: Pooled-DNA sequencing identifies novel causative variants in PSEN1, GRN and MAPT in a clinical early-onset and familial Alzheimer's disease ibero-American cohort. Alzheimer's Res. Ther. **4**(4), 1 (2012)
11. Kossinets, G., Watts, D.J.: Empirical analysis of an evolving social network. Science **311**(5757), 88–90 (2006)
12. Lee, W.C., Kang, D., Causevic, E., Herdt, A.R., Eckman, E.A., Eckman, C.B.: Molecular characterization of mutations that cause globoid cell leukodystrophy and pharmacological rescue using small molecule chemical chaperones. J. Neurosci. **30**(16), 5489–5497 (2010)
13. Lieshout, R.J.V., MacQueen, G.: Psychological factors in asthma. Allergy Asthma Clin. Immunol. **4**(1), 1 (2008)
14. Liu, L., Zhang, S., Diao, L., Yan, S., Cao, C.: Automatic verification of "isa" relations based on features. In: Proceedings of the Sixth International Conference on Fuzzy Systems and Knowledge Discovery, vol. 2, pp. 70–74. IEEE Press (2009)
15. Newcomb, T.M.: An approach to the study of communicative acts. Psychol. Rev. **60**(6), 393–404 (1953)
16. Rapoport, A.: Spread of information through a population with socio-structural bias: Iii. Suggested experimental procedures. Bullet. Math. Biophys. **16**(1), 75–81 (1954)
17. Richardet, R., Chappelier, J.C., Telefont, M., Hill, S.: Large-scale extraction of brain connectivity from the neuroscientific literature. Bioinformatics **31**(10), 1640–1647 (2015)
18. Soffer, S.N., Vazquez, A.: Network clustering coefficient without degree-correlation biases. Phys. Rev. E **71**(5), 057101 (2005)
19. Zeng, D., Liu, K., Lai, S., Zhou, G., Zhao, J.: Relation classification via convolutional deep neural network. In: Proceedings of the 25th International Conference on Computational Linguistics, pp. 2335–2344 (2014)
20. Zeng, Y., Wang, D., Zhang, T., Xu, B.: Linked neuron data (lnd): a platform for integrating and semantically linking neuroscience data and knowledge. In: Frontiers in Neuroinformatics. Conference Abstract: The 7th Neuroinformatics Congress (Neuroinformatics 2014), Leiden, the Netherlands (2014)
21. Zhu, H., Zeng, Y., Wang, D., Xu, B.: Brain knowledge graph analysis based on complex network theory. In: Selvaraj, R., Meyer, V. (eds.) BIH 2016. LNAI, vol. 9919, pp. 211–220. Springer, Berlin (2016)

# New Methodologies for Brain and Mental Health

# A Simple Distance Based Seizure Onset Detection Algorithm Using Common Spatial Patterns

Sina Khanmohammadi[1]($\boxtimes$) and Chun-An Chou[2]

[1] Department of Systems Science and Industrial Engineering,
State University of New York at Binghamton, Binghamton, NY 13902, USA
skhanmo1@binghamton.edu
[2] Mechanical and Industrial Engineering, Northeastern University, Boston, USA
ch.chou@northeastern.edu

**Abstract.** Existing seizure onset detection methods usually rely on a large number of extracted features regardless of computational efficiency, which reduces their applicability for real-time seizure detection. In this study, a simple distance based seizure onset detection algorithm is proposed to distinguish seizure and non-seizure EEG signals. The proposed framework first applies the common spatial patterns (CSP) method to enhance the signal-to-noise ratio and reduce the dimensionality of EEG signals, and then uses the autocorrelation of the averaged spatially filtered signal to classify incoming signals into a seizure or non-seizure state. The proposed approach was tested using CHB-MIT dataset that contains continuous scalp EEG recordings from 23 patients. The results showed ~95.87 % sensitivity with an average latency of 2.98 s and 2.89 % false detection rate. More interestingly, the average process time required to classify each window (1–5 s of EEG signals) was 0.09 s. The outcome of this study has a high potential to improve the automatic seizure onset detection from EEG recordings and could be used as a basis for developing real-time monitoring systems for epileptic patients.

**Keywords:** Epilepsy · Seizure onset detection · Common spatial patterns · Anamoly detection

## 1 Introduction

Epilepsy is the second most common neurological disorder that affects approximately 70 million people in different age groups (1 % of world population) [1]. Epilepsy is characterized by recurrent seizure onsets described as the sudden brief excessive electrical discharge of neurons. The seizure onset is generally detected by visual inspection of the Electroencephalogram (EEG) recordings of epileptic patients. However, this task is time-consuming, prone to human error, and subject to availability of expert neurophysiologist who can interpret the EEG signals. Therefore, efficient automated real-time seizure detection is necessary to improve

© Springer International Publishing AG 2016
G.A. Ascoli et al. (Eds.): BIH 2016, LNAI 9919, pp. 233–242, 2016.
DOI: 10.1007/978-3-319-47103-7_23

the quality of life for epileptic patients. There is a significant amount of research regarding automatic seizure detection from EEG signals. Many algorithms have been proposed in the literature (for a survey of current methods readers can refer to [2–6]). The proposed seizure detection methods can be grouped into seizure onset detection (with the objective of minimizing detection latency) and seizure event detection (with the aim of maximizing the sensitivity). Nevertheless, most of these methods suffer from the computational burden and are not suitable for real-time seizure detection (online seizure detection). Hence, there is considerable interest in developing online seizure detection methods that could provide satisfactory performance using the minimum amount of computational power [7].

In this regard, many dimensionality reduction methods such as Principal Component Analysis (PCA), Singular Value Decomposition (SVD), and Independent Component Analysis (ICA) have been used in seizure onset detection literature [8–10]. However, the applications of common spatial patterns (CSP) for seizure onset detection is less explored. CSP is a mathematical procedure that separates multivariate signals into additive subcomponents that have the maximum difference of variance between different classes. To the best of our knowledge, the seizure onset detection methods that take advantage of CSP are limited to Alotaiby and his colleagues work [11], which combines CSP and SVM to detect seizure onset from scalp EEG signals, and Qaraqe and her team's work [12], which uses CSP as a feature enhancement step to improve the extracted energy features. These two methods proposed in the literature are based on support vector machines that require a large number of features to classify a EEG signals into a seizure or non-seizure state. Extracting and processing large feature space increases the computational time and decreases the applicability of these methods for real-time classification. Furthermore, these methods have been only tested on a limited number of subjects which makes it hard to validate their generalizability.

In this paper, we propose a simple distance based seizure onset detection framework to classify signals into a seizure and non-seizure state. First, the signal is decomposed into one of the well-known frequency bands of $(\delta, \theta, \alpha, \beta)$, and then, CSP algorithm is applied to reduce the dimensionality of data. Next, the autocorrelation of the averaged spatially filtered signal (CSP results) at zero-lag/fs is used to classify signals in a sliding window into a seizure and non-seizure state. The main advantage of the proposed algorithm is its low computational cost and simplicity, which makes it ideal for real-time seizure onset detection using EEG signals.

## 2    Methodology

The overall framework (shown in Fig. 1) consists of three steps including data preprocessing, feature extraction, and classification. The details of each step are provided in the following sections:

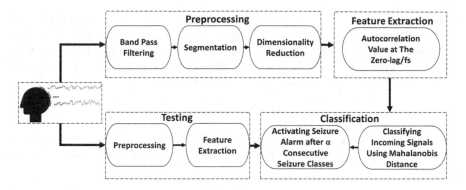

**Fig. 1.** Overview of the proposed distance based seizure onset detection framework.

## 2.1 Data Preprocessing

**Band Pass Filtering.** The first step of the proposed method includes bandpass filtering the EEG signal into one of the four broad sub-bands that have been proven to provide useful information for clinical applications. The four sub-bands include Delta (0–4 Hz), Theta (4–8 Hz), Alpha (8–16 Hz), and Beta (16–32 Hz). In this study, a third order Butterworth IIR filter is employed to filter the signal into one of the four predefined sub-bands. The frequency response of the Butterworth filter is given by [13]:

$$P_{LR}(\omega) = 1 + \frac{1}{\Delta^2}(\frac{\omega}{\omega_0} - \frac{\omega_0}{\omega})^2 \tag{1}$$

$$\Delta = \frac{\omega_2 - \omega_1}{\omega_0}, \tag{2}$$

where $\omega_1$ is the lower cut-off frequency, $\omega_2$ is the upper cut-off frequency, and $\omega_0$ is the center frequency.

**Signal Segmentation.** A baseline of seizure and non-seizure signals for each patient is required to calculate the CSP weights (details provided in the following section). Therefore, the seizure epochs and the comparative non-seizure epochs with the same length are extracted from EEG recordings of each subject. At the end of this step, two three-dimensional matrices of $A = (a_{ijk})$ and $B = (b_{ijk})$ are obtained for each subject, where $i = 1, ..., M$, $j = 1, ..., N$, and $k = 1, ..., P$. Here $M$ is the total number of time points, $N$ is the total number of channels, and $P$ is the total number of seizure epochs for one of the subjects. The elements of matrices $A$ and $B$ represent EEG signal values in the seizure and non-seizure states, respectively.

**Dimensionality Reduction and Spatial Filtering.** CSP is a method that transforms the data such that the difference of variance in two groups of data is maximized. More specifically, CSP identifies a weight matrix ($W$) by simultaneously diagonalizing the covariance matrices of two groups of data ($\Sigma_{x|c_1}$ and $\Sigma_{x|c_2}$). The CSP transformation can be summarized as:

$$CSP(X) = W^T X, \tag{3}$$

where $X$ is the input signal and $W$ is the CSP weight matrix (also know as spatial filter matrix). $W$ can be calculated by solving the following optimization problem:

$$W^* = arg \max_{W \in R^N} \left\{ \frac{W^T \Sigma_{x|c_1} W}{W^T \Sigma_{x|c_2} W} \right\} \tag{4}$$

As Eq. 4 corresponds to the well-known Rayleigh quotient, the solution of this optimization problem can be obtained by solving a generalized eigenvalue problem as:

$$\Sigma_{x|c_1} W = \lambda \Sigma_{x|c_2} W \tag{5}$$

The calculated eigenvectors correspond to CSP weights (spatial filters), and the eigenvalues represent the quality of the calculated spatial filters (the ratio of variance between two classes of data). In practice, the top $q$ eigenvectors corresponding to smallest/largest eigenvalues are selected as the CSP weights. Hence, CSP can also be used to reduce the dimensionality of data to $q$ dimensions.

### 2.2   Feature Extraction

Countless EEG signal features have been proposed for online seizure onset detection [14,15]. However in this study we have used one of the less explored EEG features (autocorrelation), which has been shown to be effective for seizure onset detection [16]. The rationale behind using autocorrelation is that the number and height of peaks of the autocorrelation function could differ in seizure and non-seizure states [17]. Hence, after spatially filtering and reducing the dimension of data, we first take average of the EEG signals across all the remaining channels and then calculate the autocorrelation of averaged signal $X$ by:

$$R(X) = \sum_{i=0}^{M-L-1} x_i^* x_{(l+i)}, \tag{6}$$

where $i$ is the time index (rows of $X$), $L$ is the maximum lag, and $*$ denotes the complex conjugate (Not to be confused with optimal value notation in Eq. 4). In this study, we have used the autocorrelation value at zero-lag/fs as our feature value. Figure 2, represents the extracted features for one of the subjects in CHB-MIT dataset. As it can be seen in the figure the autocorrelation at zero-lag/fs significantly differs between the seizure ($Y = +1$) and non-seizure states ($Y = -1$).

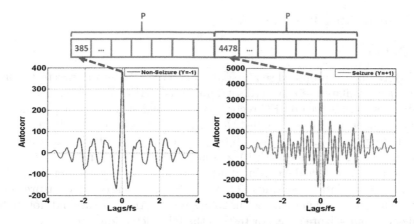

**Fig. 2.** Illustration of the feature extraction method used in this study.

Recalling that we have a total of $P$ seizure epochs for one subject, the output of feature extraction is a vector of length $2P$, where the first $P$ elements correspond to extracted features from seizure epochs and the second $P$ elements correspond to the extracted features from non-seizure epochs.

## 2.3 Classification

The classification method used in this study is a very simple classifier where the observations are assigned to the most probable class based on Mahalanobis distance. More specifically, after prepossessing the EEG signals in a moving window of length $z$ and calculating the autocorrelation feature, the Mahalanobis distance of the extracted feature to the training set (i.e. feature values of two groups of seizure and non-seizure state) is calculated and the class label of the closest group of data is assigned as the class label of the moving window of EEG signals. Mahalanobis distance is the distance between a point and a centroid of a group of observations, and is calculated as follows [18]:

$$DM = \sqrt{\sum_{d=1}^{D} \frac{(f_d - \mu_d)}{\sigma_d}}, \qquad (7)$$

where $f_d$ correspond to the current feature value at dimension $d$, $\mu$ is centroid of the group of data (i.e. seizure or non-seizure) and $\sigma$ is the standard deviation. Mahalanobis distance is a statistical measure that provides the distance of one observation from the mean of a certain probability distribution. Hence, we are basically calculating the probability that new feature value $f$ belongs to seizure or non-seizure state. Finally, when the class label of $\alpha$ consecutive windows is classified as seizure state, the seizure detection alarm is triggered to indicate seizure onset.

# 3   Results and Discussion

## 3.1   Dataset

The performance of proposed seizure onset detection framework was tested using the publicly available seizure dataset known as CHB-MIT [19–21]. The CHB-MIT dataset contains scalp EEG recordings of 24 pediatric epileptic patients. The dataset includes approximately 9–42 h of EEG signals for each patient recorded at a sampling rate of 256 Hz with 16-bit resolution. Most of the recordings have been done using 23 channels with 10–20 sensor positioning standard. In few cases, the recordings have been done using different number of channels and channel settings. Overall the dataset contains 129 files that include one or more seizure onsets. Experiments in this paper carried on 23 cases since the last case did not include any files without seizure onset for testing the false detection rate.

## 3.2   Evaluation Method

The performance of the proposed seizure onset detection framework is estimated using leave-one-record-out cross-validation scheme. More specifically, for each subject, one recording that contains seizure onset is left aside for testing and the seizure onset detection framework uses the $K - 1$ remaining seizure records for training. Next, the sensitivity, latency, and run time are calculated using the seizure recording that was withheld from the training set. For each seizure recording that is withheld from the classifier, one seizure free recording from the same subject is used to test the false detection performance of the classifier. This process is repeated until each of the seizure recordings for that subject has been tested once. The provided results are the average of all testing instances. Table 1 provide the details of the four performance metrics used in this study.

**Table 1.** Performance metrics used for evaluating the proposed seizure onset detection framework.

| Performance measure | Equation |
|---|---|
| Average sensitivity | $\mu_\gamma = \left(\frac{1}{H} \sum_{h=1}^{H} S_h\right) * 100$ |
| Average latency | $\mu_\tau = \frac{1}{V} \sum_{v=1}^{V} \tau_v$ |
| Average false detection Rate | $\mu_\varphi = \left(\frac{1}{W} \sum_{w=1}^{W} E_w\right) * 100$ |
| Average run time | $\mu_\delta = \frac{1}{W} \sum_{w=1}^{W} \delta_w$ |

* $E$ is a binary variable where $E = 1$ represents false seizure detection.
* $H$ is the total number of seizure onsets in one subject.
* $S$ is a binary variable where $S = 1$ represents seizure detection.
* $V$ is the total number of correctly detected seizure onsets.
* $W$ is the total number of tested windows.
* $\delta$ is the time required to analyze each window.
* $\tau$ is the detection delay.

It should be noted that while most studies report the average false detection rate per hour for evaluating false detection performance, this measure is biased because it depends on the size of the moving window. In other words, the larger window size selection can decrease the false detection rate. Hence, in this study, we have defined false detection rate as the number of false detections per total number of tested windows and reported the results in a percentage format.

## 3.3  Seizure Detection Results

The proposed framework requires some patient specific parameter settings. The details of required parameters are provided in Table 2. The optimum value of these parameters for each patient is identified using sensitivity analysis on the training set.

**Table 2.** List of free parameters required by the proposed seizure onset detection framework.

| Parameter | Description |
|---|---|
| $k$ | Number of CSP components |
| $\alpha$ | Alarm threshold |
| $\beta$ | Amount of overlap between consecutive windows |
| $\theta$ | Moving window size |
| $\omega$ | Frequency range (i.e. frequency band) |

After obtaining the optimum parameter settings, the proposed framework was tested using the testing procedure described in the previous section. All the implementations were done in MATLAB programming environment. Table 3 provides the average testing performance of the proposed distance based seizure onset detection algorithm using the optimum parameter settings for each patient. Except for five subjects (5, 12, 13, 16, 17), the seizure detector was able to identify 100 % of the seizure occurrences. Furthermore, the average detection latency was less than seven seconds for most of the patients (except subjects 9 and 18). Regarding false detection rate, the proposed method did not perform well on subject 13, which is consistent with previous results in Shoeb's original paper [20]. The poor false detection performance in subject 13 is most likely caused by extreme sensor location changes during the EEG signal recordings of this patient. Finally, regarding the average run time, the proposed framework took on average 0.9 s to classify a new window into a seizure and non-seizure states. The run-time is perhaps comparable to using KNN method for seizure onset detection. In the simplest form of KNN (via linear search), the complexity is $O(dN)$ where $N$ corresponds to the size of the training set, and $d$ represents dimensionality of the training dataset. Compared to KNN, the complexity of proposed framework is bounded by the complexity of Mahanbois distance calculation $O(d^2)$. Hence, when using only one feature, the complexity of the proposed framework is reduced to $O(1)$, whereas the complexity of KNN becomes $O(N)$.

More generally, because the number of samples is much larger than the dimensionality of data in EEG signals ($N \gg d$), the complexity of proposed method is much less than KNN ($O(d^2) < O(dN)$).

Comparing different seizure onset detection methods in the literature is not feasible considering the diversity of tested datasets, the difference in performance evaluation criteria, and dissimilarity of model evaluation methods (such as cross-validation, hold-out, etc.). Having said that, Fig. 3 provides a quick comparison between the proposed framework and Shoeb's original results using CHB-MIT dataset [20]. The false detection results were not compared with Shoeb's paper since they only included the false alarm rate per hour, which is not comparable with false alarm percentage measure used in this study. Regarding sensitivity, the performance of proposed method was very close to Shoeb's results and could detect one less seizure occurrence in two of the subjects. However, regarding latency, on average our method was able to detect seizure onset 1.5 s earlier.

**Table 3.** Detailed results of the performance of proposed seizure onset detection framework.

| Subject # | Sensitivity (%) | Latency (s) | False alarm rate (%) | Run time (s) |
|---|---|---|---|---|
| 1 | 100.00 % | 0.94 | 2.22 % | 0.08 |
| 2 | 100.00 % | 6.77 | 1.68 % | 0.11 |
| 3 | 100.00 % | 4.01 | 1.61 % | 0.11 |
| 4 | 100.00 % | 1.44 | 5.18 % | 0.12 |
| 5 | 75.00 % | 0.94 | 1.19 % | 0.06 |
| 6 | 100.00 % | 1.49 | 2.20 % | 0.07 |
| 7 | 100.00 % | 2.44 | 1.48 % | 0.09 |
| 8 | 100.00 % | 1.34 | 0.45 % | 0.12 |
| 9 | 100.00 % | 11.77 | 1.30 % | 0.10 |
| 10 | 100.00 % | 0.94 | 1.83 % | 0.10 |
| 11 | 100.00 % | 3.60 | 0.96 % | 0.06 |
| 12 | 91.67 % | 4.63 | 0.31 % | 0.09 |
| 13 | 91.67 % | 0.64 | 20.22 % | 0.15 |
| 14 | 100.00 % | 5.72 | 0.86 % | 0.10 |
| 15 | 100.00 % | 4.59 | 1.32 % | 0.10 |
| 16 | 80.00 % | 0.82 | 5.00 % | 0.10 |
| 17 | 66.67 % | 1.44 | 1.35 % | 0.11 |
| 18 | 100.00 % | 9.44 | 1.78 % | 0.06 |
| 19 | 100.00 % | 0.94 | 0.27 % | 0.09 |
| 20 | 100.00 % | 0.79 | 12.22 % | 0.07 |
| 21 | 100.00 % | 1.44 | 1.19 % | 0.11 |
| 22 | 100.00 % | 1.94 | 1.03 % | 0.10 |
| 23 | 100.00 % | 0.40 | 0.81 % | 0.06 |
| Average | 95.87 % | 2.98 | 2.89 % | 0.09 |

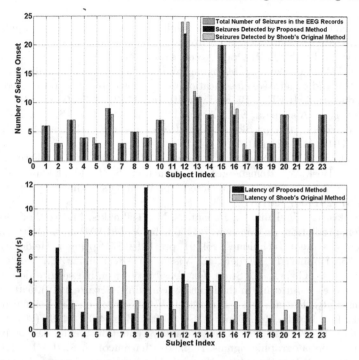

**Fig. 3.** Comparing results with Shoeb's original paper

## 4   Conclusion

This paper presents a simple distance based seizure onset detection algorithm, which is suitable for real-time monitoring of epileptic patients. The proposed method takes advantage of common spatial patterns to reduce the dimensionality of input data and uses a simple distance based classifier to detect seizure onset based on the autocorrelation value at the zero-lag/fs. The main advantage of proposed method is its computational efficiency, which enables it to classify a window of EEG signals in less than 0.1 s, and its robustness to the number of sensors used for recording EEG signals. The proposed method can be employed to reduce the time spent on offline detection of seizure onsets by experienced neurophysiologists and automatic real-time detection of seizures in epileptic patients. Nevertheless, an automatic artifact removal is essential for optimal performance in real-world settings. Furthermore, the proposed method requires patient-specific parameter settings and therefore is patient dependent. In this regard, a feature extension of this work is to modify the proposed method to automatically determine the patient specific parameters or develop a comparable parameter free algorithm for detecting seizure onsets.

## References

1. World Health Organization (WHO). Epilepsy (2015). http://www.who.int/media centre/factsheets/fs999/en/. Accessed 09 01 2016

2. Tzallas, A.T., Tsalikakis, D.G., Karvounis, E.C., Astrakas, L., Tzaphlidou, M., Tsipouras, M.G., Konitsiotis, S.: Automated Epileptic Seizure Detection Methods: A Review Study. INTECH Open Access Publisher, Rijeka (2012)

3. Thomas, E.M., Temko, A., Marnane, W.P., Boylan, G.B., Lightbody, G.: Discriminative and generative classification techniques applied to automated neonatal seizure detection. IEEE J. Biomed. Health Inf. **17**(2), 297–304 (2013)

4. Alotaiby, T.N., Alshebeili, S.A., Alshawi, T., Ahmad, I., El-Samie, F.E.A.: EEG seizure detection and prediction algorithms: a survey. EURASIP J. Adv. Sig. Process. **2014**(1), 1–21 (2014)

5. Ramgopal, S., Thome-Souza, S., Jackson, M., Kadish, N.E., Fernández, I.S., Klehm, J., Bosl, W., Reinsberger, C., Schachter, S., Loddenkemper, T.: Seizure detection, seizure prediction, and closed-loop warning systems in epilepsy. Epilepsy Behav. **37**, 291–307 (2014)

6. Giannakakis, G., Sakkalis, V., Pediaditis, M., Tsiknakis, M.: Methods for seizure detection, prediction: an overview. In: Sakkalis, V. (ed.) Modern Electroencephalographic Assessment Techniques, vol. 91, pp. 131–157. Springer, Heidelberg (2015)

7. Ponten, S., Ronner, H., Strijers, R., Visser, M., Peerdeman, S., Vandertop, W., Beishuizen, A., Girbes, A., Stam, C.: Feasibility of online seizure detection with continuous eeg monitoring in the intensive care unit. Seizure **19**(9), 580–586 (2010)

8. Lakshmi, M.R., Prasad, D.T., Prakash, D.V.C.: Survey on EEG signal processing methods. Int. J. Adv. Res. Comput. Sci. Softw. Eng. **4**(1), 84–91 (2014)

9. Harikumar, R., Kumar, P.S.: Dimensionality reduction techniques for processing epileptic encephalographic signals. Biomed. Pharmacol. J. **8**, 103–106 (2015)

10. Birjandtalab, J., Pouyan, M.B., Nourani, M.: Nonlinear dimension reduction for EEG-based epileptic seizure detection. In: 2016 IEEE-EMBS International Conference on Biomedical and Health Informatics (BHI), pp. 595–598. IEEE (2016)

11. Alotaiby, T.N., Abd El-Samie, F.E., Alshebeili, S.A., Aljibreen, K.H., Alkhanen, E.: Seizure detection with common spatial pattern and support vector machines. In: 2015 International Conference on Information and Communication Technology Research (ICTRC), pp. 152–155. IEEE (2015)

12. Qaraqe, M., Ismail, M., Serpedin, E.: Band-sensitive seizure onset detection via CSP-enhanced EEG features. Epilepsy Behav. **50**, 77–87 (2015)

13. Butterworth, S.: On the theory of filter amplifiers. Wirel. Eng. **7**(6), 536–541 (1930)

14. Jerger, K.K., Netoff, T.I., Francis, J.T., Sauer, T., Pecora, L., Weinstein, S.L., Schiff, S.J.: Early seizure detection. J. Clin. Neurophysiol. **18**(3), 259–268 (2001)

15. Logesparan, L., Casson, A.J., Rodriguez-Villegas, E.: Optimal features for online seizure detection. Med. Biol. Eng. Comput. **50**(7), 659–669 (2012)

16. Lai, Y.-C., Osorio, I., Harrison, M.A.F., Frei, M.G.: Correlation-dimension and autocorrelation fluctuations in epileptic seizure dynamics. Phys. Rev. E **65**(3), 031921 (2002)

17. Varsavsky, A., Mareels, I., Cook, M.: Epileptic Seizures and the EEG: Measurement, Models, Detection and Prediction. CRC Press, Boca Raton (2010)

18. Rajaraman, A., Ullman, J.D.: Mining of Massive Datasets. Cambridge University Press, Cambridge (2012)

19. Shoeb, A., Edwards, H., Connolly, J., Bourgeois, B., Treves, S.T., Guttag, J.: Patient-specific seizure onset detection. Epilepsy Behav. **5**(4), 483–498 (2004)

20. Shoeb, A.H.: Application of machine learning to epileptic seizure onset detection and treatment. Ph.D. dissertation, Massachusetts Institute of Technology (2009)

21. PhysioBank, PhysioToolkit. Physionet: components of a new research resource for complex physiologic signals. Circulation 101(23), e215–e220 (2000)

# A Conversational Agent for an Online Mental Health Intervention

Danielle Elmasri[1] and Anthony Maeder[2(✉)]

[1] School of Computing, Engineering and Mathematics,
Western Sydney University, Penrith, Australia
d.elmasri@westernsydney.edu.au
[2] School of Health Sciences, Flinders University, Bedford Park, Australia
anthony.maeder@flinders.edu.au

**Abstract.** This study investigated suitability of chatbots for a mental health intervention, specifically alcohol drinking habits assessment. The target group was young adults 18–25 years, the highest consumers of alcohol per capita in Australia. A chatbot program was developed to perform a standard assessment of alcohol drinking habits (AUDIT-C, 3 items rated on 5-point scale) to determine the level of health risk. Additionally, the chatbot provided information and education on responsible alcohol use, giving recommendations and feedback post-assessment using a pre-populated database of factual response contents. Usability and user-satisfaction were determined by a cohort study of 17 volunteer participants. Overall, the trial indicated strong positive reception of the intervention by users.

## 1 Introduction

Mental health conditions in Australia are on an upward spiral with around 7.3 million or 45 % of Australians aged between 16 and 85 experiencing a common mental health illness such as depression, anxiety or substance use disorder [1]. With mental health illnesses comes many barriers to receiving treatment (such as social stigma) and whilst substance abuse disorders are one of the most common mental health problems in the Western World, there are many individuals not receiving treatment [2].

The prevalence of mental health disorders is the highest in people aged up to 25 years old with 13 % having a substance use disorder [3]. The three common mental health disorders amongst young adults include anxiety disorders which affect 14.4 % of the population, affective disorders affecting 6.2 % and substance use disorders which affects 5.1 %. In Australia, it has been found that the 27 % of 18–25 year old age group suffers a mental health disorder [4]. Alarmingly a substantial proportion of these young adults consume alcohol at high risk levels.

Comorbidity of mental health disorders and substance abuse is common and the two occur together very frequently while impacting negatively on one another [5]. A common form of comorbidity includes conditions whereby substance abuse issues co-occur with other mental health disorders such as depression, bipolar disorder or anxiety [6].

© Springer International Publishing AG 2016
G.A. Ascoli et al. (Eds.): BIH 2016, LNAI 9919, pp. 243–251, 2016.
DOI: 10.1007/978-3-319-47103-7_24

Online health is a rapidly expanding alternative to orthodox medical consultation for consumers to seek professional health services and advice. In recent years, there has been an increase in the use of interactive real-time online health interventions to improve psychological functioning and well-being of clients [7]. This approach is becoming more widely accepted as it can provide the client with anonymity, security, immediate access to information, reliability and non-biased recommendations.

Conversational agents (such as chatbots and avatars) are an effective means to counteract the barriers for young adults requiring professional treatment and advice relating to mental health illnesses. Conversational agents have existed since ELIZA which was created in 1966 and more recently the ALICEbot which was introduced in 1995 [8]. Conversational agents have been used successfully in a range of areas such as education, information retrieval, business and e-commerce [9]. An example of a chatbot in health has been developed to support interpersonal skills-training components of depression treatment programs [10].

This work is focused on development of a simple chatbot to address substance abuse via alcohol misuse by young adults. Simplicity was a primary criterion, to allow ease of implementation. The chatbot has two main functionalities, namely providing alcohol education and performing an alcohol risk assessment on the user. The risk assessment is based on the three item questionnaire used by therapists internationally known as the AUDIT-C [11], which assesses drinking habits via alcohol consumption levels and frequency of drinking.

The conversational approach by the chatbot accentuates an interview style of questions which in turn has the capability to mimic a pragmatic consultation or session with a health care professional. The assessment is based on an individuals' pre-existing drinking behaviour and on conclusion the chatbot is able to distinguish a persons' level of risk based on their responses. The relevant recommendation and information is then relayed to the user as a form of feedback.

While a chatbot can be seen as convenient, reliable and accessible, our intervention was not designed with the potential or intention of replacing medical practitioners such as counsellors or therapists. Instead, it would more plausibly act as an initial encounter and direct the user to seek medical assistance if they are deemed to be at risk of a mental health illness.

## 2  Methods

The purpose of this research was to investigate whether a simple chatbot can be used as a suitable delivery mechanism for creating an effective online mental health intervention for alcohol abuse. The significance of the chatbot developed here is the approach of logically structuring conversations to allow the user to determine whether they need to seek additional professional advice, as well as providing immediate information to the user. This approach offers a means to limit the barriers which currently exist between an individual and a health care professional as it provides confidentiality, anonymity and a wide array of information and data regardless of the physical location or state of the user [12].

User requirements for the chatbot were determined by an expert panel to be as follows:

(a) A secure, anonymous and immediate advice and/or information exchange on a users' alcohol related issues which is derived from a trusted and non-biased source;

(b) A personality whereby the chatbot is seen as a friendly adviser or mentor to the user rather than a therapist or health care professional;

(c) A unique and logical conversation based on individual inputs;

(d) A simple means to communicate with an artificially intelligent agent, structuring the conversation to require little input from a user to carry on a conversation.

(e) A mechanism that provides feedback and/or advice based on their alcohol assessment and web links to relevant government agencies and private organizations for more information on how to seek help with alcohol misuse.

A prototype chatbot was implemented using AIML as for ALICE [13]. The emphasis of the research was on creating a structured conversation that allowed the user to converse with a chatbot in a human-like manner. The chatbot conversation structure was realised in four modules:

(i) initiating the conversation,

(ii) providing alcohol education information and advice exchange,

(iii) performing an AUDIT-C risk-assessment and

(iv) concluding the conversation.

The overall intention was to test the chatbot competency in achieving acceptable levels of:

(i) sophistication,

(ii) structure and flow of conversation,

(iii) logic and reasoning.

Initiating and concluding the conversation are achieved with simple predefined greeting utterances and questions to determine user name and personal; profile details. The Alcohol Education module would normally be entered first and commences by asking the user to set a topic, after which the chatbot prompts the user to ask a question to which it gives an appropriate response, and then encourages further questions to be asked. Three main alcohol education topics were implemented: Standard Drinks, Managing Drinking and Consequences of Alcohol, as shown in Fig. 1 below.

The Alcohol Risk Assessment module has three core components: (i) brief introduction to the risk assessment; (ii) administering the AUDIT-C questions; and (iii) providing the user with feedback, which are executed sequentially as shown in Fig. 2.

The purpose of the chatbot knowledge base used to manage conversational utterances in this module is to allow the user to receive information on their drinking habits, patterns and possible alcohol misuse after receiving alcohol education. The chatbot has been designed in such a way to make the user feel like the conversation is remembered and that the chatbot is behaving with context awareness. This functionality is achieved by the chatbot performing one of two actions:

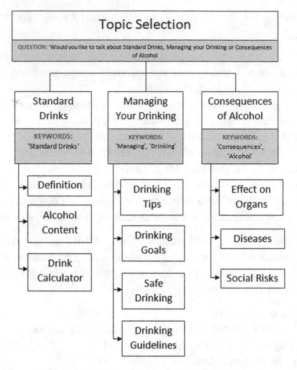

**Fig. 1.** Alcohol education conversation map

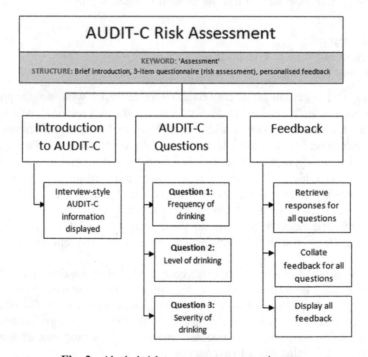

**Fig. 2.** Alcohol risk assessment conversation map.

(a) Storing the response the user has given if the chatbot believes it a sufficient answer. This is determined on the basis that the AUDIT-C is a multiple choice questionnaire, thus a sufficient answer will be deduced once the chatbot is able to map a response back to one of the possible multiple choice answers. If this process is successful then the chatbot will prepare and collate the relevant feedback for the response.

(b) If the answer is not sufficient then the chatbot will attempt to collect the appropriate response from the user. If the question being asked is open ended then the chatbot will clarify that question by re-wording the question in a way that simplifies what is being asked. In contrast, if the question is close-ended then the chatbot will re-pose the question so that the user can re-read what is being asked and then ask them to say 'Yes' or 'No' as their answer. Once this process is complete then step (a) is repeated for the next question and so forth.

## 3 Results

User testing was conducted on 17 participants aged 18–25 (10 male, 7 female) who passed a pre-screening to establish them as low to medium risk <5 drinks per day). The sample sized was due to availability of volunteers rather than statistical powering, and there was no control group.

Each participant was allocated a 30 min session, with 12 min allocated to user testing based on their interaction with the chatbot. The first step in the user testing process involved introducing the chat interface to the user. The interface of the chatbot is very similar to many interfaces that are commonly used on mobile phones devices and online social media websites. This meant that most users readily understood and accepted how to use it. Next, the user was given a brief demonstration on how the a conversational interaction between the chatbot and individual takes place. This introductory phase took approximately 2 min. Thereafter, the user was allowed to freely interact with the chatbot at their own will. They were given no specific conversations or words to say but instead were told to interact with the chatbot in a way they feel would be suitable for them to use for the purpose of exploring the topic of their alcohol consumption, It was anticipated that they would spend approximately 5 min for the alcohol education part and a further 5 min for the AUDIT-C assessment part. All individuals had the opportunity to ask questions during user testing and interrupt the process if assistance was required.

At the conclusion of the user testing, the individual was then asked to complete an 8 item questionnaire and undergo an interview in the remaining 15 min of the session. The purpose of the questionnaire was to assess the users' overall satisfaction with the chatbot responses in the alcohol education and alcohol risk assessment functions. Additionally, the questionnaire was also designed to investigate the effectiveness of the conversation structure in influencing user satisfaction. The questionnaire was designed based on the well known Client Satisfaction Survey which was created in 1979 to assess client satisfaction with health and mental health services [14]. The questions from the original Client Satisfaction Survey were altered to suit the context of an online service being delivered in the form of a conversational agent. This was achieved by substituting words from the original survey such as 'our service' with the phrases more relevant to the project such as 'the chatbot's questions and answers'.

Interviews were undertaken after the questionnaire completion and allowed further information to be gathered on the users' level of satisfaction with the chatbot. There was an emphasis placed specifically on determining any elements that contributed to dissatisfaction in the chatbots' conversation structure. The interview was structured with four questions:

*Question 1:* The level of user satisfaction, including what aspects of the conversational agent influenced satisfaction or dissatisfaction.

*Question 2:* The overall experience with using the chatbot in terms of the terminology and conversational reasoning/understanding; this includes identifying and explaining any undesirable results and/or outcomes that the chatbot may have produced during the user testing.

*Question 3:* The degree of simplicity and ease of use of the chatbot; this includes user friendliness, terminology and navigating through the conversation.

*Question 4:* To provide any suggestions and/or comments on how to improve the chatbot conversational structure and ability to converse.

User responses to the questionnaire are summarised in Table 1, and when converted to positive-high scores on a 4 point scale, the corresponding statistics are shown in Table 2. As can be seen, user satisfaction is generally high (mean 3.29–3.76) and

**Table 1.** Questionnaire results summary

| | Responses | | | |
|---|---|---|---|---|
| | Excellent | Good | Fair | Poor |
| Q1 | 12 | 9 | 0 | 0 |
| | No, definitely | No, not really | Yes, Generally | Yes, Definitely |
| Q2 | 0 | 0 | 13 | 8 |
| | Almost all needs | Most needs | Only a few needs | None of my needs |
| Q3 | 15 | 5 | 1 | 0 |
| | No, definitely | No, I don't think so | Yes, I think so | Yes, Definitely |
| Q4 | 0 | 2 | 9 | 10 |
| | Quite dissatisfied | Indifferent or mildly dissatisfied | Mostly satisfied | Very satisfied |
| Q5 | 0 | 0 | 6 | 15 |
| | Yes helped great deal | Yes helped somewhat | No they didn't really help | No they seemed to make things difficult |
| Q6 | 8 | 11 | 2 | 0 |
| | Very satisfied | Mostly satisfied | indifferent/mildly | quite dissatisfied |
| Q7 | 15 | 6 | 0 | 0 |
| | No definitly not | No I don't think so | Yes I think so | Yes, Definitely |
| Q8 | 0 | 2 | 11 | 8 |

**Table 2.** Questionnaire results statistics

| Responses | Mean | Std | Variance |
|---|---|---|---|
| Q1 | 3.57 | 0.51 | 0.26 |
| Q2 | 3.38 | 0.50 | 0.25 |
| Q3 | 3.67 | 0.58 | 0.33 |
| Q4 | 3.38 | 0.67 | 0.45 |
| Q5 | 3.67 | 0.48 | 0.23 |
| Q6 | 3.29 | 0.64 | 0.41 |
| Q7 | 3.76 | 0.51 | 0.26 |
| Q8 | 3.29 | 0.64 | 0.41 |
| Total | 3.55 | 0.57 | 0.33 |

consistent (std 0.50–0.67), but an absolute conclusion on the significance of these values cannot be drawn without controls. It is also not possible to validate the accuracy of the AUDIT-C assessment in this case.

The overall results of the interview are shown in Table 3 and have been grouped using topic analysis into four categories: professional as it provides confidentiality, anonymity and a wide array of information and data regardless of the physical location or state of the user [12].

**Table 3.** Interview results summary

| All Participants Interview Topic Analysis | | | |
|---|---|---|---|
| Keywords and topics | | | |
| Positives | Negatives | Comments | Suggestions |
| Knowledge base was informative | Too much information | Personalisation was Good | Suggestion Pictures |
| 15 | 5 | 2 | 2 |
| Simple-Guided Conversation | Conversation caused confusion | Humanlike Conversation | Recognising more keywords |
| 15 | 3 | 5 | 6 |
| Quick Response Time | Undesirable Interface | Reliability and Accuracy | Suggestion Voice Recognition |
| 8 | 5 | 3 | 1 |
| Clear to comprehend | Incorrect/Inappropriate Response | Simple Language | |
| 4 | 1 | 9 | |
| Ease of use | | | |
| 4 | | | |

(a) *Positives:* these are any factors that were mentioned by participants as elements of the chatbot that contributed to user satisfaction;
(b) *Negatives:* these are any factors that were mentioned by participants as elements of the chatbot that produced undesirable effects and contributed to user dissatisfaction;
(c) *Comments:* these are general comments which have been made by participants;
(d) *Suggestions:* these are any suggestions that participants offered to improve the usability, reliability or accuracy of the chatbot.

It can be seen that there is good agreement with the findings of the questionnaire, with many strong positive reasons offered for user satisfaction. However a major source of user dissatisfaction was the nature of the user interface: users were frustrated by the need to type their utterances rather than speak naturally: this could be overcome by a speech recognition interface variant. Some users criticized the inability of the chatbot to recognize different keywords that those with which it had been programmed, and more generally that there was too much information, resulting from use of the highly structured conversation maps. This would require a far more sophisticated artificial intelligence approach to be used to drive the system, such as reinforcement learning or natural language processing.

## 4   Conclusion

The intention of the trial was not to determine the accuracy of the assessment or measure subsequent behaviour change, rather it was to assess the suitability of having a relatively real and believable conversation with a simple online chatbot as a human surrogate for a health professional. Overall, the trial indicated positive reception of the intervention by users and that availability of chatbot variants with different behavior and sophistication in their conversational ability would further enhance user satisfaction and perceived usefulness. Further work could explore this more complex modeling of the conversational agent's reasoning. In addition, a larger sample size and inclusion of controls would enable richer statistical analysis.

## References

1. Australian Institute of Health and Welfare: Prevalance, impact and burden (2012) [Online]
2. Copeland, J., Martin, G.: Web-based interventions for substance use disorders: a qualitative review. J. Subst. Abuse Treat. **26**(2), 109–116 (2004)
3. Tait, R.J., Christensen, H.: Internet-based interventions for young people with problematic substance use: a systematic review. Med. J. Aust. **192**(11), 15–21 (2010)
4. Rickwood, D.J., Deane, F.P., Wilson, C.J.: When and how do young people seek professional help for mental health problems? Med. J. Aust. **187**(7), 35–39 (2007)
5. Gordon, A.: Comorbidity of mental disorders and substance use: a brief guide for the primary care clinician. Australian Government Department of Health and Ageing Monograph Series, vol. 71 (2008) [Online]

6. Saisan, J., Smith, M., Segal, J.: Substance Abuse and Mental Health (2015) [Online]
7. Wade, S.L., Wolfe, C.R.: Telehealth interventions in rehabilitation psychology: postcards from the edge. Rehabil. Psychol. **50**(4), 323–324 (2005)
8. Schumaker, R.P., Liu, Y., Ginsburg, M., Chen, H.: Evaluating mass knowledge acquisition using the ALICE chatterbot. Intl. J. Hum. Comput. Stud. **64**(11), 1132–1140 (2006)
9. Shawar, B., Atwell, E.: Different measurements metrics to evaluate a chatbot system. In: Bridging the Gap: Academic and Industrial Research in Dialog Technologies Workshop Proceedings, pp. 89–96 (2007)
10. Mohr, D.C., Burns, M.N., Schueller, S.M., Clarke, G., Klinkman, M.: Behavioral intervention technologies: evidence review and recommendations for future research in mental health. Gen. Hosp. Psychiatry **35**(4), 332–338 (2013)
11. Bush, K., Kivlahan, D.R., McDonell, M.B., Fihn, S.D., Bradley, K.A.: The AUDIT alcohol consumption questions (AUDIT-C): an effective brief screening test for problem drinking. Arch. Intern. Med. **158**(16), 1789–1795 (1998)
12. Fogg, B.: Overview of captology, in persuasive technology. In: Fogg, B. (ed.) Using Computers to Change What We Think and Do, pp. 15–21. Morgan Kaufmann, San Francisco (2003)
13. Wallace, R.S.: The anatomy of A.L.I.C.E. In: Epstein, R.B. (ed.) Parsing the Turing Test, pp. 181–210. Springer Science+Business Media B.V, Berlin (2008)
14. Larsen, D.L., Attkisson, C.C., Hargreaves, W.A., Nguyen, T.D.: Assessment of client/patient satisfaction: development of a general scale. Eval. Program Plann. **2**(3), 197–207 (1979)

# Acute Stress Detection Using Recurrence Quantification Analysis of Electroencephalogram (EEG) Signals

Miaolin Fan[3](✉), Mohammad Samie Tootooni[1],
Rajesh Sharma Sivasubramony[1], Vladimir Miskovic[1], Prahalada K. Rao[2],
and Chun-An Chou[3]

[1] State University of New York, Binghamton, NY, USA
{mfan4,mtootoo1,rsivasu1,miskovic}@binghamton.edu
[2] Mechanical and Materials Engineering Department,
University of Nebraska-Lincoln, Lincoln, NE, USA
prao@binghamton.edu
[3] Mechanical and Industrial Engineering Department,
Northeastern University, Boston, MA, USA
cachou@binghamton.edu

**Abstract.** In the present work we intend to classify the brain states under physical stress and experimental control conditions based on the nonlinear features of electroencephalogram (EEG) dynamics using support vector machine (SVM) and least absolute shrinkage and selection operator (LASSO). Recurrence Quantification Analysis (RQA) method was employed to quantify the nonlinear features of high-density electroencephalogram (EEG) signals recorded either during instances of acute stress induction or comparison conditions. Four RQA measures, including determinism (DET), entropy (ENTR), laminarity (LAM) and trapping time (TT) were extracted from the EEG signals to characterize the deterministic features of cortical activity. Results revealed that LASSO was highly efficient in classifying the conditions using any one of the selected RQA measures, while SVM achieved accurate classification based solely on ENTR and TT. Among all four measures of non-linear dynamics, ENTR yielded the best overall classification accuracy.

**Keywords:** Electroencephalography · Stress · Recurrence quantification analysis · LASSO · SVM

## 1 Introduction

Large-scale recordings of brain electrical activity provide a classical example of a non-linear dynamical system which reflects the myriad interactions among thousands of cortical neurons [9,10]. In recent years, there has been burgeoning interest in applying advanced quantitative tools for characterizing non-linear dynamics of electroencephalographic (EEG) recordings [19]. As a non-linear dynamics analysis approach, *Recurrence plot* (RP) visualizes the recurrence patterns of time series signals in 2-dimensional squared matrix [5]. Recurrence quantification analysis (RQA) of brain signals has been applied with great success to the

© Springer International Publishing AG 2016
G.A. Ascoli et al. (Eds.): BIH 2016, LNAI 9919, pp. 252–261, 2016.
DOI: 10.1007/978-3-319-47103-7_25

problem of seizure detection – in particular, it has been demonstrated that the RP based methods are more efficient than many other approaches in detecting transitions from normal to epileptic states [1,3,16]. Such advances in the nonlinear dynamical analysis of EEG signals, combined with machine learning algorithms developed in recent decades, provide increased opportunities for multivariate classification based on non-invasively collected EEG data.

Although not as successful as in seizure detection, RP based methods can also be used for other EEG-based states classification tasks, including: (1) the monitoring or evaluation of responses to anesthesia [2,11]; (2) evaluating the effect of treatment on patients with major depression using EEG recorded at various sleep stages [7], and (3) the burst suppression patterns detection [12]. While these studies focus on that classifying distinct patterns which are related to neurophysiological disorders or levels of consciousness, whether if a mild transition of states can be detected using this approach remains to be explored. In our study, a non-linear data analysis framework was adopted based on the metrics extracted from RP with a selection of machine learning algorithms. The feasibility of using RQA for analyzing nonlinear dynamics in EEG signals is tested, with the goal of identifying to what extent physical stress states can be detected by pattern recognition with machine learning techniques.

## 2    Methods

### 2.1    Data Collection and Pre-processing

**Experimental Settings.** In this study, we conducted two experiments in order to perform acute stress detection. In the setup of Dataset 1, 32 participants were randomly assigned to either an acute stress (cold presser challenge) or a comparison condition (lukewarm water hand immersion). The procedure was conducted as follows: resting-state EEG signals were recorded for approximately 2 min before, during and after stress induction (or comparison state) – these are referred to as *pre*, *press* and *post* conditions from this point onward. In the *pre* and *post* conditions, participants were asked to close their eyes for the first minute (*EC* condition) and then open their eyes for the second minute (*EO* condition). During *press* phase, participants were instructed to immerse their right hand, up to the wrist, either into a container of chilled water ($0$–$3\,°C$) or lukewarm water (depending on their random assignment). Participants were then asked to keep their hand immersed and to sit still for 2 min (though some participants in the acute stress condition were not able to maintain their hand in ice water for the entire duration).

In the setup for Dataset 2, we recorded EEG signals from two participants, where we manipulated the stress versus comparison condition on a within-subject basis. In this experiment, the two participants first completed hand immersion into lukewarm water followed by chilled water hand immersion. High-density EEG signals were recorded continuously during the *cold*, *warm* and *pre* conditions, with eyes opened.

**EEG Recording and Artifact Correction.** After reading and signing an informed consent form, participants were ushered into a dimly lit, EEG recording room equipped with a white noise generating sound screen. The nasion-inion and pre-auricular anatomical measurements were assayed to locate and mark each individual's vertex site. Each participant was fitted for placing an electrode net, which was then soaked in electrolyte. The dense-array EEG net application then followed, which consisted of a 128 electrode (plus average reference) Electrical Geodesics, Inc. (EGI) HydroCel Geodesic Sensor Net with sponge inserts. The target sensor impedances were at or below 60 kOhm at recording onset. The signal was amplified by an EGI Net Amps 400, digitized at 1 kHz, and recorded using Net Station 4.5.6 software running on a Mac Pro. The EEG recordings were digitally downsampled to 500 Hz to speed subsequent computational steps.

We retained only sensors located on the scalp. The artifact correction process was as follows: in a first step, we performed a spatial principal components analysis (sPCA) for each participant, treating sensors as variables and time points as observations to identify a reduced number of orthogonal components capable of accounting for 98 % of variance in spatial topography. Next, we performed a reduced-rank independent components analysis (ICA) using the Infomax algorithm implemented in the EEGLAB toolbox (version 12.0.2.5b) for MATLAB to extract as many independent components as there were spatial principal components. A conservative approach was adopted with the goal of retaining as much brain activity as possible; thus independent components were removed before backprojecting only in cases where they were deemed near-exclusively artifactual based on manual inspection of the temporal, spatial, and spectral properties or in cases where they possessed a rhythmic nature that was expected to seriously distort subsequent analyses (i.e., heartbeats). Temporally discrete artifacts of even large amplitude were retained in cases where the component included any amount of plausible brain signals.

## 2.2 Recurrence Quantification Analysis

**Recurrence Plot.** Been originally proposed by Eckmann in 1987, RP provides a visualization of recurrence patterns with a binary matrix [5]. It was rediscovered in later years when several metrics were defined based on RP to quantify the complexity and deterministic behaviors of dynamic systems [15,21,23].

Assume that the time series data of a dynamic system at fixed time $t$ is given by an n-dimensional vector $v_t = (v_1(t), v_2(t), \ldots, v_n(t))^T$. Having defined the embedding dimension $m$ and time delay $\tau$, the trajectories of selected system can be reconstructed in phase space such that the $i^{th}$ state of the system is represented by a vector $x_i$ with $m$ components, and $x_i = (v_{1+(i-1)\tau}, v_{2+(i-1)\tau}), \ldots, v_{m+(i-1)\tau})^T$, $i \in 1, \ldots, N$. The original RP, which is a *thresholded* version, is defined as follows:

$$\mathbf{R}_{i,j} = \Theta(\varepsilon - \|x_i - x_j\|), \; x_i \in \mathbb{R}^m, \; i,j = 1, \ldots, N, \tag{1}$$

where $\Theta(\cdot)$ is the Heaviside function. In this formulation, $\| \cdot \|$ is a norm which defines the measure of distances between any two points on the trajectory of attractor, and $\varepsilon$ is a threshold to be applied to the distance matrix. A squared binary matrix is obtained sequentially to represent which time points on the trajectory are sufficiently close to each other. Figure 1 shows an example of RP in each experiment condition in our study.

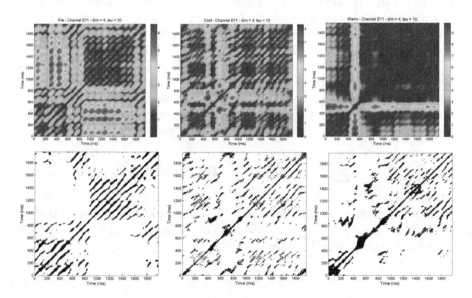

**Fig. 1.** An illustrative example of single-electrode RPs ($m = 4$, $\tau = 10$, using fixed amount of neighborhood method with $RR \approx 1\%$) in *pre*, *cold* and *warm* conditions from Participant 1 in Dataset 2.

**Parameter Estimation.** Previous literature suggested that the RQA method relays strongly on the appropriate selection of parameters, including the embedding dimension $m$, the time delay $\tau$, and the recurrence threshold $\varepsilon$ [13,14,22]. In our study, we employed identical parameters for all subjects. The nearest-neighbor methodology was used for estimating $m$, which determines $m$ as the maximum integer steps until the false nearest neighbors become unchanging [8]. Moreover, $\tau$ was selected as the first local minimum in the mutual information function of time series data [6]. Finally, the fixed amount of nearest neighbors approach was utilized in our study to estimate the threshold, resulting in various $\varepsilon$ for every point on the trajectory with the Recurrence Rate (RR) fixed to $1\%$ [24]. The advantage of this approach is the consistency of recurrence point density, which allows for a comparison between systems without the necessity of normalization of time series signals.

The type of norm in Eq. (1) is also critical as it defines the geometrical shape of neighborhood surrounding each point on RP, even though it is not strictly a parameter [13]. Typical options include minimum norm, maximum norm and Euclidean norm. Although the maximum norm is a common choice, we selected Euclidean norm in our study because it yields an intermediate number of neighbors compared to the other two options [14].

**Quantification Measures.** For Dataset 1, before applying a non-overlapping sliding window (size $= 1$ s) to the signals to extract RQA measures, a fraction (2.5 %) of the whole signals was discarded from both ends of each condition. For Dataset 2, the window size is 2 s and the entire recordings were used.

In our selected RQA measures, *determinism* (DET) and *entropy* (ENTR) are computed based on the diagonal structures of RP, while the *laminarity* (LAM) and *trapping time* (TT) are based on the vertical lines.

Assume that a constant threshold $\varepsilon$ is used for defining neighborhood in $\mathbf{R}_{i,j}$. The histogram of diagonal lines of length $l$ is then defined as:

$$P(l) = \sum_{i,j=1}^{N} (1 - \mathbf{R}_{i-1,j-1})(1 - \mathbf{R}_{i+l,j+l}) \prod_{k=0}^{l-1} \mathbf{R}_{i+k,j+k}. \tag{2}$$

Denote the minimum length of diagonal line as $l_{min}$. DET measures the predictability of system by computing the percentage of diagonal lines in RP. The formula for computing DET is given as follows:

$$DET = \frac{\sum_{l=l_{min}}^{N} l P(l)}{\sum_{l=1}^{N} l P(l)}. \tag{3}$$

ENTR is the Shannon entropy [18] of the probability that a diagonal line has exact length of $l$ in the distribution of all diagonal lines in RP. It is obvious that this probability $p(l) = P(l)/N_l$ and thus ENTR is defined as:

$$ENTR = -\sum_{l=l_{min}}^{N} p(l) \ln p(l), \tag{4}$$

which measures the complexity from the distribution lengths of diagonal lines. Similar to Eq. (2), the histogram of vertical lines of length $v$ is computed by the following equation:

$$P(v) = \sum_{i,j=1}^{N} (1 - \mathbf{R}_{i,j})(1 - \mathbf{R}_{i,j+v}) \prod_{k=0}^{v-1} \mathbf{R}_{i,j+k}. \tag{5}$$

Analogous to DET, LAM measures the percentage of vertical lines in RP, which is closely related to the intermittency of a dynamic system. The mathematical definition of LAM is as follows:

$$LAM = \frac{\sum_{v=v_{min}}^{N} v P(v)}{\sum_{v=1}^{N} v P(v)}, \tag{6}$$

where $v_{min}$ is the minimum length of vertical lines as in the case of DET.

TT is the average length of vertical lines which indicates how long the system remains in a specific state. The formula is as follows:

$$TT = \frac{\sum_{v=v_{min}}^{N} vP(v)}{\sum_{v=v_{min}}^{N} P(v)}. \tag{7}$$

## 2.3  Pattern Classification

Suppose a dataset is collected through $p$ sensors, and the total number of time windows is $n$. Then for each RQA measure, there is an $n \times p$ data matrix whose rows represent the observations (windows) and columns represent the sensors. Each observation is labeled with the corresponding experimental condition. For Dataset 1, we defined 2 scenarios which contain 3 classes in each. Scenario 1 includes eyes-closed ($EC$) and eyes-open ($EO$) in control conditions, and *stress* condition. Scenario 2 includes pre-stimulus (*pre*), stress (*press*) and post-stimulus (*post*) conditions. For Dataset 2, each participant has 3 conditions: *pre*, *cold* and *warm*, so the 3-class classification was performed as well as pair-wise binary classifications.

For each subject, the entire dataset was divided evenly (50/50 hold out cross-validation) into training and test set with balanced classes. Least absolute shrinkage and selection operator (LASSO) [20] and support vector machine (SVM) [4] with linear kernel were used as classifiers. A brief introduction of each algorithm is given in the following sections.

**Least Absolute Shrinkage and Selection Operator.** LASSO is a regularization method that can be applied to both regression and classification problems [20]. In a regression problem, suppose the model is given by $f(x) = w^T x + b$, the mathematical formulation is as follows:

$$\arg\min_{w,b} |f(x_i) - t_i|^2, \tag{8}$$

$$s.t. \sum |w| \leq \lambda, \tag{9}$$

where $f(x_i)$ and $t_i$ are the prediction and target value for the $i^{th}$ data point, $w$ is the coefficient vector and $b$ is the intercept in regression model. $\lambda$ is a tuning parameter that controls the shrinkage, which is commonly selected using cross-validation. In the case of our study, the formulation is generalized to solve multi-class classification problems by replacing Eq. (8) with the objective function of the multinomial logistic regression model.

**Support Vector Machine.** SVM was originally proposed as a binary classification model which minimizes the geometrical margin between two classes [4]. The objective of linear kernel SVM classifier is to find the decision boundary, a hyperplane represented by $f(x)$ as the same function in LASSO, which is equivalent to solving the following optimization problem:

$$\arg \min_{w,b} \quad \frac{1}{2}\|w\|^2 + C\sum_{i=1}^{n}(\xi_i), \tag{10}$$

$$s.t. \quad t_i(w^T x_i + b) \geq 1 - \xi_i, \tag{11}$$

$$\xi_i \geq 0 \quad \forall\, i \in \{1, ..., n\}, \tag{12}$$

where $\xi_i$ are slack variables introduced to tolerant misclassified data points lying in between support vectors (soft-margin SVM). $C$ is the tuning parameter to control the tolerance level. It should be noted that, as suggested by previous work, nonlinear classification algorithms may suffer from the risk of overfitting issues when the features are more than the examples [17]; therefore, only linear classifiers were employed in our study.

## 3    Results and Discussions

For Dataset 1, LASSO is able to perform classification with a good accuracy (71.20 % to 99.01 % in Scenario 1, 72.11 % to 100 % in Scenario 2). On average, the classification using ENTR yields the best accuracy (90.50 % and 93.43 % for two scenarios respectively). As shown in Fig. 2, the classification for all RQA measures seems to be influenced by individual variation in both scenarios. On the other hand, while SVM performed at a comparable level as LASSO using ENTR and TT, it completely failed to classify the patterns using DET and LAM that are two analogous measures representing the percentage of points lying on diagonal and vertical lines in RP. In particular, DET indicates the deterministic pattern of signals; the periodic signals have higher DET because they have longer diagonal lines.

Similar patterns are also observed in the classification of Dataset 2 (see Table 1). One probable reason may be the automatic feature selection procedure in LASSO, in which a subset of sensors (typical size is around 20 to 30) is selected for the majority classification task. In this case, it may suggest a sparse recurrence pattern, characterized by DET and LAM, to be best captured by these selected channels.

However, these results are still preliminary and need to be further investigated. First, one of the major limitations of this approach is its high computational cost, which is approximately 200 ms for each time window of 1 s length. The computational cost is extremely expensive especially when using high-density recording arrays as we did and if the end-goal is real-time classification. Therefore, a sensor selection or signal fusion procedure might be considered to reduce the computational cost as well as to remove some sensors which do not carry critical information about the pattern of interest. Another important consideration is the parameter selection in RP. On the other hand, as no standard criterion has been established for selecting $\varepsilon$ and window length, a systematic

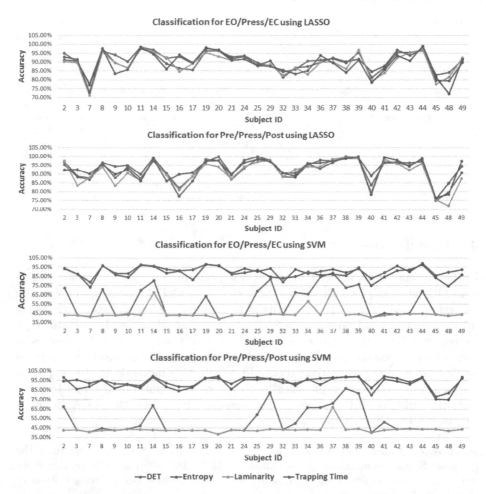

**Fig. 2.** The classification performance of four RQA measures using EEG signals recorded in the first experiment. The color of curves indicates the type of RQA measure. It was suggested that the accuracy of LASSO does not vary with the type of RQA measure in both scenarios, while the accuracy of SVM drops with LAM (green curves) and DET (blue curves). (Color figure online)

approach can be developed to select these parameters. On the other hand, an adaptive algorithm can be implemented to estimate the parameters for each window or participant individually. Finally, the four RQA measures were selected based on previous studies, but other RQA metrics can be explored as features as well. Narrow frequency bands of EEG signals can also be used for comparison, because it was suggested [3] that decomposing the EEG signals into such bands night improve the classification accuracy in seizure detection.

**Table 1.** The details of performance in Dataset 2. The classification task with best performance of each row is highlighted in bold. As shown below, the *Cold/Pre* yields the highest accuracy of the majority cases.

| Classifier | Feature | Participant 1 | | | | Participant 2 | | | |
|---|---|---|---|---|---|---|---|---|---|
| | | All | Warm/Cold | Warm/Pre | Cold/Pre | All | Warm/Cold | Warm/Pre | Cold/Pre |
| LASSO | DET | 97.78 % | 98.33 % | 98.33 % | **100.00 %** | 90.43 % | 95.16 % | 90.32 % | **98.41 %** |
| | ENTR | **96.67 %** | 93.33 % | **96.67 %** | **96.67 %** | 89.36 % | **100.00 %** | 93.55 % | 90.48 % |
| | LAM | 97.78 % | 98.33 % | 96.67 % | **100.00 %** | 94.68 % | 96.77 % | **98.39 %** | 93.65 % |
| | TT | 97.78 % | 98.33 % | 96.67 % | **100.00 %** | 89.36 % | 98.39 % | 95.16 % | **100.00 %** |
| SVM | DET | 67.78 % | 60.00 % | **95.00 %** | 88.33 % | 50.00 % | 51.61 % | 50.00 % | **60.32 %** |
| | ENTR | 97.78 % | **100.00 %** | 96.67 % | **100.00 %** | 96.81 % | 98.39 % | 96.77 % | **98.41 %** |
| | LAM | 90.00 % | 63.33 % | 90.00 % | **96.67 %** | 32.98 % | 51.61 % | 50.00 % | **60.32 %** |
| | TT | 96.67 % | 98.33 % | **100.00 %** | 98.33 % | 90.43 % | 98.39 % | 95.16 % | **100.00 %** |

## 4 Conclusion

In the present study, LASSO and SVM was performed to classify physical stress states based on RQA measures derived from ongoing EEG recordings. Our results indicate that the recurrence patterns of resting-state EEG signals under stressful and control conditions can be characterized and identified by certain RQA measures utilizing the entire sensor array, while for some other RQA measures, it seems more promising to pre-select a subset of sensors. Future work should focus on developing more sophisticated parameter selection methods and/or advanced sensor selection/fusion approaches to reduce the computational costs. In addition, the utility of EEG frequency band decomposition and other RQA measures can be systematically explored.

**Acknowledgment.** This research is made possible through the funding from the National Science Foundation (grant number CMMI - 1538059), and the Transdisciplinary Area of Excellence (TAE) exploratory research grant provided by State University of New York, Binghamton.

## References

1. Acharya, U.R., Sree, S.V., Ang, P.C.A., Yanti, R., Suri, J.S.: Application of nonlinear and wavelet based features for the automated identification of epileptic EEG signals. Int. J. Neural Syst. **22**(02), 1250002 (2012)
2. Becker, K., Schneider, G., Eder, M., Ranft, A., Kochs, E.F., Zieglgänsberger, W., Dodt, H.U.: Anaesthesia monitoring by recurrence quantification analysis of EEG data. PloS ONE **5**(1), e8876 (2010)
3. Chen, L.L., Zhang, J., Zou, J.Z., Zhao, C.J., Wang, G.S.: A framework on wavelet-based nonlinear features and extreme learning machine for epileptic seizure detection. Biomed. Signal Process. Control **10**, 1–10 (2014)
4. Cortes, C., Vapnik, V.: Support-vector networks. Mach. Learn. **20**(3), 273–297 (1995)
5. Eckmann, J.P., Kamphorst, S.O., Ruelle, D.: Recurrence plots of dynamical systems. EPL (Europhys. Lett.) **4**(9), 973 (1987)

6. Fraser, A.M., Swinney, H.L.: Independent coordinates for strange attractors from mutual information. Phys. Rev. A **33**(2), 1134 (1986)
7. Helland, V.C.F., Postnova, S., Schwarz, U., Kurths, J., Kundermann, B., Hemmeter, U., Braun, H.A.: Comparison of different methods for the evaluation of treatment effects from the sleep EEG of patients with major depression. J. Biol. Phys. **34**(3–4), 393–404 (2008)
8. Kennel, M.B., Brown, R., Abarbanel, H.D.: Determining embedding dimension for phase-space reconstruction using a geometrical construction. Phys. Rev. A **45**(6), 3403 (1992)
9. Koch, C., Laurent, G.: Complexity and the nervous system. Science **284**(5411), 96–98 (1999)
10. Korn, H., Faure, P.: Is there chaos in the brain? II. Experimental evidence and related models. C. R. Biol. **326**(9), 787–840 (2003)
11. Li, X., Sleigh, J.W., Voss, L.J., Ouyang, G.: Measure of the electroencephalographic effects of sevoflurane using recurrence dynamics. Neurosci. Lett. **424**(1), 47–50 (2007)
12. Liang, Z., Wang, Y., Ren, Y., Li, D., Voss, L., Sleigh, J., Li, X.: Detection of burst suppression patterns in EEG using recurrence rate. Sci. World J. **2014**, 1–11 (2014)
13. Marwan, N.: How to avoid potential pitfalls in recurrence plot based data analysis. Int. J. Bifurcat. Chaos **21**(04), 1003–1017 (2011)
14. Marwan, N., Romano, M.C., Thiel, M., Kurths, J.: Recurrence plots for the analysis of complex systems. Phys. Rep. **438**(5), 237–329 (2007)
15. Marwan, N., Wessel, N., Meyerfeldt, U., Schirdewan, A., Kurths, J.: Recurrence-plot-based measures of complexity and their application to heart-rate-variability data. Phys. Rev. E **66**(2), 026702 (2002)
16. Murali, L., Chitra, D., Manigandan, T., Sharanya, B.: An efficient adaptive filter architecture for improving the seizure detection in EEG signal. Circuits Syst. Signal Process. **35**, 1–18 (2015)
17. Pereira, F., Mitchell, T., Botvinick, M.: Machine learning classifiers and fMRI: a tutorial overview. Neuroimage **45**(1), S199–S209 (2009)
18. Shannon, C.E.: A mathematical theory of communication. ACM SIGMOBILE Mob. Comput. Commun. Rev. **5**(1), 3–55 (2001)
19. Stam, C.J.: Chaos, continuous EEG, and cognitive mechanisms: a future for clinical neurophysiology. Am. J. Electroneurodiagn. Technol. **43**(4), 211–227 (2003)
20. Tibshirani, R.: Regression shrinkage and selection via the lasso. J. R. Stat. Soc.: Ser. B (Methodol.) **58**, 267–288 (1996)
21. Webber, C.L., Zbilut, J.P.: Dynamical assessment of physiological systems and states using recurrence plot strategies. J. Appl. Physiol. **76**(2), 965–973 (1994)
22. Webber Jr., C.L., Zbilut, J.P.: Recurrence quantification analysis of nonlinear dynamical systems. In: Tutorials in Contemporary Nonlinear Methods for the Behavioral Sciences, pp. 26–94 (2005)
23. Zbilut, J.P., Webber, C.L.: Embeddings and delays as derived from quantification of recurrence plots. Phys. Lett. A **171**(3), 199–203 (1992)
24. Zbilut, J.P., Zaldivar-Comenges, J.M., Strozzi, F.: Recurrence quantification based Liapunov exponents for monitoring divergence in experimental data. Phys. Lett. A **297**(3), 173–181 (2002)

# Prediction of Seizure Spread Network via Sparse Representations of Overcomplete Dictionaries

Feng Liu[1]([⊠]), Wei Xiang[2], Shouyi Wang[1], and Bradley Lega[3]

[1] Department of Industrial, Manufacturing and Systems Engineering,
University of Texas at Arlington, Arlington, TX 76019, USA
feng.liu@mavs.uta.edu, shouyiw@uta.edu
[2] Department of Computer Science and Engineering,
University of Texas at Arlington, Arlington, TX 76019, USA
wei.xiang@mavs.uta.edu
[3] Neurological Surgery, University of Texas Southwestern, Dallas, TX 75253, USA
bradley.lega@utsouthwestern.edu

**Abstract.** Epilepsy is one of the most common brain disorders and affect people of all ages. Resective surgery is currently the most effective overall treatment for patients whose seizures cannot be controlled by medications. Seizure spread network with secondary epileptogenesis are thought to be responsible for a substantial portion of surgical failures. However, there is still considerable risk of surgical failures for lacking of priori knowledge. Cortico-cortical evoked potentials (CCEP) offer the possibility of understanding connectivity within seizure spread networks to know how seizure evolves in the brain as it measures directly the intracranial electric signals. This study is one of the first works to investigate effective seizure spread network modeling using CCEP signals. The previous unsupervised brain network connectivity problem was converted into a classical supervised sparse representation problem for the first time. In particular, we developed an effective network modeling framework using sparse representation of over-determined features extracted from extensively designed experiments to predict real seizure spread network for each individual patient. The experimental results on five patients achieved prediction accuracy of about 70 %, which indicates that it is possible to predict seizure spread network from stimulated CCEP networks. The developed CCEP signal analysis and network modeling approaches are promising to understand network mechanisms of epileptogenesis and have a potential to render clinicians better epilepsy surgical decisions in the future.

**Keywords:** Brain connectivity · Sparse representation · Feature selection · CCEP · Seizure spread network

## 1 Introduction

The human brain is among the most complex systems known to mankind [2]. There has been a great deal of neurophysiological researching attempting to

© Springer International Publishing AG 2016
G.A. Ascoli et al. (Eds.): BIH 2016, LNAI 9919, pp. 262–273, 2016.
DOI: 10.1007/978-3-319-47103-7_26

understand brain functions and networks through detailed analysis of neuronal excitability and synaptic transmission [9,10]. Though the advances in brain imaging techniques have enabled many studies to investigate brain functional connectivity with widely variable spatial and temporal resolution using different neurophysiology and neuroimaging modalities including electroencephalography (EEG), magnetoencephalography (MEG), functional near-infrared spectroscopy (fNIRS), and functional MRI (fMRI) approaches [16,20]. However, most of current work on brain functional connectivity analyzes at a relatively coarse level of connectivity of the intrinsic dynamic brain network. The results are often at odds with the longstanding neuroscientific theory [7]. In this paper, we employ cortico-cortical evoked potentials (CCEPs) which directly measure the local neural activity inside brain to map effective brain connectivity via stimulation. The major advantage of mapping brain connectivity via stimulation is the ability to assess directed dynamical spread networks and discover functional cortical connections in vivo, which is not possible using MRI-based tract tracing nor with the fMRI-based covariance methods [6].

To understand pathology of epilepsy, more researchers are focusing on abnormal brain network connectivity. Historically speaking, there are two opposing perspective to view brain functionality: integration and segregation. The former views different areas of cortex collaborate together to perform certain tasks, such as attention, memory processing, etc. However the latter perspective think the "segregated" area of cortex is responsible for certain functionality of the brain, such as language, emotion etc. A good discussion of integration and segregation can be found in the Nature Review paper [3]. The advantage of the former one is to investigate brain in a more systematic view by searching distinction of functional and effective connectivity among patients and controls. Moreover, the emerging interdisciplinary area of complex network theory can offer a systematic measurement of network characteristics with great capability to model networks in nature and man-made complex systems [1,8,19,26]. Recently, an increasing number of theoretical and empirical studies approach the function of the human brain from a network perspective, i.e., the integration paradigm. The aim of human connectomics is to uncover the underlying dynamics associated with their connectivity. Disturbed interaction among brain areas is associated with brain and mental disorder [21,22]. Many researchers have verified that a large amount of brain diseases arise from dysfunction of brain network [24,28,30]. CCEP offers the possibility of understanding effective connectivity within seizure networks to improve diagnosis and identify resection candidates for seizure surgery to a finer spatial resolution. In our paper, CCEP signals are used to construct connectivity of epilepsy patients in order to predict the ictal onset spreading network. The rest of paper is organized as follows: data description and preprocessing is presented in Sect. 2. The presented supervised sparse feature selection formulation is given in Sect. 3. The experimental result of spread network prediction is given in Sects. 4 and 5 concludes this paper and future research is also described.

# 2    Data Processing and Visualization

## 2.1    Data Acquisition

Patients were drawn from the surgical epilepsy program at University of Texas Southwestern Medical Center (UTSW), the preeminent surgical epilepsy program in a metropolitan area of 7 million people. We have also analyzed subset of our existing database of intracranial electrode implantations [15] (as described in Table 1) that have both structural MRI and CCEP mapping. Prior to electrode implantation, patients undergo resting-state fMRI as well as detailed structural MRI including diffusion-tensor imaging (DTI).

**Table 1.** Information of 5 patients studied in this paper, who undergo the surgical epilepsy program at UTSW.

| Subject ID | Sex | Age | Duration (years) | Total seizures | Early spread | Late spread | Seizure analyzed | Onset pattern | Onset site | Early site | Late site |
|---|---|---|---|---|---|---|---|---|---|---|---|
| 1 | M | 59 | 8 | 4 | 0.2 | 30 | 4 | 4 | R entorhinal | MTG | Insula |
| 2 | F | 38 | 8 | 7 | 2 | 13 | 5 | 4 | R amygdala | Para hippocampu | STG |
| 3 | M | 30 | 21 | 3 | 0.3 | 12 | 3 | 1 | L precuneus | Fusiform | Lingula |
| 4 | F | 63 | 54 | 14 | 0.3 | 9 | 5 | 4 | L angular g. | MTG | Fusiform |
| 5 | F | 42 | 15 | 5 | 0.6 | 10 | 5 | 4 | R planum polare | STG | Supramarginal |

## 2.2    Stimulation Polarity

Stimulations (conducted using the Grass S88 stimulator (Warwick, RI, USA) [15]) show switched polarity pattern due to the bipolar stimulation was applied between adjacent electrodes by switching anode and cathode electrodes. The reason we prefer bipolar stimulation as opposed to unipolar stimulation where the stimulation is performed between an area of interest and a distant site, is that bipolar stimulation allows for more localized current flow in the cortex beneath electrodes, thereby minimizing the spatial spread of stimulation and increasing its spatial resolution [12,18]. In this paper, we show that stimulation responses categorized based on polarity of stimulus are related to the CCEPs measured and thereof we suggest to divide signals into groups based on polarity of stimulus and then choose those from positive and negative group separately for further analysis, as explained later.

In most studies [11] CCEPs at each site were averaged before any task of data mining to be done, however, in this paper we separate them out and term the responses resulted from stimulus showing positive polarity as the *Positive Group*, and that from stimulus of negative polarity as the *Negative Group*. For comparison, we also average all CCEPs despite of its source and name it as the *Mixed Group*. In this paper, we refer to the averaged response from three different groups using positive/negative/mixing averaged response. Figure 1 illustrates two examples of the comparison between responses from three groups.

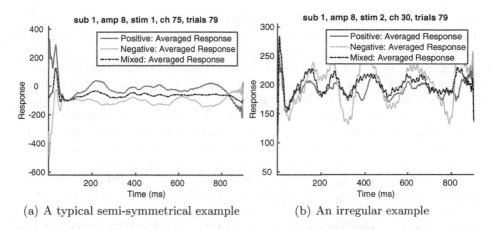

(a) A typical semi-symmetrical example       (b) An irregular example

**Fig. 1.** Comparison of positive, negative and mixing averaged signals categorized according to the polarity of stimulus signals. Most paper studied on signals drawn with the black dotted line while in this paper, we think polarity factor should be taken into account when doing further data analysis.

It is worth noting that in Fig. 1(a), the positive and negative averaged response demonstrate a *semi*-symmetrical structure where the momentum on the first 80ms is affected by a dynamic force. We believe such dynamics were caused by neuronal activities of those attempting to recover to its normal state. Besides, some averaged responses like Fig. 1(b) can be treated as irregular ones since positive and negative averaged responses do not follow a similar trend (i.e. increase/decrease at different phases).

With both groups, it is not wise to average signals over all trials (i.e., analyzing on the black dotted signals shown in Fig. 1). The underlying tissue (which may be more sensitive to one polarity) will show averaged response in one group that have larger amplitude at all phases comparing to the other's. If we compare mixing averaged response with either positive or negative one, most likely we will see some prominent features weakened due to a distinguishable profile of the averaged response signal, including (1) semi-symmetry and (2) sensitivity to different polarity of stimulus. Therefore, we need to extract signals whose averaged response is stronger with respect to the polarity of its source of stimulus.

## 2.3 Data Preprocessing

In this paper, to simplify further data analysis using averaged signals, we extract and only work with the positive group (exemplified by Fig. 3). To remove post-stimulation artifacts which occur nondeterminately at various times between 85 ms to 95 ms, peak and valley detection algorithm is applied following which we retrieve signals from +1 ms till +900 ms (for some sites, there exist strong response immediately after the timing of post-stimulation artifact). After that, Savitzky-Golay filter is applied to smooth all signals without greatly distorting the signals. Many of stimulus signals jitter with sine waves whose frequency is found fixed at 49 Hz. To alleviate this problem, we apply a specific designed band-pass filter to attenuate artifact-induced frequency at 49 Hz, as well as those frequencies from 1 to 3 Hz and outside 100 Hz. Besides, by analyzing patterns of the stimulus signals, we find it necessary to remove outlier trials as they give rise to much stronger and longer CCEPs. To this end, all trials were further taken care of statistically using the approach of trimmed mean, i.e. for all trials stimulated on the same pair of sites, we remove those generated from stimulus signals whose trimmed means are two standard deviations away from mean of the distribution of trimmed means over all stimulus signals at the two stimulation sites (with 25 % of the ends discarded). This guarantees all trials are generated from similar stimulations. Afterwards, trimmed mean approach is also used for every channel in order to get rid of outlier trials. Take for example subject 1: during four stimulations with amplitude 8 mA on CP1-CP2, UP2-UP3, UP5-UP6 and UP7-UP8 respectively, there are 80 trials among all the 140 channels. Trimmed mean approach based on stimulus signals helps get rid of 10, 13, 9, 10 trials for each of the four stimulations respectively, while the trimmed mean approach based on channels removes 2 trials per channel. The signal responses over all trials on one channel can be visualized using event-related potential (ERP) plot [4], by which the visualization of expected stimulation along trials should have a clear curve belonging to similar colormap (shown in Fig. 2). Finally, we convert signals to Z-scores so that for most signals their strengths are fixed from −5 to +5 as in Fig. 3.

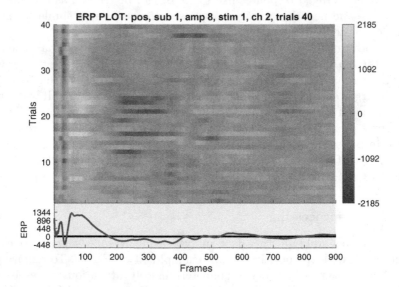

**Fig. 2.** An example of ERP plot, where the signal responses can be visualized clearly with similar colormap along trials. (Color figure online)

pos, sub 1, amp 8, stim 3, chs 140, trials 36

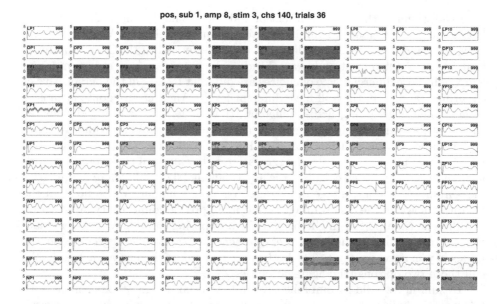

**Fig. 3.** Normalized Z-scores from positive averaged responses on 140 channels for patient 1. The signals were averaged over 36 repetitive 8 mA stimulations on channel UP3 and UP4. Magenta colored regions indicate stimulus sites, cyan indicates seizure onset zone, and red and green indicate EARLY and LATE ictal spread respectively [15]. For e.g., UP5, UP6 are both stimulus site and seizure onset zone. (Color figure online)

## 3 Supervised Sparse Feature Selection

### 3.1 Experimental Design of Features

When it comes to modeling the brain connectivity based on the measurement of how similar two channels' time series signals are, there are many options to be chosen. The most popular ones can be categorized as linear and nonlinear measurements [14,23], linear ones include cross correlation, coherence, and nonlinear measurements include mutual information, transfer entropy, Granger causality, phase synchronization, etc.

Different measurement will usually result in different networks, combined with the lack of ground truth information, it's hard to determine which one is more reasonable and accurate. However our case is different since we have a supervised label that was generated from the spread network, which makes it possible to compare prediction accuracy from different methodologies. The other choices come from the data preprocessing step and an appropriate frequency band need to be selected, the band pass filter level includes. Moreover, according to our analysis, we want to explore the effected network from both positive stimulus and negative stimulus, we also want make a contrast without considering the positive and negative stimulus. Another experimental design consideration includes the epoch signal length after the stimulus, we assume that after the stimulus, there is a transient period and it's hard to measure that exact length since every channel exhibits different temporal behavior. We picked 0.3 s, 0.5 s, 0.7 s and 0.8 s as different levels of the time series length. Other options is that we have different stimulus amplitude, which are 2 mA, 4 mA, 6 mA and 8 mA. All those different type of choices are different factors in the perspective of experimental design, they all have different levels. Another antagonistic choices comes when aggregating across different trials under the same conditions, as the impulsive stimulus signals were applied to the same channel about 40 times under the condition of the same stimulus amplitude, the same stimulus sites for the same person. One way of aggregation is to calculate the averaged epoch time series first and then calculate the adjacency matrix using different similarity measurement. The advantage of average first is to eliminate white noise in the channels, however the disadvantage is that more precise connectivity information at different time period might be lost. The opposing paradigm is to calculate the neural synchrony similarity measurement first and then aggregate on the adjacency matrix, we try to use both ways to predict the spread network. We call those two options trial aggregation design.

To sum up, we did a comprehensive full factorial design of experiment with 6 factors, including (1) similarity measurements, (2) positive, negative vs overall stimulus, (3) stimulus amplitude, (4) epoch signal length following stimulus, (5) frequency band-pass design, (6) trial aggregation design. The frequency band-pass have 6 levels, which are 4–100 Hz, 4–8 Hz, 8–13 Hz, 13–25 Hz, 25–40 Hz, 30–100 Hz; the neural time series similarity measurements used in our research include cross correlation, coherence, mutual information, transfer entropy, phase synchronization and dynamic time warping. In Table 2, a summary of level counts for each factor is given.

**Table 2.** Number of levels of different factors. The number of features here in our exploration is the number of full factorial of all the six factors in our design, which is 3456 features.

| Factor | Number of levels |
| --- | --- |
| Similarity measurements | 6 |
| Positive, negative vs. overall stimulus | 3 |
| Stimulus magnitude | 4 |
| Epoch signal length | 4 |
| Band pass frequency | 6 |
| Trial aggregation design | 2 |

### 3.2   Sparse Feature Selection

In order to select the most useful features, we used a sparse feature selection method procedure regularized with $L_1$ norm. The idea behind of the sparse representation is that we want to represent connection vector $y$ as a linear combination of the fewest features from the overcomplete dictionary [27], which becomes a powerful tool for biomedical data [29]. Here we use a sparse feature selection model which allows certain degree of noise, and the goal function is given below:

$$J_1(x; \lambda) = \|y - Ax\|_2^2 + \lambda \|x\|_1 \tag{1}$$

where $A \in R^{n \times k}$ is the overcomplete dictionary with each column being the prediction results using our factorial experimental design of 6 factors, $n$ is the number of nodes and $k$ is the number of features, $y \in R^n$ is the supervised connection vector. The first part of Eq. (1) is to measure the sparse representation error and the second term is trying to make the selected features to be sparse compared to the over-complete dictionary. By minimizing the goal function, we will get the selected ensemble of prediction methodologies. Unlike the traditional ensemble method [25], our learned vector $x$ signifies the supervised weighted version of an ensemble of weak classifiers. As a result, our problem becomes a classic $\ell_1$-penalized least-squares problem. There are plenty of algorithms to solve it available [5,17,27], here in our research, we use Homotopy algorithm proposed in [5]. For more detailed description of Homotopy algorithm, please refer to Donoho and Tsaig's paper [5].

## 4   Network Connectivity Modeling and Prediction

### 4.1   Spread Network Construction and Prediction

Like our previous work [15], in this paper we refined CCEP paradigm to analyze the seizure spread from ictal onset zones to EARLY and LATE sites of seizure propagation, defined as spread from onset site before or after 3 s.

By better understanding the epilepsy ictal onset spread network, we can resect pathological path and reduce the potential destruction of functionality in other cortical region. Promising clinical results from [13] show that 42 % of patient are seizure free after resective epilepsy surgery based on seizure ictal onset spreading network.

In every similarity measurement, it's nontrivial to select the threshold to get the connected network with appropriate density. Take the calculation of cross correlation for each trial as an example, we observed a time variant adjacency matrix. If the same threshold is used, sometime, a very densely connected network is generated, for another stimulus trial, a very sparsely connected network is generated. Furthermore, we observed that if we average time series from all epoch trials first and then compute the cross correlation, the resulting correlation coefficients are much higher than directly calculating correlation for each trial. To solve that problem, a dynamically adjusted threshold is used in the paper. The dynamically adjusted threshold is based on the priori knowledge of average degree on brain network, which has been extensively studies in the literature.

The predesignated percentage is calculated based on the following equation:

$$p = \frac{k}{(N - 1)} * 100 \% \tag{2}$$

Using $p$ to get the percentile in the correlation matrix, we can generate a network with the average degree to be $k$.

## 4.2   Experimental Result

Based on the framework mentioned, We conducted the sparse feature selection of the first two patients' seizure onset spreading network, and test the learned features on the next three patients and achieved 72.3 % accuracy. Since we have 6 factors, it's impossible to give a comprehensive accuracy result. We illustrate 2 factors, namely, the similarity measurements and band pass frequency design in the following table. The training accuracy is 80.5 % and the testing accuracy is 72.3 %. Generally speaking, the correlation and mutual information measurement perform better than the other 4 measurements (Table 3).

**Table 3.** Accuracy summary.

| | Training | | | | | | Testing | | | | | |
|---|---|---|---|---|---|---|---|---|---|---|---|---|
| | Corr | Cohe | MI | TE | PS | DTW | Corr | Cohe | MI | TE | PS | DTW |
| 4–100Hz | 72.3 % | 69.3 % | 74.3 % | 73.5 % | 68.8 % | 62.3 % | 71.3 % | 68.6 % | 74.6 % | 72.7 % | 68.4 % | 60.8 % |
| 4–8Hz | 68.7 % | 66.1 % | 67.4 % | 70.2 % | 69.2 % | 59.3 % | 66.6 % | 67.5 % | 68.2 % | 68.8 % | 70.0 % | 61.2 % |
| 8–13Hz | 65.2 % | 54.0 % | 68.3 % | 64.2 % | 67.3 % | 61.8 % | 65.9 % | 63.0 % | 68.1 % | 63.4 % | 64.7 % | 62.1 % |
| 13–25Hz | 71.4 % | 67.4 % | 69.7 % | 69.0 % | 66.2 % | 63.0 % | 69.9 % | 66.6 % | 68.8 % | 70.2 % | 65.9 % | 63.4 % |
| 25–40Hz | 70.5 % | 69.3 % | 70.2 % | 71.1 % | 65.4 % | 65.9 % | 71.4 % | 67.9 % | 70.3 % | 72.1 % | 65.2 % | 72.0 % |
| 30–100Hz | 71.8 % | 72.5 % | 73.9 % | 68.5 % | 71.7 % | 64.8 % | 71.1 % | 71.5 % | 74.5 % | 68.3 % | 71.9 % | 63.9 % |
| Sparse | 80.5 % | | | | | | 72.3 % | | | | | |

Abbreviations– Corr: correlation, Cohe: coherence, MI: mutual information, TE: transfer entropy, PS: phase synchronization, DTW: dynamic time warping.

Take patient 1 as an illustrative example, the predicted spread network is given in Fig. 5 compared to Fig. 4, which is the real seizure spread network. To the best of our knowledge, we are among the first to investigate prediction of seizure spread network using CCEP signals processing and data mining analytic

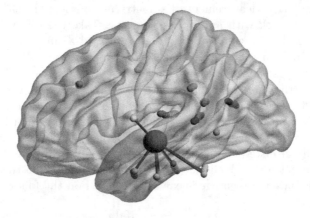

**Fig. 4.** Spread network of Patient 1: the large red node is the seizure onset area, and the connected nodes to the large red node are the cortical sites where seizure arrives within 3 s. (Color figure online)

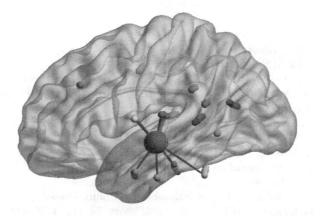

**Fig. 5.** Predicted Spread network of Patient 1: the large red node is the seizure onset area, and the connected nodes to the large red node are the predicted cortical sites that should receive seizure attack from the origin sites. (Color figure online)

approaches. The prediction accuracy of more than 70 % achieved in this preliminary study is promising to confirm that it is possible to predict fast seizure spread locations from CCEP signals. Such information will be of great importance for neurosurgeons to make better surgery plan and improve success rate for patients with epilepsy.

## 5    Conclusion

In this paper, we proposed to predict seizure ictal onset spread network which is a missing part in literature. In our work, we implemented an extensive experimental design using 6 factors. We separately investigated both positive and negative stimulated signals, thus giving us additional information when extracting features. A sparse learning framework of over complete dictionary is presented, the framework is scalable that more effecting factors can be added. We converted unsupervised brain network connectivity problem into a classical supervised sparse representation problem, which there exist a plenty of algorithms to solve. The proposed framework achieved satisfactory result.

Through CCEP mapping, we can develop new network generation scheme and scalable efficient algorithms for directed brain connectivity analysis. The scope of this study is planned as a step forward to understand neural circuits of epilepsy and provide a new computational framework to understand seizure focus, initiating seizure circuits, paths of spread, neuromodulatory centers, and to develop a system's view of epilepsy. It will establish valuable knowledge of seizure-spread networks and their relationship with some critical factors in presurgery assessment. The brain network analysis methods can also be generalized to analyze other brain disorders or cognitive functions of the brain with immediate clinical implications. In our future research, the sensitivity and specificity error rate will also taking into account in the goal function formulation instead of the overall accuracy as we studied here.

# References

1. Barabási, A.L., Albert, R.: Emergence of scaling in random networks. Science **286**(5439), 509–512 (1999)
2. Bullmore, E., Sporns, O.: Complex brain networks: graph theoretical analysis of structural and functional systems. Nat. Rev. Neurosci. **10**(3), 186–198 (2009)
3. Deco, G., Tononi, G., Boly, M., Kringelbach, M.L.: Rethinking segregation and integration: contributions of whole-brain modelling. Nat. Rev. Neurosci. **16**(7), 430–439 (2015)
4. Delorme, A., Makeig, S.: EEGLAB: an open source toolbox for analysis of single-trial EEG dynamics including independent component analysis. J. Neurosci. Methods **134**(1), 9–21 (2004)
5. Donoho, D.L., Tsaig, Y.: Fast solution of-norm minimization problems when the solution may be sparse. IEEE Trans. Inf. Theory **54**(11), 4789–4812 (2008)
6. Enatsu, R., Piao, Z., OConnor, T., Horning, K., Mosher, J., Burgess, R., Bingaman, W., Nair, D.: Cortical excitability varies upon ictal onset patterns in neocortical epilepsy: a cortico-cortical evoked potential study. Clin. Neurophysiol. **123**(2), 252–260 (2012)
7. Friston, K.J.: Functional and effective connectivity: a review. Brain Connect. **1**(1), 13–36 (2011)
8. Guan, Z.H., Liu, F., Li, J., Wang, Y.W.: Chaotification of complex networks with impulsive control. Chaos: Interdisc. J. Nonlinear Sci. **22**(2), 023137 (2012)
9. Snead, O.C.: Basic mechanisms of generalized absence seizures. Annals. Neurol. **37**(2), 146–157 (1995)
10. Jefferys, J.G.: Advances in understanding basic mechanisms of epilepsy and seizures. Seizure **19**(10), 638–646 (2010)
11. Keller, C.J., Honey, C.J., Entz, L., Bickel, S., Groppe, D.M., Toth, E., Ulbert, I., Lado, F.A., Mehta, A.D.: Corticocortical evoked potentials reveal projectors and integrators in human brain networks. J. Neurosci. **34**(27), 9152–9163 (2014)
12. Keller, C.J., Honey, C.J., Mégevand, P., Entz, L., Ulbert, I., Mehta, A.D.: Mapping human brain networks with cortico-cortical evoked potentials. Phil. Trans. R. Soc. B **369**(1653), 20130528 (2014)
13. Kim, D.W., Kim, H.K., Lee, S.K., Chu, K., Chung, C.K.: Extent of neocortical resection and surgical outcome of epilepsy: intracranial EEG analysis. Epilepsia **51**(6), 1010–1017 (2010)
14. Kreuz, T.: Measures of neuronal signal synchrony. Scholarpedia **6**(12), 11922 (2011). (Revision 152249)
15. Lega, B., Dionisio, S., Flanigan, P., Bingaman, W., Najm, I., Nair, D., Gonzalez-Martinez, J.: Cortico-cortical evoked potentials for sites of early versus late seizure spread in stereoelectroencephalography. Epilepsy Res. **115**, 17–29 (2015)
16. Letzen, J.E., Craggs, J.G., Perlstein, W.M., Price, D.D., Robinson, M.E.: Functional connectivity of the default mode network and its association with pain networks in irritable bowel patients assessed via lidocaine treatment. J. Pain **14**(10), 1077–1087 (2013)
17. Liu, J., Ji, S., Ye, J., et al.: SLEP: sparse learning with efficient projections. Ariz. State Univ. **6**, 491 (2009)
18. Nathan, S.S., Sinha, S.R., Gordon, B., Lesser, R.P., Thakor, N.V.: Determination of current density distributions generated by electrical stimulation of the human cerebral cortex. Electroencephalogr. Clin. Neurophysiol. **86**(3), 183–192 (1993)

19. Newman, M.E.: The structure and function of complex networks. SIAM Rev. **45**(2), 167–256 (2003)
20. Otti, A., Guendel, H., Henningsen, P., Zimmer, C., Noll-Hussong, M.: Functional network connectivity of pain-related resting state networks in somatoform pain disorder: an exploratory fMRI study. J. Psychiatry Neurosci.: JPN **38**(1), 57 (2013)
21. Sporns, O.: Structure and function of complex brain networks. Dialogues Clin. Neurosci. **15**(3), 247–262 (2013)
22. Sporns, O., Tononi, G., Kötter, R.: The human connectome: a structural description of the human brain. PLoS Comput. Biol. **1**(4), e42 (2005)
23. Uddin, L.Q., Clare Kelly, A., Biswal, B.B., Xavier Castellanos, F., Milham, M.P.: Functional connectivity of default mode network components: correlation, anticorrelation, and causality. Hum. Brain Mapp. **30**(2), 625–637 (2009)
24. Vecchio, F., Miraglia, F., Curcio, G., Della Marca, G., Vollono, C., Mazzucchi, E., Bramanti, P., Rossini, P.M.: Cortical connectivity in fronto-temporal focal epilepsy from EEG analysis: a study via graph theory. Clin. Neurophysiol. **126**(6), 1108–1116 (2015)
25. Wang, H., Fan, W., Yu, P.S., Han, J.: Mining concept-drifting data streams using ensemble classifiers. In: Proceedings of the Ninth ACM SIGKDD International Conference on Knowledge Discovery and Data Mining, pp. 226–235. ACM (2003)
26. Watts, D.J., Strogatz, S.H.: Collective dynamics of small-world networks. Nature **393**(6684), 440–442 (1998)
27. Wright, S.J., Nowak, R.D., Figueiredo, M.A.: Sparse reconstruction by separable approximation. IEEE Trans. Signal Process. **57**(7), 2479–2493 (2009)
28. Yaffe, R.B., Borger, P., Megevand, P., Groppe, D.M., Kramer, M.A., Chu, C.J., Santaniello, S., Meisel, C., Mehta, A.D., Sarma, S.V.: Physiology of functional and effective networks in epilepsy. Clin. Neurophysiol. **126**(2), 227–236 (2015)
29. Ye, J., Liu, J.: Sparse methods for biomedical data. ACM SIGKDD Explor. Newsl. **14**(1), 4–15 (2012)
30. Zhou, J., Seeley, W.W.: Network dysfunction in Alzheimers disease and frontotemporal dementia: implications for psychiatry. Biol. Psychiatry **75**(7), 565–573 (2014)

# A Novel Mutual-Information-Guided Sparse Feature Selection Approach for Epilepsy Diagnosis Using Interictal EEG Signals

Shouyi Wang[1](✉), Cao Xiao[2], Jeffrey J. Tsai[3], Wanpracha Chaovalitwongse[2], and Thomas J. Grabowski[4]

[1] Department of Industrial, Manufacturing and Systems Engineering, University of Texas at Arlington, Arlington, TX 76019, USA
shouyiw@uta.edu
[2] Department of Industrial and Systems Engineering, University of Washington, Seattle, WA 98195, USA
{xiaoc,artchao}@uw.edu
[3] Department of Neurology and Harborview Medical Center, University of Washington, Seattle, WA 98104, USA
jjtsai@uw.edu
[4] Departments of Radiology and Neurology, University of Washington, Seattle, WA 98195, USA
tgrabow@uw.edu

**Abstract.** Diagnosing people with possible epilepsy has major implications for their health, occupation, driving and social interactions. The current epilepsy diagnosis procedure is often subject to errors with considerable interobserver variations by manually observing long-term lengthy EEG recordings that require the presence of seizure (ictal) activities. It is costly and often difficult to obtain long-term EEG data with seizure activities that imped epilepsy diagnosis for many people, in particular in areas that lack of medical resources and well-trained neurologists. There is a desperate need for a new diagnostic tool that is capable of providing quick and accurate epilepsy-screening using short-term interictal EEG signals. However, it is challenging to analyze interictal EEG recordings when patients behaviors same as normal subjects. This research is dedicated to develop new automatic data-driven pattern recognition system for interictal EEG signals and design a quick screening process to help neurologists diagnose patients with epilepsy. In particular, we propose a novel information-theory-guided spare feature selection framework to select the most important EEG features to discriminate epileptic or non-epileptic EEG patterns accurately. The proposed approach were tested on an EEG dataset with 11 patients and 11 normal subjects, achieved an impressive diagnostic accuracy of 90 % based on visually-evoked potentials in a human-computer task. This preliminary study indicates that it is promising to provide fast, reliable, and affordable epilepsy diagnostic solutions using short-term interictal EEG signals.

G.A. Ascoli et al. (Eds.): BIH 2016, LNAI 9919, pp. 274–284, 2016.
DOI: 10.1007/978-3-319-47103-7_27

# 1 Introduction

Epilepsy is the most common neurological brain disorders next to strokes, and about 1 % of human population (40 million people) suffer from epilepsy [1]. An accurate diagnosis of people with possible epilepsy has big implications for their health, occupation, driving and social interactions, and an inaccurate diagnosis may have fatal consequences, especially in operating rooms and intensive care units. However, false diagnosis of epilepsy is unfortunately common in every-day practice. The estimates of the misdiagnosis rate of epilepsy varies greatly, from 5 % in a prospective childhood epilepsy study, 23 % in a British population-based study [2], to as high as 41 % in a Swedish study [3]. One reason for the misdiagnosis of epilepsy is that many other diseases or medical conditions can result in abnormal changes in brain behavior, or even cause seizure-like episodes and thus can be confused with epilepsy [1]. Among commonly used medical tests such as blood tests, magnetic resonance imaging (MRI), positron emission tomography (PET), electroencephalogram (EEG) recording play a central role in epilepsy diagnosis because it directly detects electrical activity in the brain. The epileptic diagnosis heavily relies on a tedious visual screening process by neurologists from lengthy EEG recordings that require the presence of seizure (ictal) activities. Thus, a prolonged (24-h) EEG monitoring are often necessary. In the past decades, there have been many quantitative analysis systems to help neurologists identify epileptiform patterns from long-term EEG recordings for seizure detection and seizure prediction. However, it is costly and often diffi-cult to obtain long-term EEG data with seizure activities for epilepsy patients, especially in the areas that lack of medical resources and well-trained neurolo-gists. There have been very few studies that using short-term interictal EEG for more convenient and affordable epilepsy diagnosis. There is a desperate need for a new medical diagnostic tool that is capable of providing quick and accurate epilepsy-screening using short-term interictal EEG signals.

This study is designed to investigate the application of short-term interic-tal EEG signals for epilepsy diagnosis using machine learning techniques. In particular, we propose an information-theory-guided feature selection and pre-diction framework to identify epilepsy-specific EEG patterns in a fast screen-ing process in a human-computer interaction task using visually-evoked poten-tials (VEP). The proposed method has a potential to be applied to determine whether a patient is epileptic or non-epileptic in a quick screening process. The organization of the paper is as follows. Section 2 presents the information-guided sparse feature selection framework with regularization. The experimental design, data acquisition, and method implementation and validation procedure are pre-sented in Sect. 3. The experimental results are provided in Sect. 4, and concluding remarks are given in Sect. 5.

# 2 Information-Theory-Guided Sparse Feature Selection

We propose a novel sparse feature selection approach that interactively integrates information theory with a sparse learning optimization framework with regular-ization to identify optimal feature subset to discriminate patterns of two classes.

**Feature Selection.** Feature selection techniques have been widely used to identify most important decision variables, to avoid overfitting and improve model performance, and to gain a deeper insight into the underlying processes or problem. Feature selection techniques generally can be categorized into three categories: embedded methods, wrapper methods, and filter methods [4]. Both embedded methods and wrapper methods rely on an employed classifier or model for feature subset selection. Thus, the feature selection performance is specific to the selected model. Typical approaches include Pudi's floating search [5], stepwise selection [6]. Filter techniques assess the relevance of features by looking only at the intrinsic properties of the data. Some popular examples include correlation-based feature selection [7], Fast correlation-based feature selection [8], and minimum redundancy maximum relevance (mRMR) [9]. However, most current filter techniques select high-ranked features and do not consider feature dependency fully in feature selection. Several individually low-scored features can be combined to form a strong discriminative feature subset for classification. To address this problem, we propose a novel feature selection framework that combines mutual information feature filtering and sparse-learning method interactively to capture feature dependencies and identify the most informative feature subset efficiently.

**Mutual Information-Based Feature Ranking.** In information theory, mutual information (MI) is a measure of inherent dependence between two independent variables [10]. MI measures how much information a feature contains about the class without making any assumptions about the nature of their underlying relationships. The mutual information of two variables X and Y, denoted by $I(X, Y)$, can be calculated by:

$$I(X;Y) = \sum_{y \in Y} \sum_{x \in X} p(x,y) \log \left( \frac{p(x,y)}{p(x)\,p(y)} \right), \tag{1}$$

where p(x) and p(y) are the marginal probability distribution and $p(X, Y)$ is the joint probability distribution of the variable X and Y. MI can capture nonlinear dependency among random variables and can be applied to rank features in feature selection problems [9]. The basic idea is to keep the more informative features (with higher MI) and remove the redundant or less-relevant features (with low MI) in filter-based approaches. These approaches can work well in many cases. However, they are subject to issues of missing some important features by just excluding low MI-ranked features. The interactions and dependencies among features are insufficiently considered in the current MI-based feature selection approaches. Some low-ranked weak features may be integrated with high-ranked features to produce stronger discrimination power for classification. Based on this consideration, we propose a novel feature selection framework that can consider both high-ranked and low-ranked features to discover the most important features efficiently.

**Interactive Feature Selection Framework.** The key idea of the proposed approach is to take into account feature dependency while keeping the searching process computational efficient. The proposed mutual-information-guided feature selection framework is built on the three steps: MI-based feature ranking, sparse feature learning on low MI-ranked features, and integration of high- and low-ranked features. In the feature ranking step, we use MI to rank features and identify a subset of high MI features that have the best informative power individually to class labels. Among those features, the highly correlated features are considered as redundant features and removed in a way similar to the MRMR approach. Given a number of features $k$, the subset of top $k$ features ranked by MI is denoted by $S$, and the subset of the remaining features is denoted by $W$. In the second step, we employ the most popular sparse learning algorithm, (least absolute shrinkage and selection operator) lasso, to select potentially important feature subset from the low-ranked features in set $W$. The formulation of lasso with a $l_1$-norm penalty is as follows:

$$\sum_{i=1}^{n} (y_i - \beta x_i)^2 + \lambda ||\beta||_1. \tag{2}$$

The lasso method can effectively select a sparse model by penalizing and forcing coefficients of some variables to be zero. Assume $k_2$ features are selected by the lasso algorithm. The third step is to find the optimal feature subset by exploring the $k_1$ high-MI-ranked features and $k_2$ lasso selected low-MI-ranked features. Within a small set of $(k_1 + k_2)$ features, it is possible to enumerate different combinations of feature subsets with a small feature pool. Feature subset evaluation is based on leave-one-out cross-validation classification performance using logistic regression. We propose to evaluate feature subset in an ascending order of feature set size. In particular, we start with one feature, then combinations of two features, combinations of three features, etc. The subset evaluation stops when the cross-validation accuracy cannot be further improved. Then we report the best prediction model with optimal feature subset. The proposed mutual-information-guided sparse feature selection framework is shown in Fig. 1.

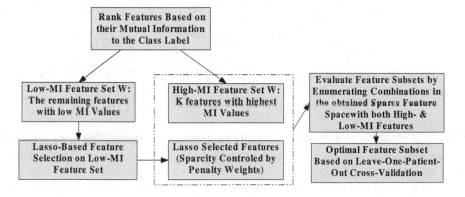

**Fig. 1.** The framework of the mutual information-guided feature selection approach.

Compared with other feature selection, the proposed framework combines information theoretic criteria and sparse learning method to supervise feature selection and discover the most important features efficiently.

## 3    Experimental Design for Epilepsy Diagnosis

**EEG Data Acquisition.** In this study, EEG was recorded from a 128-channel electrode array using a geodesic sensor net and Electrical Geodesics, Inc. (EGI; Eugene, OR) amplifier system with signal amplified at a gain of 1000 and band-pass filtered between 0.1 Hz and 100 Hz. During recording, EEG was referenced to the vertex electrode and digitized continuously at 500 Hz. The placement of the 128 scalp EEG electrodes is shown in Fig. 2.

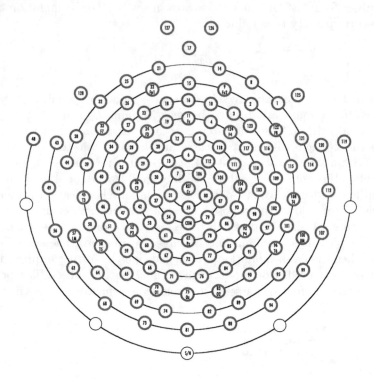

**Fig. 2.** The placement of the 128 EEG electrodes in the experimental setup.

**Visually Evoked Potentials.** Visually evoked potentials (VEPs) are electrical potentials (usually EEG) recorded in presence of visual stimuli, and are distinct from spontaneous EEG potentials recorded without stimulation. In particular, the steady-state visually evoked potentials (SSVEPs) have been widely investigated in the past 40 years and have been shown to be useful to analyze many brain cognitive paradigms (visual attention, binocular rivalry, working memory, and brain rhythms) and clinical neuroscience (epilepsy, aging, schizophrenia, migraine, autism, depression, anxiety, and stress). SSVEPs are evoked responses induced by long stimulus trains with flickering visual stimuli. The steady-state potentials are periodic with a stationary distinct spectrum showing stable characteristic SSVEPs peaks over a long time period. It has been found that photosensitivity is found to be common in patients with epilepsy, and visual stimulation may engage the mechanism underlying hyperexcitability in the patients. A series of experiments by Wilkins et al. indicated that spatial properties of visual patterns can elicit epileptiform EEG abnormalities [11]. The epileptic response was reported to be sensitive to luminance, with higher luminance inducing a higher risk of epilepsy [12]. People with migraine or epilepsy are especially prone to symptoms of visual perceptual distortions and visual stress on viewing flicking striped patterns. In a recent study, Birca et al. showed that SSVEP harmonics in the gamma range (50–100 Hz) have significantly stronger amplitudes and greater phase alignment for patients with febrile seizures. In children with focal epilepsy, a similar effect in the gamma range was shown by Asano et al. [13]. As patient with epilepsy are prone to exhibit abnormal EEG responses to repetitive modulated flicking patterns, the resulting SSVEPs can be employed to discriminate epileptic and non-epileptic patients in a short EEG test rather than a long-term EEG monitoring often around or longer than 24 h. The experimental design of this study is based on this observation. We make an attempt to test the hypothesis that epileptic and non-epileptic EEG recordings during steady state visual stimulation can be classified.

**Experimental Design.** Eleven patients with epilepsy and eleven healthy subjects were recruited in this experiment. The 11 patients had been diagnosed with idiopathic generalized epilepsy (IGE) at University of Washington (UW) Medicine Regional Epilepsy Center at Harborview. The patients with history of photic-induced seizure or photoparoxysmal responses (PPR) were exclude in order to minimize the risk of inducing seizures during the experiment. The 11 healthy subjects were selected from those who did not have a history of neurological or psychiatric diagnoses such as migraine or schizophrenia. All the patients and normal subjects had normal or corrected-to-normal visual acuity.

Each subject underwent the same experimental protocol during EEG recording. Visual stimuli were consisted of a high contrast strip pattern presented on a 19-inch LaCie Electron Blue IV monitor at a resolution of $800 \times 600$ pixels, with a 72 H vertical refresh rate and a mean luminance of $34 \, cd/m^2$. The strip contrast pattern flickering (condition 1) or switching (condition 2) at 7.5 Hz and the contrast level were temporally modulated by 10 levels from lowest contrast (level 1) to highest contrast (level 10) periodically. Each contrast level lasted for 1.067 s with 16 reversals of the flicker pattern. Thus, each stimulus of 10 contrast levels was 10.67 s. Each subject performed 20 trials for condition 1 and 20 trials for condition 2 with brief breaks between trials. A typical session of each subject is about 10–15 min.

**Signal Processing and Feature Extraction.** The visual stimulation flicking at a constant frequency can evoke harmonic oscillations and the SSVEPs were found to have the same fundamental frequency (rst harmonic) as the visual stimulating frequency [14]. A recent study showed that the higher SSVEP harmonics can also play an important role in studying brain functions [15]. In this study, we extracted frequency features of SSVEPs by Discrete Fourier Transform (DFT) with a 0.5 Hz resolution for each EEG channel of each trial with a time length of 1.067 s. The frequency components obtained from DFT are subject to signal variations. If signal strengths are different, the DFT coefficients are also different even the two time series signals share similar wave patterns. EEG signal is known to have significant inter-individual variability [16], and the signal amplitudes can vary considerable from one person to another. Thus, the extracted DFT frequency components can be problematic in feature selection and model construction across subjects. To tackle this problem, we introduced an normalization step based on Parseval's Theorem. Parsevals Theorem states that the power spectrum summed over all frequencies is equal to the variance of the signal. Based on this rule, we take standard deviation of a signal as a normalization factor and normalize the signal to unit variance before applying DFT.

From the normalized DFT frequency components, the components at stimulation frequency (7.5 Hz) and multiple of stimulation frequency (up to 9th harmonics) were selected as signal features. Then a segment of EEG signal is represented by nine features that include nine harmonic frequency components that may be informative. The feature extraction was applied to each EEG channel of each trial for each subject. For each subject, the features from trials with the same contrast level were averaged to be the features of the contrast level. In summary, there are 128 (channel) × 10 (contrast level) × 9 (frequency component) = 11520 features for each subject. In the next, we will present a new feature selection approach to select the most informative features to discriminate epileptic patients from normal subjects.

**Assessment and Validation.** The feature subset assessment was based on leave-one-out cross-validation procedure as shown in Fig. 3. In order to reduce the bias of training and testing data, cross validation techniques have been extensively to assess a classification model. In this study, we employed a leave-one-patient-out cross-validation methodology in order to avoid the potential bias of having EEG samples from the same patients in both the training and testing data. We measured model classification accuracy by the average of sensitivity and specificity. Sensitivity and specificity are widely used in the medical domain as classification performance measures. We labeled the EEG samples from epileptic patients as positive and those from non-epileptic patients as negative. The sensitivity measures the fraction of positive cases that are classified as positive; the specificity measures the fraction of negative cases classified as negative.

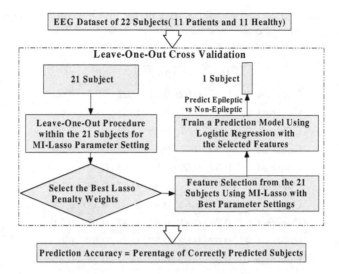

**Fig. 3.** The leave-one-patient-out cross-validation procedure for model assessment.

## 4 Computational Results

We performed our feature selection and classification approach for each of the 10 contrast level and each of the 9 harmonic frequencies independently. This experimental setup is specially designed to find out which contrast and which harmonic frequency are most prominent to discriminate epileptic patients from normal subjects. In the feature selection step, we selected the top ten highest MI feature set first, and performed Lasso to select additional features from the remaining features with relative-low MI values. Once we finalize the feature candidates (lasso-selected low-MI features and top 10 high-MI features), we enumerate feature subset starting from one feature. The feature combination with the highest cross-validation classification accuracy was selected as the as the optimal feature subset. The classification accuracies for each contrast level and harmonic frequency are shown in Table 1. We notice that the contrast level 7 and the 5th harmonic frequency generated the best validation accuracy of 90 %. There were six selected channels: 53, 54, 56, 75, 114, 119. Using prior knowledge guided feature selection have very good interpretability to physicians and neurologist.

We also compared three popular feature selection approaches, regular Lasso feature selection [17], stepwise feature selection using statistical significance test [6], Pudil's floating search [5]. Table 2 shows the classification performance comparisons of our method with the three popular feature selection methods. The feature subset picked up by our approach generated the highest cross-validation accuracy of 90 %, followed by the Pudil's floating search with an accuracy of 85 %. Both regular Lasso and stepwise selection got the validation accuracy of 80 %. Also for the overall performance cross the 10 contrast levels and 6 harmonic

**Table 1.** The classification accuracies for 10 contrast and 9 harmonic frequency levels using leave-one-patient-out cross-validation. The contrast level 7 and the 5th harmonic frequency generated the best testing classification accuracy of 90 %.

|  | 1F | 2F | 3F | 4F | 5F | 6F |
|---|---|---|---|---|---|---|
| Contrast 1 | 0.57 | 0.62 | 0.71 | 0.62 | 0.57 | 0.62 |
| Contrast 2 | 0.57 | 0.57 | 0.67 | 0.48 | 0.48 | 0.67 |
| Contrast 3 | 0.62 | 0.57 | 0.48 | 0.62 | 0.57 | 0.52 |
| Contrast 4 | 0.90 | 0.76 | 0.57 | 0.62 | 0.71 | 0.86 |
| Contrast 5 | 0.57 | 0.52 | 0.67 | 0.62 | 0.52 | 0.48 |
| Contrast 6 | 0.67 | 0.71 | 0.48 | 0.57 | 0.48 | 0.57 |
| Contrast 7 | 0.76 | 0.62 | 0.81 | 0.52 | **0.90** | 0.48 |
| Contrast 8 | 0.76 | 0.81 | 0.67 | 0.57 | 0.57 | 0.71 |
| Contrast 9 | 0.67 | 0.62 | 0.57 | 0.48 | 0.57 | 0.62 |
| Contrast 10 | 0.62 | 0.52 | 0.52 | 0.71 | 0.57 | 0.52 |

frequencies, the proposed approach achieved an overall accuracy of 61 % while performance of other methods were around 50 % with larger standard deviation. This indicates that the feature subset selected by the proposed approach had better discriminative power than the feature subsets selected by the comparing approaches. The experimental results confirmed that the proposed feature selection framework indeed works effectively to capture feature dependencies and discover optimal feature subset. We combined high-MI features with promising low-MI features indeed generated stronger discriminative features that may be ignored by most of the current feature selection algorithms. The proposed information-guided sparse feature selection framework is capable of generating a spare model with good interpretability while preserving the most informative feature combinations to improve classification performance.

**Table 2.** The performance comparison of the proposed method with three popular feature selection algorithms. The feature subset selected by the proposed approach generated the best cross-validation performance cross 9 contrast and 10 harmonic frequency levels.

|  | Classification performance comparison of best feature subset | | | | Accuracy statistics over contrast & freq. levels | |
|---|---|---|---|---|---|---|
|  | Testing accuracy | Contrast level | Harmonic freq. ($\times 7.5$ Hz) | Selected channels | Mean accuracy | Std. |
| MI-Lasso | **0.9048** | 7 | 5 | 53, 54, 56, 75, 114, 119 | **0.62** | **0.10** |
| Regular Lasso | 0.8095 | 7 | 2 | 10, 14, 105, 114 | 0.49 | 0.17 |
| Stepwise selection | 0.8095 | 3 | 2 | 32, 40, 61, 78, 97 | 0.48 | 0.17 |
| Pudi's floating search | 0.8571 | 8 | 2 | 62 | 0.48 | 0.15 |

# 5 Conclusions and Discussions

A quick and accurate epilepsy-screening tool could enormously reduce associated healthcare costs and improve the current diagnosis procedure. To reliably recognize if a patient has epilepsy, we developed a novel mutual-information-guided sparse feature selection and classification framework to identify epilepsy-specific patterns from visually-evoked potentials in a human-computer task. The experimental results confirmed that the proposed method achieved the best diagnostic accuracy compared with several popular methods. The proposed method has a potential to help physicians to determine whether a patient is epileptic or non-epileptic in a quick screening process. More importantly, the proposed information-theory-guided sparse feature selection is an generally framework. It is also promising to help physicians and neurologists in recognizing abnormal brainwave patterns in huge medical dataset with different brain imaging techniques (such as EEG, MEG, and fMRI). The long-term goal of this study is to develop a fast, reliable, and affordable epilepsy diagnostic system using short-term interictal EEG signals. Such a system can revolutionize the current epilepsy diagnosis practice with wide and convenient applications.

# References

1. Epilepsy Foundation: Epilepsy foundation: not another moment lost to seizures (2006). http://www.epilepsyfoundation.org
2. van Donselaar, C.A., Stroink, H., Arts, W.-F.: How confident are we of the diagnosis of epilepsy? Epilepsia **47**(S1), 9–13 (2006)
3. Forsgren, L.: Prospective incidence study and clinical characterization of seizures in newly referred adults. Epilepsia **31**, 292–301 (1990)
4. Saeys, Y., Inza, I., Larranaga, P.: A review of feature selection techniques in bioinformatics. Bioinformatics **23**(19), 2507–2517 (2007)
5. Pudil, P., Novoviov, J., Kittler, J.: Floating search methods in feature selection. Pattern Recogn. Lett. **15**(11), 1119–1125 (1994)
6. Draper, N., Smith, H.: Applied Regression Analysis, 2nd edn. Wiley-Interscience, Hoboken (1998)
7. Hall, M.: Correlation-based feature selection for machine learning. Ph.D. thesis, Department of Computer Science, Waikato University, New Zealand (1999)
8. Yu, L., Liu, H.: Efficient feature selection via analysis of relevance and redundancy. J. Mach. Learn. Res. **5**, 1205–1224 (2004)
9. Peng, H., Long, F., Ding, C.: Feature selection based on mutual information: criteria of max-dependency, max-relevance, and min-redundancy. IEEE Trans. Pattern Anal. Mach. Intell. **27**(8), 1226–1238 (2005)
10. Cover, T.M., Thomas, J.A.: Elements of Information Theory (Wiley Series in Telecommunications and Signal Processing), 2nd edn. Wiley-Interscience, Hoboken (2001)
11. Wilkins, A., Nimmo-Smith, I., Tait, A., McManus, C., Sala, S.D., Tilley, A., Arnold, K., Barrie, M., Scott, S.: A neurological basis for visual discomfort. Brain **107**, 989–1017 (1984)

12. Vialatte, F., Maurice, M., Dauwels, J., Cichocki, A.: Steady-state visually evoked potentials: focus on essential paradigms and future perspectives. Prog. Neurobiol. **90**(4), 418–438 (2010)
13. Asano, E., Nishida, M., Fukuda, M., Rothermel, R., Juhasz, C., Sood, S.: Differential visually-induced gamma-oscillations in human cerebral cortex. NeuroImage **45**(2), 477–489 (2009)
14. Regan, D.: Human Brain Electrophysiology: Evoked Potentials and Evoked Magnetic Fields in Science and Medicine. Elsevier Science Ltd., New York (1989)
15. Muller-Putz, G.R., Scherer, R., Brauneis, C., Pfurtscheller, G.: Steady-state visual evoked potential (SSVEP)-based communication: impact of harmonic frequency components. J. Neural Eng. **2**(4), 123–130 (2005)
16. Smith, S.: EEG in the diagnosis, classification, and management of patients with epilepsy. J. Neurol. Neurosurg. Psychiatry **76**, ii2–ii7 (2005)
17. Tibshirani, R.: Regression shrinkage and selection via the lasso. J. R. Stat. Soc. Ser. B **58**, 267–288 (1994)

# Clique Identification and Propagation for Multimodal Brain Tumor Image Segmentation

Sidong Liu[1]($\boxtimes$), Yang Song[1], Fan Zhang[1], Dagan Feng[1], Michael Fulham[2,3], and Weidong Cai[1]

[1] School of Information Technologies, University of Sydney, Sydney, Australia
sidong.liu@sydney.edu.au
[2] Sydney Medical School, University of Sydney, Sydney, Australia
[3] Department of PET and Nuclear Medicine, Royal Prince Alfred Hospital, Sydney, Australia

**Abstract.** Brain tumors vary considerably in size, morphology, and location across patients, thus pose great challenge in automated brain tumor segmentation methods. Inspired by the concept of clique in graph theory, we present a clique-based method for multimodal brain tumor segmentation that considers a brain tumor image as a graph and automatically segment it into different sub-structures based on the clique homogeneity. Our proposed method has three steps, neighborhood construction, clique identification, and clique propagation. We constructed the neighborhood of each pixel based on its similarities to the surrounding pixels, and then extracted all cliques with a certain size $k$ to evaluate the correlations among different pixels. The connections among all cliques were represented as a transition matrix, and a clique propagation method was developed to group the cliques into different regions. This method is also designed to accommodate multimodal features, as multimodal neuroimaging data is widely used in mapping the tumor-induced changes in the brain. To evaluate this method, we conduct the segmentation experiments on the publicly available Multimodal Brain Tumor Image Segmentation Benchmark (BRATS) dataset. The qualitative and quantitative results demonstrate that our proposed clique-based method achieved better performance compared to the conventional pixel-based methods.

## 1 Introduction

Gliomas are the most common primary tumors in adults. The median survival for patients with high-grade gliomas is <2 years and these gliomas account for a disproportionate loss of potential years of life. A patient with a high-grade glioma loses, on average, 12 years of potential life, which is one of the highest for any type of cancer. There is also a high economic cost to families and the community [1,2]. Neuroimaging is a fundamental component of routine clinical care and research for gliomas. The routine radiological assessment of magnetic

© Springer International Publishing AG 2016
G.A. Ascoli et al. (Eds.): BIH 2016, LNAI 9919, pp. 285–294, 2016.
DOI: 10.1007/978-3-319-47103-7_28

resonance (MR) studies in patients with gliomas includes the delineation of the enhancing rim, regions of cystic/necrotic change, the degree of tumor infiltration and surrounding edema. These routine assessments can have large inter-rater variation, which can relate to the reader's experience, and could be enhanced by accurate and reproducible measurements of the relevant tumor sub-components such as edema, tumor edge etc. Such indices offer the opportunity to improve image interpretation and assist treatment planning. Delineation of glioma sub-components, however, relies heavily on segmentation techniques. The aim of brain tumor segmentation is to extract the pathologic regions from healthy tissues. Manual segmentation is a slow process and so automated approaches have been explored over the past decade [3–5].

A main challenge for automated methods is that gliomas vary considerably in size, morphology, and location across patients. Intensity gradient between normal and abnormal tissues is the key factor for identifying the glioma. All brain tumor segmentation algorithms assume that if a pixel is similar to its immediate neighbors, then these pixels should be grouped together to represent the same structure. Current brain tumor segmentation algorithms can be categorized as *generative* or *discriminative* models [6]. Generative approaches encode the prior knowledge learned from existing data, such as tumor-specific appearance, or the spatial distribution of different tissues, and then infer the most likely segmentation of the tumor for a given set of brain images based on the tissue spatial distribution patterns [7,8]. Generative methods need image registration to model the tissue spatial distributions, and it is difficult to transform the semantic descriptions of tumor appearances into appropriate probabilistic models. Discriminative methods avoid modeling these patterns. Instead they use local features, mostly pixel-wise features, e.g., intensity differences or intensity probability distribution of pixels within a patch to infer the segmentation of tumor structures, and classify these pixels/patches as a lesion or non-lesional area using classification algorithms such as support vector machines (SVM), or random forests [9–11]. There are also many non-pixel features, such as gray-level co-occurrence matrix (GLCM) statistics [12], 3D difference-of-Gaussian (DoG) features [13], discrete curvelets [14,15], hierarchical binary robust independent elementary features (BRIEF) [16], volumetric local binary patterns (vLBPs) [17] and Gabor wavelets [18]. Discriminative models typically require large amounts of training data to ensure accurate classification performance. This approach is now being used widely as brain tumor imaging data become increasingly available.

The local features in discriminative models are usually extracted from the neighborhoods of pixels [19]. To construct the neighborhood, a straightforward way is to use the standard 4- and 8-pixel neighborhoods [20]. This approach, although widely used, restricts the adaptability to neighborhood variations. For example, a pre-defined neighborhood may contain both a tumor and a non-tumor structure. There are also other algorithms that model the local relationship based on spatial interaction between nearby pixels [21], or a wider spatial context of the pixels [22]. While they can successfully model local information, these methods are usually computationally inefficient. Hence, we present an automated method to extract the local relationship among pixels and to segment the brain tumor into different sub-structures in an effort to increase the effectiveness and efficiency of current discriminative methods. This method is inspired by the concept of clique in graph theory, i.e., a subset of nodes (pixels) in which all of them are mutually connected [23,24]. Thus, the local relationship is defined at the clique-level instead of at the pixel-level. We also propose a clique propagation scheme for image segmentation based on the inter- and intra-clique variations. Our proposed method is designed to accommodate the various sequences that are used in the MR assessment of gliomas - T2-weighted (T2), T2-weighted fluid-attenuated inversion recovery (FLAIR), T1-weighted (T1), T1-weighted contrast-enhanced with intravenous gadolinium (T1c), diffusion and perfusion sequences. We evaluated our method on the publicly available Multimodal Brain Tumor Image Segmentation Benchmark (BRATS) dataset [6]. The BRATS dataset provides high-quality multimodal MR data for each patient, including T1, T1c, T2 and FLAIR, which can be used to test the capability of our proposed method in accommodating different imaging sequences. In addition, this dataset contains both low-grade and high-grade gliomas, allowing us to evaluate the proposed method with varying tumors in different sizes, morphologies and locations [25]. To demonstrate the effectiveness of the proposed method, we compared it to the conventional methods that use pixel-wise features.

## 2   Methods

Our proposed method has three steps. Step 1 is feature extraction and neighborhood construction. Local features are extracted for individual pixels, and used to calculate the similarities between neighboring pixels to construct the neighborhood represented by a pixel adjacency matrix. Step 2 is clique identification. A set of $k$-clique, each containing $k$ connected pixels, are identified based on the pixel adjacency matrix, and a weighted clique transition matrix is further built to show the connectivity between different cliques. Step 3 is clique propagation, which groups the connected cliques into different tumor sub-structures. The overall flow of the proposed method is illustrated in Fig. 1.

**Feature Extraction and Neighborhood Construction.** Features are firstly extracted from the multi-sequence imaging data to describe the pixels numerically and further to construct the pixel adjacency matrix. Without overemphasizing the feature design, we used the first order texture features in this study. Specifically, mean, variance, skewness and kurtosis were computed from the local patches around the pixels in each of the scans. In this study, each subject had undertaken T1, T1c, T2 and FLAIR sequences. Along with the original multimodal intensities, each pixel $p$ is represented as a 20-dimensional feature vector $V(p)$, as in Eq. (1):

$$V(p) = V_{v \in \{T1,T1c,T2,FLAIR\}}(I(p), M(p), V(p), S(p), K(p)) \qquad (1)$$

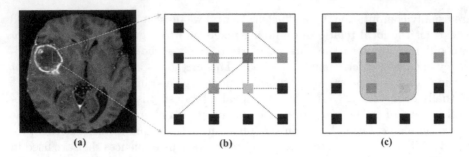

**Fig. 1.** Outline of the proposed method. (a) The axial slice of one MR scan; (b) 3-clique extraction based on the local neighbourhood construction (triangles formed by the colored nodes); (c) segmentation result given the clique propagation. (Color figure online)

where $I, M, V, S, K$ indicate intensity, mean, variance, skewness and kurtosis for the pixel $p$. A pixel adjacency matrix $PM$ is constructed to represent the neighborhood information, with $pm(p_i, p_j) = 1$ indicating the two pixels are neighbors. Instead of connecting all pixels within the local patch, a thresholding scheme was adopted to eliminate some dissimilar items for the target pixel. Specifically, cosine similarity was applied to calculate the similarity between pixels based on the feature vectors, and the threshold $s_{low}$ was used to regulate the size of neighborhood for a target pixel $p_t$, as in Eq. (2):

$$pm(p_t, p_j) = 1, \; if \; cos(V(p_t), V(p_j)) > s_{low} \tag{2}$$

where $p_j$ belongs to the local patch defined for $p_t$. In our experiments, a $5 \times 5$ window with the target pixel in the center was selected as the local patch, which was also used for computing the feature vector. The threshold was set at 0.99 since the pixels are highly similar in terms of the extracted feature vectors.

**Clique Identification and Connection.** The aim of brain tumor segmentation is to find the regions where the pixels are highly homogeneous. The thresholding scheme described above helps to eliminate heterogeneous pixels from the surroundings. However, the direct similarity between pixels is not sufficient to measure the homogeneity without considering the neighbors. So for our method we would like to build the relationship between pixels by further utilizing the neighborhood information. Specifically, the clique is used as the underlying unit to define how the pixels are related.

The concept of clique is introduced in graph theory as a subset of vertices such that every two vertices in this subset are connected. In our study, treating the pixel adjacency matrix as a graph, a $k$-clique $C_k$ is a group of $k$ pixels that are neighbors to each other, as in Eq. (3):

$$C_k = \{p(1), p(2), ..., p(k)\}, \forall i, j \in [1, k], s.t., pm(p(i), p(j)) = 1 \tag{3}$$

The pixels in a clique (triangle) are fully connected, sharing common neighbors with each other, thus these pixels are reinforced mutually and regarded as highly coherent. On the other hand, with the local patch approach, only the most related items are incorporated such that the influence of unrelated pixels in the patch is eliminated. While the pixels in the same clique are considered in the same class, the next step was to identify how pixels from different cliques are related. Specifically, we defined that two cliques are connected if they share common pixels. Supposing there are $h$ ($0 < h < k$) common pixels, the two cliques are $h$-connected. According to this, the pixels are considered to be related if the located cliques are connected.

**Clique Propagation.** The relationship of all cliques can be represented as a weighted transition matrix $TM$ in which the weight indicates the connectivity according to $h$, i.e., $tm(C(i), C(j)) = h$. Starting from a certain clique, clique propagation is conducted by traversing the whole transition matrix to find the connected cliques, which represent one of the regions for the segmentation result. The weights in the transition matrix are used to control the coherence of the connected cliques by reserving connection above the threshold $h_{low}$, i.e.,

$$tm(C(i), C(j)) = 1, \text{ if } h > h_{low} \tag{4}$$

The clique size $k$ and the threshold $h_{low}$ are two major parameters to determine the segmented region's size. Lowering $k$ and $h_{low}$ will relax the coherence, leading to larger segmented regions. In this study, we selected $h_{low}$ as $k - 1$ so that two cliques were highly connected. The influence of $k$ is discussed in Sect. 3. Finally, the segmentation result is obtained by finding all connected subsets of cliques.

## 2.1 Performance Evaluation

As previously indicated we used the publicly available BRATS dataset [6] to evaluate the methods. The dataset contained 30 sets of multi-sequence MR scans from 10 patients with low-grade (astrocytomas or oligoastrocytomas) and 20 with high-grade (anaplastic astrocytomas and glioblastoma multiforme tumors) gliomas. All subjects had T1, T1c, T2 and FLAIR imaging sequence carried out. Each subject's images were rigidly registered to the T1c scan, and resampled to $1mm$ isotropic resolution in a standardized axial orientation. All scans were manually annotated by up to four human expert raters. Five tumor sub-structures (classes) were labeled for each patient - 'edema' (class 1), 'non-enhancing core' (class 2), 'necrotic core' (class 3), 'active core' (class 4) and others (class 0).

In our experiments, each subject's data were processed at the axial slice-level, and the segmentation result was obtained by combining all slices. Each slice was segmented into different regions with the clique propagation algorithm. The size of clique $k$ was selected manually for each subject. Then, the SVM classifier was used to identify the label of each region based on the average pixel feature within each region. The SVM model was trained using LibSVM [26] with linear kernel by $C$-$SVC$ [27] (with the default parameters, i.e., $gamma = 1/$number of features, $coef0 = 0$, and $degree = 3$). In addition, evaluation was performed from intra- and inter-patient perspectives. For the intra-patient evaluation, the

SVM classifier was trained on one slice that crosses the center of the tumor such that all classes were included. For the inter-patient evaluation, the leave-one-subject-out cross-validation was performed.

## 3   Results

For our method the relationship between pixels was established based on cliques. According to the definition of a clique, a larger clique is composed of multiple small cliques, e.g., a 4-clique contains four 3-cliques. Thus, two pixels are definitely in the same region with 3-clique propagation if they are together with 4-clique propagation, but not vice-versa. In other words, the parameter $k$ can be used to control the size of the segmented regions. The segmentation results of the proposed clique propagation algorithm on an example slice before labeling using the SVM classifier, with $k = 3$ and 4 (shown in the second and third row), is shown in Fig. 2. Compared to the expert segmentation (shown in the first row), the 3-clique propagation can recognize the outline of edema, but it also includes some unexpected tissues, such as necrosis (as indicated with the light green circle in (b)) and a non-tumor region (at bottom). Increasing the clique size to 4, i.e.,

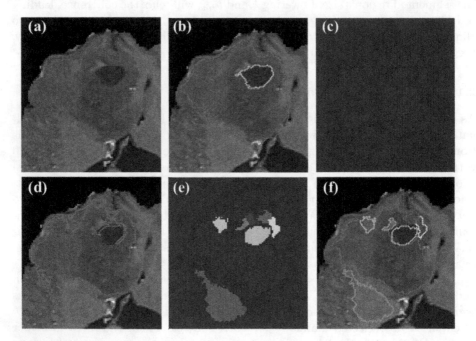

**Fig. 2.** Comparisons of the clique propagation method with different parameter $k$. Ground truth: (a) original cropped MR scan, (b) expert segmentation; 3-clique propagation: (c) region map, (d) segmentation result; 4-clique propagation: (e) region map, (f) segmentation result. The segmented regions are indicated with various colors. (Color figure online)

only 4-cliques are extracted to build the transition matrix, the 4-clique propagation can segment the edema, which is a better segmentation result. Thus, a smaller clique size will lead to an excessively smooth segmentation. On the other hand, while the larger clique size would be helpful to discriminate different structural details, it would also result in over-segmentation. In the experiments, based on our visual inspection, most of subjects in BRATS dataset under study were analyzed with $k = 4$; $k = 5$ was used for a few subjects where the tumors were difficult to identify.

Figure 3 shows the results of our method, compared to the expert segmentation on two slices from a low-grade and a high-grade tumor. For the low-grade

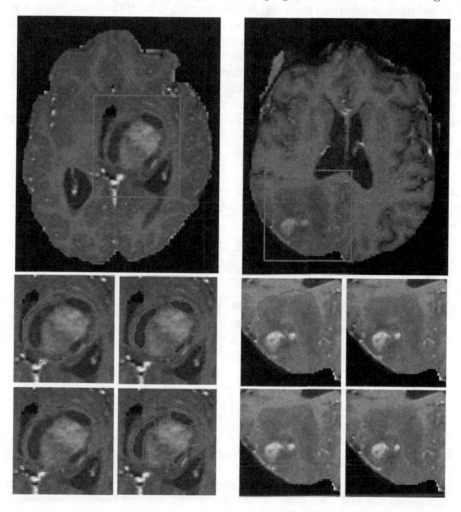

**Fig. 3.** Transaxial images from a low-grade glioma (left) and a high-grade glioma (right). The expert segmentation results are given in the second row. In the low-grade glioma, contours of the tumor with minimal surrounding edema and cystic elements are shown; in the high-grade glioma, the edema and tumor core contours are displayed. Our segmentation results are shown in the third row. (Color figure online)

tumor, the whole tumor outline and necrosis are shown in the first row, and the corresponding segmentation results using our method are given in the second row. For the high-grade case, the whole tumor and tumor core are shown. Visually, it can be seen that our results are reasonably close to the expert labeling.

Quantitative results from the comparison are summarized in Table 1. As suggested by Menze et al. [6], the Dice coefficient was computed to describe the performance from three levels: whole tumor (comprising tissue classes 1–4), tumor core (classes 1, 3, and 4) and active core (class 4). The second and the third columns show the intra-patient and inter-patient evaluation results. Overall, our method outperformed the SVM approach with a higher Dice coefficient. Since the SVM approach is based on the pixel feature extracted from the local patch, the improvement indicates the advantage of constructing the enforced neighborhood relationship, i.e., the clique. While relatively small improvement was obtained at the whole tumor level, Dice values were better at the tumor and active core levels compared to the SVM approach. This shows that our method is able to identify the small structures that are usually difficult to identify. However, these small regions, such as the high-grade active cores, are also more sensitive to the clique relationship, and may be merged to the surrounding structures. This potentially leads to compromised performance, as demonstrated in the intra-patient AC HG segmentation.

**Table 1.** Average DICE coefficient for the 10 patients with low-grade (LG) and 20 with high-grade (HG) gliomas for whole tumor (WT), tumor core (TC) and active core (AC).

|        | Intra-patient | | Inter-patient | |
|--------|------|----------|------|----------|
|        | SVM  | Proposed | SVM  | Proposed |
| WT LG  | 0.821 | **0.825** | 0.710 | **0.757** |
| WT HG  | 0.678 | **0.708** | 0.607 | **0.619** |
| TC LG  | 0.625 | **0.705** | 0.388 | **0.536** |
| TC HG  | 0.569 | **0.653** | 0.358 | **0.469** |
| AC LG  | 0.622 | **0.699** | 0.176 | **0.512** |
| AC HG  | **0.661** | 0.641 | 0.199 | **0.410** |

## 4   Conclusions and Future Works

In this paper, we present a clique-based algorithm for brain tumor segmentation in multi-sequence MR scan data. All cliques were identified based on the neighborhood of each pixel and the relationship between pixels was built from intra- and inter-clique perspectives in terms of the connections among cliques. The clique propagation algorithm was used to finalize the segmentation. We applied it to a publicly available glioma dataset (BRATS). Our approach was superior to the SVM-based approach. Since our method does not specifically depend on any features, we used the simplest features, such as mean and variance in the imaging data. We would expect a better performance when using customized features for different imaging modalities.

A potential research direction based on this study is to design novel features to capture the complex characteristics of human gliomas. Currently, the weight for transition matrix, the selection of $h_{low}$, and clique size $k$ are determined empirically, so it would be interesting to investigate intelligent methods to select these parameters and then evaluate them. Another potential direction would be incorporating other pixel-based region labeling methods rather than SVM alone.

# References

1. Holland, E.C.: Progenitor cells and glioma formation. Curr. Opin. Neurol. **14**, 683–688 (2001)
2. Angelini, E.D., Clatz, O., Mandonnet, E., Konukoglu, E., Capelle, L., Duffau, H.: Glioma dynamics, computational models,: a review of segmentation, registration, and in silico growth algorithms and their clinical applications. Curr. Med. Imaging Rev. **3**(4), 262–276 (2007)
3. Bauer, S., Wiest, R., Nolte, L.P., Reyes, M.: A survey of MRI-based medical image analysis for brain tumor studies. Phys. Med. Biol. **58**(13), 97–129 (2013)
4. Liu, S., Cai, W., Liu, S.Q., Zhang, F., Fulham, M.J., Feng, D., et al.: Multimodal neuroimaging computing: a review of the applications in neuropsychiatric disorders. Brain Inform. **2**(3), 167–180 (2015)
5. Liu, S., Cai, W., Liu, S.Q., Zhang, F., Fulham, M.J., Feng, D., et al.: Multimodal neuroimaging computing: the workflows, methods, and platforms. Brain Inform. **2**(3), 181–195 (2015)
6. Menze, B., Jakab, A., Bauer, S., Kalpathy-Cramer, J., Farahani, K., Kirby, J., et al.: The multimodal brain tumor image segmentation benchmark (BRATS). IEEE Trans. Med. Imaging **34**(10), 1993–2024 (2014)
7. Corso, J.J., Sharon, E., Dube, S., El-Saden, S., Sinha, U., Yuille, A.: Efficient multilevel brain tumor segmentation with integrated bayesian model classification. IEEE Trans. Med. Imaging **27**(5), 629–640 (2008)
8. Pohl, K.M., Fisher, J., Levitt, J.J., Shenton, M.E., Kikinis, R., Grimson, W.E.L., Wells, W.M.: A unifying approach to registration, segmentation, and intensity correction. In: Duncan, J.S., Gerig, G. (eds.) MICCAI 2005. LNCS, vol. 3749, pp. 310–318. Springer, Heidelberg (2005). doi:10.1007/11566465_39
9. Parisot, S., Duffau, H., Chemouny, S., Paragios, N.: Graph-based detection, segmentation & characterization of brain tumors. In: CVPR, pp. 988–995. IEEE (2012)
10. Wels, M., Carneiro, G., Aplas, A., Huber, M., Hornegger, J., Comaniciu, D.: A discriminative model-constrained graph cuts approach to fully automated pediatric brain tumor segmentation in 3-D MRI. In: Metaxas, D., Axel, L., Fichtinger, G., Székely, G. (eds.) MICCAI 2008. LNCS, vol. 5241, pp. 67–75. Springer, Heidelberg (2008). doi:10.1007/978-3-540-85988-8_9
11. Pohl, K.M., Bouix, S., Kikinis, R., Grimson, W.E.L.: Anatomical guided segmentation with non-stationary tissue class distributions in an expectation-maximization framework. In: ISBI, pp. 81–84. IEEE (2004)

12. Liu, S., Cai, W., Wen, L., Eberl, S., Fulham, M.J., Feng, D.: A robust volumetric feature extraction approach for 3D neuroimaging retrieval. In: EMBC, pp. 5657–5660. IEEE (2010)

13. Cai, W., Liu, S., Song, Y., Pujol, S., Kikinis, R., Feng, D.: A 3D difference-of-Gaussian-based lesion detector for brain PET. In: ISBI, pp. 677–680. IEEE (2014)

14. Liu, S., Jing, L., Cai, W., Wen, L., Eberl, S., Fulham, M.J., et al.: Localized multiscale texture based retrieval of neurological image. In: CBMS, pp. 243–248. IEEE (2010)

15. Liu, S., Cai, W., Wen, L., Eberl, S., Fulham, M.J., Feng, D.: Localized functional neuroimaging retrieval using 3D discrete curvelet transform. In: ISBI, pp. 1877–1880. IEEE (2011)

16. Ng, G., Song, Y., Cai, W., Zhou, Y., Liu, S., Feng, D.: Hierarchical and binary spatial descriptors for lung nodule image retrieval. In: EMBC, pp. 6463–6466. IEEE (2014)

17. Liu, S., Cai, W., Wen, L., Feng, D.: Volumetric congruent local binary patterns for 3D neurological image retrieval. In: International Conference on Image and Vision Computing New Zealand, pp. 272–276 (2011)

18. Liu, S., Cai, W., Wen, L., Feng, D.: Multiscale and multiorientation feature extraction with degenerative patterns for 3D neuroimaging retrieval. In: ICIP, pp. 1249–1252. IEEE (2012)

19. Pham, D.L., Xu, C., Prince, J.L.: Current methods in medical image segmentation 1. Ann. Rev. Biomed. Eng. **2**, 315–337 (2000)

20. Li, S.Z., Singh, S.: Markov Random Field Modeling in Image Analysis. Springer, London (2009)

21. Subbanna, N.K., Precup, D., Collins, D.L., Arbel, T.: Hierarchical probabilistic Gabor and MRF segmentation of brain tumours in MRI volumes. In: Mori, K., Sakuma, I., Sato, Y., Barillot, C., Navab, N. (eds.) MICCAI 2013. LNCS, vol. 8149, pp. 751–758. Springer, Heidelberg (2013). doi:10.1007/978-3-642-40811-3_94

22. Bauer, S., Nolte, L.-P., Reyes, M.: Fully automatic segmentation of brain tumor images using support vector machine classification in combination with hierarchical conditional random field regularization. In: Fichtinger, G., Martel, A., Peters, T. (eds.) MICCAI 2011. LNCS, vol. 6893, pp. 354–361. Springer, Heidelberg (2011). doi:10.1007/978-3-642-23626-6_44

23. West, D.B.: Introduction to Graph Theory. Prentice Hall, Upper Saddle River (2001)

24. Zhang, F., Cai, W., Song, Y., Young, P., Traini, D., Morgan, L., et al.: Beating cilia identification in fluorescence microscope images for accurate CBF measurement. In: ICIP, 4496–4500. IEEE (2015)

25. Weizman, L., Sira, L.B., Joskowicz, L., Constantini, S., Precel, R., Shofty, B., et al.: Automatic segmentation, internal classification, and follow-up of optic pathway gliomas in MRI. Med. Image Anal. **16**(1), 177–188 (2012)

26. Chang, C.C., Lin, C.J.: LIBSVM: a library for support vector machines. ACM Trans. Intell. Syst. Technol. **2**, 1–27 (2011)

27. Boser, B.E., Guyon, I.M., Vapnik, V.N.: A training algorithm for optimal margin classifiers. In: The Fifth Annual Workshop on Computational Learning Theory, pp. 144–152 (1992)

# Cross Subject Mental Work Load Classification from Electroencephalographic Signals with Automatic Artifact Rejection and Muscle Pruning

Sajeev Kunjan[1(✉)], T.W. Lewis[1], T.S. Grummett[1], D.M.W. Powers[1],
K.J. Pope[1], S.P. Fitzgibbon[2], and J.O. Willoughby[3]

[1] School of Computer Science, Engineering and Mathematics,
Flinders University, Adelaide, SA 5001, Australia
{chat0068,trent.lewis,tyler.grummett,david.powers,
kenneth.pope}@flinders.edu.au
[2] Oxford Centre for Functional MRI of the Brain, University of Oxford, Oxford, UK
sean.fitzgibbon@ndcn.ox.ac.uk
[3] School of Medicine, and Centre for Neuroscience,
Flinders University, Adelaide, SA, Australia
john.willoughby@flinders.edu.au

**Abstract.** Purpose of this study was to understand the effect of automatic muscle pruning of electroencephalograph on cognitive work load prediction. Pruning was achieved using an automatic Independent Component Analysis (ICA) based component classification. Initially, raw data from EEG recording was used for prediction, this result was then compared with mental work load prediction results from muscle-pruned EEG data. This study used Support Vector Machine (SVM) with Linear Kernel for cognitive work load prediction from EEG data. Initial part of the study was to learn a classification model from the whole data, whereas the second part was to learn the model from a set of subjects and predict the mental work load for an unseen subject by the model. The experimental results show that an accuracy of nearly 100 % is possible with ICA and automatic pruning based pre-processing. Cross subject prediction significantly improved from a mean accuracy of 54 % to 69 % for an unseen subject with the pre-processing.

## 1 Introduction

Recently there is an increased focus on researches to predict mental work load automatically for human operators involved in critical tasks like surgery, driving, critical plant operation etc. Additional mental work load could be from distraction, unplanned work load and other sources. This could impact operators capacity to pay sustained attention, store information in working memory, and switch between concurrent tasks [6]. This situation could potentially compromise execution of the primary task which could result in catastrophic incidents.

© Springer International Publishing AG 2016
G.A. Ascoli et al. (Eds.): BIH 2016, LNAI 9919, pp. 295–303, 2016.
DOI: 10.1007/978-3-319-47103-7_29

Human physiological measures have been effectively used to predict the mental work load of people in various researches. Electroencephalographic (EEG) is one of the important physiological measure used for this purpose. Electrocardiography, Electromyography, Electrooculography, Galvanic skin response, pupillometry and body temperature are the other important physiological measures. These techniques mostly focus on electrical activity in heart/skeletal muscles, eye movement, skin electrical properties, pupil diameter and body temperature. EEG is a technique that measures the brain electrical activity. This makes EEG an excellent measure to base mental work load estimation when compared with other physiological measures [8]. This study focuses on mental work load prediction from EEG data.

Machine learning is defined as a 'Field of study that gives computers the ability to learn without being explicitly programmed' [15]. The application of machine learning is wide spread in areas such as spam filtering, optical character recognition, search engines, computer vision etc. Machine learning is classified into two major categories: supervised learning and unsupervised learning. In supervised learning, algorithms are provided with a set of inputs and outputs to learn generalized rule which maps given inputs to output. In unsupervised learning, the machine is not provided with any example data to learn from, algorithm need to find a structure in the input without being guided with any example. This study focuses on supervised learning. A model is trained by the algorithms using labeled data. The labeled data has set of input features along with the actual output, which algorithm uses to develop a general model to predict output for any unseen input data. For this study, classifiers are trained to predict mental work load on various subjects. The EEG data used for this current study were taken from a previous study investigating gamma rhythms under different conditions, including mental work load [7].

This study focuses on the cognitive work load predictive power of EEG data. The discriminative power of EEG features significantly improves by incorporating pre-processing in the machine learning. Novelty of this study is that the pre-processing is achieved by de-noising and *automatic (no human expert)* muscle pruning of the EEG using ICA based component classification [5]. Classification is performed using SVM with linear kernel on two different data sets, one being pruned through pre-processing and the other relatively raw in nature. SVM with linear kernel is used as primary learning algorithm in this study. In addition unreported results using Logistic Regression, ANN and SVM with Gaussian kernel reiterate the improvement when using automatic muscle pruning. Second part of the study focuses on generating a general model which could be applied to the EEG data from an unseen subject and predict the cognitive work load. High level of accuracy achieved in predicting mental work load using a model trained with all subjects and improvement in accuracy for unseen subject in case of cross subject classification sets this study apart from the current literature.

## 2    Background and Related Works

EEG is a clinical method that records the electrical signals generated by brain structures through the electrodes. EEG recording can be done through non invasive and invasive methods. In case of non invasive method, electrodes are attached to the scalp surface, whereas implanted in case of invasive. Literature indicates that cerebral activity measured through EEG recordings using non invasive method is more contaminated with signals from eye movements, head movements and muscle activities [1,19]. It is widely used because of its non-invasive nature, high-temporal resolution, and comparative low-cost. Signal classification and reproducibility is very important for brain computer interfaces [12] and this demands precise positioning and repositioning of the electrodes. Precise positioning of electrodes on the scalp are achieved through EEG caps. Various regions of the brain produce different kinds of waves based on the activity happening in the brain [13]. An EEG signal captured by each electrodes placed on the scalp consists of many waves with different characteristics [16].

Mental work load assessment from EEG Power Spectral Density bands is a well-researched field of study. A variety of cognitive tasks and classification methods were used to determine mental work load in related studies. Some of the prior studies published in the area of automatic mental work load prediction from EEG data are listed below.

Wilson et al. [20] study used multiple psychophysiological features such as heart rate, heart rate variability, eye blinks, electrodermal activity, topographically recorded electrical brain activity for the analysis of mental work load in pilots during flight. Artificial Neural Network (ANN) was used for classification of cognitive work load and results showed 90 % accuracy. Gevins and Smith [6] studied discrimination of three different levels of cognitive work load of subjects performing various tasks of computer interaction. Theta (4–8Hz) and alpha(8–14Hz) frequency bands of spectral power were used in the study. This spectral features are fed to neural networks for classifying the cognitive work load of users. Kohlmorgen et al. [10] measured driver work load of drivers in a car driving simulation environment. The study used Linear Discriminant Analysis on features extracted and optimized for each user from EEG for work load assessment. The experimental results show 92 % accuracy in classifying cognitive work load as low and high. Putze et al. [14] proposed a method to predict cognitive work load from data recorded from subjects performing a lane change task in a driving simulator, while solving visual and cognitive secondary tasks. EEG data, skin conductance, pulse, and respiration data were employed to learn the SVM model. Wang et al. [17] used hierarchical Bayes model to predict cross subject workload and the study used data from all subject to train the model and no pre-processing was used on the EEG data, test was not conducted on unseen subject for workload prediction.

# 3    Materials and Methods

This study consists of two experiments: In the first experiment, entire data set is provided to the learning algorithm and a cross validation technique is employed to ensure separate training and testing data. In the first experiment there is no separation between the subjects. In the second experiment the model is trained with all subjects excluding one and the resultant model is used for predicting mental work load for the excluded subject which is unseen by the model. In both experiments there are two cases: one with raw EEG data and the other with muscle pruned data. Finally, results from each case in both of the experiments are compared statistically to understand the enhancement of mental work load predictive power of EEG when pre-processing is used.

The study constitutes of following 6 major steps: raw data collection, pre-processing, feature extraction, normalization, cross validation and training the model. Based on the nature of the experiment and case, one or more steps are omitted.

## 3.1    Raw Data Collection

This study have used EEG data from research conducted by Grummett et al. [7] at Flinders University. EEG is an electrophysiological monitoring method to record electrical activity caused by neurons in the brain. It is typically non-invasive procedure with the electrodes placed along the scalp.

In this research [7] by Grummett et al., subjects (n = 9) performed easy and hard versions of an oddball task in each sensory modality (auditory, visual, tactile). For this research, subjects were selected from Flinders Medical Centre patients. As a screening exercise subjects underwent verbal, memory and spatial test to ensure their suitability for the oddball task. Hard tasks were performed such that the detection of the target stimulus was only possible if very close attention was paid to the non-target. Hard tasks were tailored to each subject in preliminary trials, to ensure adequate, effort full performance. Each oddball study consisted of eight blocks of 85 stimuli, a total of 680 stimuli. The duration of each stimulus was 70 ms with an inter-stimulus interval varying between 900 and 1100 ms. Total counts of targets and non-targets were 128 and 552, respectively. Work load scores (NASA-TLX), response times and accuracy measures were recorded and indicated that hard oddball tasks were much harder than the standard (easy) oddball tasks. For this current study only the data from the auditory modalities was considered. For the auditory oddball task, stimuli consisted of two sinusoidal tones that differed in frequency. Non-target stimuli consisted of tones at 1000 Hz. In the easy task, the target stimulus was a tone of 1500 Hz. In the hard task, the target stimuli were tones at a frequency of 1005, 1010, 1015, 1020, or 1025 Hz, depending on subject-specific perceptual ability. All tones were presented at 70 dB above hearing threshold with duration of 70 ms (rise and fall times of 10 ms). EEG was recorded digitally using a 128-channel EEG system (Compumedics, Victoria Australia) system with 59 electrodes (10:10 system placements). The Flinders

Clinical Research Ethics Committee approved the experimental studies described in [7] and all subjects signed written, informed, consent.

## 3.2   Automatic Muscle Pruning

EEG data collected through non-invasive method have high probability of contaminated with muscle (electromyography, EMG) signals and other sources of contamination. Grummett et al. [7] demonstrated a process to decontaminate the EEG data. The 500 Hz re-sampled EEG data was pre-processed using EEGLAB with two plugin toolboxes. Source information flow toolbox (SIFT) was used for de-trending and the function "clean_rawdata" [11] for automatically managing artifact. The steps were:

(1) Remove flat-line channels (threshold = 5 s).
(2) High pass filter (0.5 Hz).
(3) Remove noisy channels based on correlation (threshold = 0.8) and line-noise (threshold = 4) this step removes entire channels if (a) the correlation between the channel and its neighboring channels is less than the specified value, or (b) the channel has more line noise relative to its signal.
(4) Process noisy segments using artifact subspace reconstruction which (a) finds a clean data segment, (b) defines bad segments as having activity which is a certain number of standard deviations away from the clean data segment (threshold = 5), and (c) repairs these data segments using a mixing matrix that is computed using the clean data segment.

This data was then subjected to ICA using adaptive mixture independent component analysis(AMICA) [3]. EMG contaminated components were automatically eliminated using a heuristic [5] and surface EEG was reconstructed. The heuristic excludes independent components (ICs) with spectral gradients greater than a certain threshold. The spectral gradient was calculated by fitting a straight line to the loglog spectrum (logarithmic power vs logarithmic frequency) of each IC between 7 Hz and 75 Hz. ICs with a gradient greater than a −0.034 (i.e. power that does not decrease fast enough with frequency as determined by the threshold) were identified as ICs containing EMG (muscle IC) and discarded. The resultant data is referred as pruned data for the rest of this paper.

## 3.3   Feature Extraction

Although the original data was collected in a traditional oddball, event-related potential paradigm [7], this current study is interested in the sustained mental work load of the subject. As such, for each session of hard or easy oddball the data was divided into non overlapping, 10 s epochs, regardless of whether the events were target or non-targets. We are not interested in the subject's response to different events but their sustained work load or concentration throughout the session. Average power spectra from each 10 s epoch were estimated using the

Welchs modified periodogram method [18] with 1-s, half-overlapping blocks with a Hanning window. Average spectral band power was calculated in each of several frequency bands, namely delta $(1 - 4$ Hz$)$ theta $(4 - 8$ Hz$)$, alpha $(8 - 14$ Hz$)$, beta $(14 - 25$ Hz$)$ and gamma $(25 - 45$ Hz$)$. Average spectral power on these frequency band are the features used by the machine learning algorithm. This resulted in 295 features, 59 common electrodes across subjects and 864 instances from auditory oddball experiment.

### 3.4    Normalization

Data sets are normalized to ensure that the features have a standard scale and are distributed normally with a zero mean and standard deviation 1. This helps the algorithm to efficiently train a model, by ensuring that each feature has values that varying over a similar range.

### 3.5    Cross Validation

In order to make sure the training and validation of the model is done on different sets of data, 10-fold cross validation technique is used. In 10-fold cross validation, the data set is divided into 10 folds of roughly equal size. Then from each fold one sample is taken for validation purpose and remaining is used for training. This process is repeated for 10 times with each fold serving as test set once [4]. This method of sampling is used in the first experiment (see Sect. 3) and each fold of it contain data from every subject. For the second experiment each time one subject excluded from training set and the excluded subject used for, a leave-one (subject)-out evaluation. This process is repeated 10 times for each of 9 subjects for statistical analysis. This gives an indication of the cross-subject mental workload classification ability of the system.

### 3.6    Training Model

SVM with linear kernel was selected in this study due to its wide spread usage and simplicity. SVM performs classification tasks by constructing hyperplanes in a multidimensional space that separates cases of different class labels. The objective of the SVM algorithm is to find feature weightage to optimize the cost function [9]. The regularization parameter to prevent model from over fitting the training set was determined to be 0.05 empirically. Other standard algorithms: SVM with gaussian kernel, ANN and Logistic regression are also used to reiterate the results. MATLAB version R2015a was used for implementing the classifiers and analyzing the results.

## 4    Experimental Results and Discussion

A series of testing was done to understand the effect of the pre-processing has on EEG data in predicting the mental work load. Two sets of experiments were conducted as part of this study. First one was intended to find out how mental work load prediction improves by the automatic muslce pruning without separating out the subjects. Second experiment was aimed at training a model with EEG data from set of subjects and then testing it with a subject the model has not seen yet. T-test is used for statistically analyzing the result.

*Experiment 1: Raw EEG versus Pruned EEG*

First experiment was done to classify raw and pruned EEG with SVM linear classifier. This mental workload prediction experiment was conducted ten rounds to get a statistical analysis and mean accuracy on raw data is 85 % and pruned data is 99 %. T-test result shows that there was a significant difference in the score for pruned data (M = 99.79, SD = 0.07) and raw data (M = 85.37, SD = 0.82)conditions; t(18) = −55.27, $p < 0.05$. This indicates that the pre-processing done on the data gives a significant level of accuracy improvement. The pruned data was further experimented with other learning algorithms like Logistic Regression, Artificial Neural Network and SVM with Gaussian Kernel. All of this additional testing yielded 100 % accuracy consistently.

*Experiment 2: Generalizing to unseen Subjects*

Second experiment was to understand the effectiveness of generalizing the trained model to an unseen subject's data, or cross-subject transfer. EEG data from all subjects excluding one was used for training the model, the excluded subject was then used for, a leave-one (subject)-out evaluation. This step was repeated for each of the nine subjects for ten rounds. This experiment was done for both raw and pruned EEG to understand the difference in performance. Table 1 shows the accuracy from the executions on the raw and pruned data. Each row represents the mean accuracies from respective data set. Mean accuracy of raw data classification is 54 %, whereas pruned data yielded average accuracy of 69 %. T-test result indicates that there is a significant difference in the scores for pruned data (M = 68.80, SD = 0.87) and raw data (M = 53.70, SD = 0.05)conditions; t(18) = 19.02, $p < 0.05$. Figure 1 shows the box-plots from accuracy data for ten rounds of test execution for raw and pruned data. This shows that the pre-processing done on the data gives a significant level of accuracy improvement on unseen subject, the result improved from a mere chance to some level of confidence.

**Table 1.** Cross subject accuracy: first and second row indicates the mean accuracy for each subject for raw and pruned data respectively. Each column represent the subject which is left out from training the model and later tested with.

|        | Sub1 | Sub2 | Sub3 | Sub4 | Sub5 | Sub6 | Sub7 | Sub8 | Sub9 | Avg  |
|--------|------|------|------|------|------|------|------|------|------|------|
| Raw    | 0.52 | 0.46 | 0.57 | 0.97 | 0.52 | 0.50 | 0.50 | 0.34 | 0.46 | 0.54 |
| Pruned | 0.75 | 0.73 | 0.42 | 1.00 | 0.50 | 0.67 | 1.00 | 0.29 | 0.83 | 0.69 |

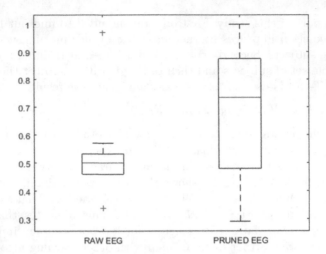

**Fig. 1.** Box plot of mean accuracies of mental workload prediction for 9 subjects using raw and pruned EEG.

## 5    Conclusion and Future Scope

This study was taken up to analyze the improvement in cognitive work load discriminative power of EEG data by the ICA based component classification and automatic (no human expert) muscle pruning. This was achieved through two set of experiments: First experiment was to learn and test the classification model through a 10 fold cross validation approach using all of the data set. Second experiment was to learn model from EEG data and test it with data from a subject that was not used for training machine learning algorithm. The experiments were executed with SVM linear classifier and other unreported standard classifier results were used to re-validate the improvement observed. The results indicate that the pre-processing improves the cognitive work load predictive power significantly with resultant accuracy nearly 100 % consistently. This suggest that further work should be undertaken to validate the technique on more real world and challenging data set. A key finding in this research is that the *cross subject* predictive power also improved significantly with mean accuracy change from 54 % to 69 %. Cross subject accuracy of 69 % shows that there is still opportunity to improve and further research need to focus in this direction, including using alternative classification models such as common spatial patterns(CSPs) algorithm [2] which is popular in brain computer interface research.

## References

1. Ball, T., Kern, M., Mutschler, I., Aertsen, A., Schulze-Bonhage, A.: Signal quality of simultaneously recorded invasive and non-invasive EEG. NeuroImage **46**(3), 708–716 (2009)
2. Blankertz, B., Tomioka, R., Lemm, S., Kawanabe, M., Muller, K.R.: Optimizing spatial filters for robust EEG single-trial analysis. IEEE Sig. Process. Mag. **25**(1), 41–56 (2008)

3. Delorme, A., Palmer, J., Onton, J., Oostenveld, R., Makeig, S.: Independent EEG sources are dipolar. PloS ONE **7**(2), e30135 (2012)
4. Domen, N., Mihelj, M., Marko, M.: A survey of methods for data fusion and system adaptation using autonomic nervous system responses in physiological computing. interact. Comput. **24**(3), 154–172 (2012)
5. Fitzgibbon, S., DeLosAngeles, D., Lewis, T., Powers, D., Grummett, T., Whitham, E., Ward, L., Willoughby, J., Pope, K.: Automatic determination of EMG-contaminated components and validation of independent component analysis using EEG during pharmacologic paralysis. Clin. Neurophysiol. **127**, 1781–1793 (2015)
6. Gevins, A., Smith, M.E.: Neurophysiological measures of cognitive workload during human-computer interaction. Theor. Issues Ergon. Sci. **4**(1–2), 113–131 (2003)
7. Grummett, T.S., Fitzgibbon, S.P., Lewis, T.W., et al.: Constitutive spectral EEG peaks in the gamma range: suppressed by sleep, reduced by mental activity and resistant to sensory stimulation. Front. Hum. Neurosci. **8**(927) (2014)
8. Heger, D., Putze, F., Schultz, T.: Online workload recognition from EEG data during cognitive tests and human-machine interaction. In: Dillmann, R., Beyerer, J., Hanebeck, U.D., Schultz, T. (eds.) KI 2010. LNCS (LNAI), vol. 6359, pp. 410–417. Springer, Heidelberg (2010). doi:10.1007/978-3-642-16111-7_47
9. Hsu, C.W., Chang, C.C., Lin, C.J., et al.: A practical guide to support vector classification (2003)
10. Kohlmorgen, J., Dornhege, G., Braun, M.L., Blankertz, B., Müller, K.R., Curio, G., Hagemann, K., Bruns, A., Schrauf, M., Kincses, W.E.: Improving human performance in a real operating environment through real-time mental workload detection. In: Towards Brain-Computer Interfacing. The MIT press (2006)
11. Kothe, C.A., Makeig, S.: Bcilab: a platform for brain-computer interface development. J. Neural Eng. **10**(5), 056014 (2013)
12. Kubler, A., Mattia, D.: Chapter 14 - Brain computer interface based solutions for end-users with severe communication disorders. In: Laureys, S., Gosseries, O., Tononi, G. (eds.) The Neurology of Conciousness, 2nd edn, pp. 217–240. Academic Press, San Diego (2016)
13. Niedermeyer, E., da Silva, F.H.L.: Electroencephalography: Basic Principles, Clinical Applications and Related Fields. Williams and Wilkins, Lippincott, Philadelphia (1993)
14. Putze, F., Jarvis, J.P., Schultz, T.: Multimodal recognition of cognitive workload for multitasking in the car. In: 2010 20th International Conference on Pattern Recognition (ICPR), pp. 3748–3751 (2010)
15. Samuel, A.L.: Some studies in machine learning using the game of checkers. IBM J. Res. Develop. **3**, 210–229 (1959)
16. Teplan, M.: Fundamentals of EEG measurement. Measur. Sci. Rev. **2**(2), 1–11 (2002)
17. Wang, Z., Hope, R.M., Wang, Z., Ji, Q., Gray, W.D.: Cross-subject workload classification with a hierarchical Bayes model. NeuroImage **59**(1), 64–69 (2012)
18. Welch, P.D.: The use of fast fourier transform for the estimation of power spectra: a method based on time averaging over short, modified periodograms. IEEE Trans. Audio Electroacoust. **15**(2), 70–73 (1967)
19. Whitham, E.M., Pope, K.J., Fitzgibbon, S.P., Lewis, T., Clark, C.R., Loveless, S., Broberg, M., Wallace, A., DeLosAngeles, D., Lillie, P., et al.: Scalp electrical recording during paralysis: quantitative evidence that EEG frequencies above 20Hz are contaminated by EMG. Clin. Neurophysiol. **118**(8), 1877–1888 (2007)
20. Wilson, G.F.: An analysis of mental workload in pilots during flight using multiple psychophysiological measures. Int. J. Aviat. Psychol. **12**(1), 3–18 (2002)

# EEG Topography and Tomography (sLORETA) in Analysis of Abnormal Brain Region for Mild Depression

Xiaowei Li, Tong Cao, Bin Hu$^{(\boxtimes)}$, Shuting Sun, and Jianxiu Li

Ubiquitous Awareness and Intelligent Solutions Lab, Lanzhou University,
Lanzhou, China
{lixwei, caotl4, bh, sunstl4}@lzu.edu.cn,
lijianx_e@l63.com

**Abstract.** Mild depression disorder affects a large number of people, and if not correctly treated, it could evolve into major depression disorder. So far, lots of studies have suggested that several abnormal brain regions are linked to major depression disorder, including prefrontal cortex (PFC), anterior cingulate cortex (ACC) etc. However mild depression disorder gained less attention. This study therefore examined whether mild depression exists dsyregulation in these brain regions. 20 subjects participated in our experiment, and affective facial expressions pictures were used as stimuli when recording EEG signals. Brain activity of theta and alpha bands were examined using EEG topography and standardized low-resolution electromagnetic tomography (sLORETA). Results suggested that mild depressed subjects exhibited higher activity in motor cortex (Brodmann area: 4, 6) and lower activity in visual cortex (Brodmann area: 18, 19) and *prefrontal* cortex (Brodmann area: 11, 47) compared to normal controls. These finding indicated that mild depressed subjects paid much more attention to negative facial expressions. Future studies should be focused on the role of brain regions played in mild depression in more detail.

**Keywords:** Mild depression · EEG · EEG topography · sLORETA

## 1 Introduction

According to the World Health Organization, depression is among the leading cause of disability worldwide with approximately 350 million people affected [1]. Major Depressive Disorder (MDD) is characterized by persistent depressed mood or loss of interest or pleasure from daily activities, and at its worst, depression can lead to suicide. Therefore, the diagnosis and treatment of depression are very important. However, in present, the way of diagnosis of depression is mainly according to the doctor's clinical experience and patient's self-report, which is subjective and could lead to misdiagnosis. Thus it is very meaningful to explore an easy, accurate and practical method of depression detection.

Davidson and coworkers suggested that depression may be seen as a disorder of the representation and regulation of mood and emotion [2]. Furthermore previous study has suggested that frontal lobe have great relationship with mood. For instance, activation

© Springer International Publishing AG 2016
G.A. Ascoli et al. (Eds.): BIH 2016, LNAI 9919, pp. 304–311, 2016.
DOI: 10.1007/978-3-319-47103-7_30

in this frontal region is associated with attempts to down regulate emotional responses to negative pictures by reframing the negative scenes as less negative (either by viewing the picture with a sense of detachment or by imagining the improvement of the depicted scenario) [3]. Thus we need an effective method to study frontal cortex of depression. To our knowledge, Electroencephalography (EEG) is an objective and reliable method for the evaluation of brain function which is often used in auxiliary diagnosis of illnesses such as depression [4], seizure and schizophrenia [5]. The advantages of EEG are sensitivity, relatively low-cost and convenience of recording. Hence we are exploring such method with EEG. EEG research has revealed that greater relative left frontal electroencephalographic (EEG) activity is related to positive emotion [6], while greater relative right frontal EEG activity is related to negative emotion. Individuals with MDD tend to exhibit relative left frontal hypoactivity [7, 8]. A number of studies have also reported that greater relative activity of right prefrontal is related to depression scores [9]. Therefore, it's may be a risk marker that relatively less EEG activity of left frontal. Although similar frontal asymmetry patterns have also been noted in other psychiatric disorders (e.g. anxiety, ADHD) [10], they have been most extensively studied and reliably altered in MDD, and most commonly increased theta has been found in patients. In addition, studies of facial emotion processing play an important role in the research of emotion and cognition in MDD. Stuhrmann's research has suggested that MDD have mood-congruent processing bias in the amygdala, insula, parahippocampal gyrus, fusiform face area and putamen [11].

Nowadays, mild depression is more prevalent than major depression, and previous research has suggested that mild depression strongly predicts MDD [12]. The risk of developing major depression in subjects with mild depression was found to be 8.0 % after 2 years [12]. So the absolute number of subjects with mild depression receiving professional help is considerable. But only few studies were engaged in mild depression research. Therefore, the aim of this study was to find out whether exist differences of mild depression brain area. So we adopted a emotion evoked paradigm using facial emotion picture, and collected their EEG signal at same time. We made use of EEG topography and sLORETA (standardized low-resolution electromagnetic tomography) to observe the abnormal brain regions of mildly depressed subjects during the viewing facial pictures, because those methods can more directly and accurately show the difference brain regions between two group. Thus, the present paper will focus on EEG topography and sLORETA data obtained in mild depression, as compared with age- and sex-matched controls.

## 2  Methods

### 2.1  Subjects

In this study, there were thirty seven students from Lanzhou university (Lanzhou, Gansu province of china) participated in. All of them were right-handed, with normal or corrected-to-normal vision and there were no prior history of psychopathology. In order to classify the emotional state of subjects, all of them were asked to complete the Beck Depression Inventory test-II (BDI-II). A BDI score of >13 and <=19 was considered to indicate a mild depressive state; <9 was considered to indicate a non-depressive state [13]. By scale scanning, only twenty subjects was selected. The number of mildly depressed subjects was ten whose ages ranged from 19 to 22 (Mean = 20.60, SD = 1.838) and BDI scores ranged from 14 to 23 (Mean = 18.40, SD = 4.526). In order to obtain an equal number of subjects in each group, we selected 10 subjects (2 females, 8 males) from the normal group, with BDI scores ranging from 2 to 9 (Mean = 6.80, SD = 2.573), and ages corresponding to those of the mildly depressed group. All volunteers gave their consent and were rewarded for their participation.

## 2.2    Task and Experiment Procedure

The stimulus materials contained 60 facial expression images selected from the Chinese Facial Affective Picture System (CFAPS) [14]. The experiment consisted of two blocks: Neu_block and Emo_Block. Each block contains 15 trials, Each trial was presented for 6 s, followed by a gray background presented for 2 s, hence, participants completed the whole experiment in approximately 5 min. Nue_block contained 15 trials with two neutral Chinese facial expressions shown simultaneously. For Emo_block each trial contained two pictures of Chinese facial expression, one neutral and one emotional (sad, angry, depressed, and terrified), the location of emotional stimuli was presented on the left or right side of the screen randomly. The pictures appear randomly in each block. Stimuli were displayed on a black background screen. At the beginning of the experiment, participants were given 5 practice trials from a separate set of images to ensure that they understood what to do.

## 2.3    EEG Data Recordings and Processing

The experiment took place in a sound-attenuated, light-dimmed, and air-conditioned room. The EEG was acquired with a 128-channel HydroCel Geodesic Sensor Net, and NetStation software, version 4.5.4. All Electrode impedances were maintained below 70 k$\Omega$ [19]. All channels were referenced to ear-linked during acquisition. The continuous EEG signals were recorded at sampling rates of 250 Hz.

A band-pass filter of 1–70 Hz and a notch filter of 50 Hz were applied to the data to reduce noise and eliminate ocular artifacts. Adaptive filter using minimum square algorithm of LMS algorithm to eliminate the power noise. We marked the raw EEG signals according to the high amplitude characteristic of EOG contaminated zone to eliminate EOG signals.

Previous research has revealed that theta and alpha bands are closely related to cognitive function and depression. Therefore, power spectrum differences between two group was using T-test in two frequency bands under two conditions (neutral expression, negative expression), and presented as topography. In addition, the differences between the groups were also compared voxel-by-voxel using independent a log-F-ratio statistic test in two frequency bands. This was facilitated by the sLORETA built-in voxel wise randomization tests (5000 permutations), based on statistical nonparametric mapping (SnPM). The levels of significance were corrected for multiple comparisons. The voxels with significant differences ($p < 0.05$). Brodmann areas (BA) as well as coordinates in the MNI-brain were also noted.

## 3 Results

### 3.1 Profile of Mood States (POMS)

Means and standard deviations for age and BDI scores for the mildly depressed and normal group are shown in Table 1. The BDI scores indicate that mildly depressed subjects suffer anxiety and affective disorders.

**Table 1.** Mild depressive disorder and control group characteristics (Means ± S.D.).

|  | N | Age | BDI |
|---|---|---|---|
| Depressed subjects | 10 | 20.60 ± 1.838 | 18.40 ± 4.526 |
| Control subjects | 10 | 20.20 ± 2.044 | 6.80 ± 2.573 |
| T-test |  | P > 0.61 | P < 0.01 |

Note: N: Number of participates. BDI: Beck Depression Inventory. The t-test is based on an independent group test comparing the means of the two groups and shows probabilities (p) of the null hypothesis. Confidence interval is at 95 % confidence level.

### 3.2 EEG Results and Analysis

The statistical differences between groups for current density at the source are shown in Tables 2 and 3. EEG results indicate that the difference between mild depressed patients and normal controls is mainly concentrated in the frontal lobe, temporal lobe, parietal lobe and occipital lobe on theta and alpha bands.

**Table 2.** sLORETA results of statistical differences in theta band of mild depression group and control group when they viewing expressional pictures and neutral pictures.

|  | Activity | Log of ratio of averages | BA | Structure | Lobe |
|---|---|---|---|---|---|
| Expressional pictures | ↑ | 0.649 | 4L | Precentral gyrus | Frontal lobe |
|  | ↓ | −0.527 | 19L | Inferior occipital gyrus | Occipital lobe |
|  | ↓ | −0.301 | 19R | Middle occipital gyrus | Occipital lobe |
| Neutral pictures | ↑ | 0.403 | 5I | Postcentral gyrus | Parietal lobe |
|  | ↓ | −0.644 | 47L | Middle frontal gyrus | Frontal lobe |
|  | ↓ | −0.630 | 47R | Inferior frontal gyrus | Frontal lobe |
|  | ↓ | −0.477 | 21L | Middle temporal gyrus | Temporal lobe |
|  | ↓ | −0.359 | 21R | Middle temporal gyrus | Temporal lobe |
|  | ↓ | −0.489 | 18L | Inferior occipital gyrus | Occipital lobe |

Note: ↑: mild depressed group has higher activity than normal group, BA: Brodmann area, r: right, l: left

**Table 3.** sLORETA results of statistical differences in alpha band of mild depression group and control group when they viewing expressional pictures and neutral pictures.

| | Activity | Log of ratio of averages | BA | Structure | Lobe |
|---|---|---|---|---|---|
| Expressional pictures | ↑ | 0.670 | 4L | Precentral gyrus | Frontal lobe |
| | ↓ | −0.452 | 47R | Inferior frontal gyrus | Frontal lobe |
| | ↓ | −0.376 | 11L | Middle frontal gyrus | Frontal lobe |
| Neutral pictures | ↑ | 0.537 | 4L | Precentral gyrus | Frontal lobe |
| | ↑ | 0.536 | 40L | Sub-gyral | Parietal lobe |
| | ↑ | 0.395 | 40R | Sub-gyral | Parietal lobe |
| | ↓ | −0.569 | 47L | Inferior frontal gyrus | Frontal lobe |
| | ↓ | −0.507 | 47R | Inferior frontal gyrus | Frontal lobe |
| | ↓ | −0.514 | 18L | Inferior occipital gyrus | Occipital lobe |

Note: ↑: mild depressed group has higher activity than normal group, BA: Brodmann area, r: right, l: left

Many studies have suggested that prefrontal cortex plays a very important role in depression. A host of brain imaging studies have found activation in the orbito frontal andor inferior frontal cortex in association with suppressing or reappraising negative emotional stimuli (e.g. BA: 11 [15, 16]; BA: 47 [16, 17]) and with suppressing the influence of negative emotional stimuli on subsequent behavior (BA: 47) [18]. In our study, left prefrontal cortex of mild depression has lower theta and alpha activity in both of two experiment blocks (Table 2, 3). According to our results, the patterns also exist in mild depressive disorder.

In addition, we found that mild depressive disorder had higher activity in left motor cortex (BA: 4L, 6L) for theta band (Table 2, Fig. 1) when they observing emotional stimulus. The same situation existed in neutral block. To our knowledge, motor cortex involved in the planning, control, and execution of voluntary movements. Moreover, according to L. Carr's study, human will automatically mirrored expressions on the face when they viewing emotional facial expressions in other activities [19]. So depressed patients are more vulnerable to the interference of picture stimulus and will tend to imitate the expression unconsciously, hence motor cortex of mild depressed patients has higher activity.

Primate studies have shown reciprocal connections between the lateral edge of the OFC and the medial prefrontal emotion-regulatory network [20]. These regions share extensive reciprocal connections with the amygdala, anterior temporal and anterior cingulate cortex [21]. In our study, results showed that the previsual (BA: 18, 19) cortex activity about visual information process of mild depression was decreased when compared with controls. Primary visual cortex activity was decreased in all bands for two blocks, except alpha band when subjects observing emotional stimulus. The decreased activity in primary visual cortex may lead to the emotion regulation disorder which is the cause of depression.

Many previous research has found that depression tend to exhibit relative left frontal and previsual cotex hypoactivity in resting state [22–24]. Thus those cortex

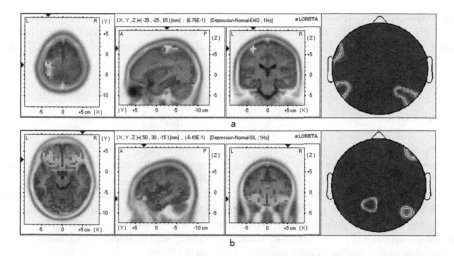

**Fig. 1.** Source localization results (left) and EEG mapping results (right), based on statistic contrast analysis in the theta band (4–8 Hz) of the mild depressed group and control group when they viewing expressional pictures (a) and neutral pictures (b). (sLORETA results: red area means that normal group has higher activity than mild depressed group in this area; EEG mapping results: red area means that there is statistic difference in this area). (Color figure online)

exists differences under emotion and neutral condition. However, there were differences between two conditions. By compared the statistical differences of left and right prefrontal cortex in alpha band, the results showed that the statistical differences at right prefrontal are more apparent than the left in emotional block (Log of ratio of averages: 0.367 (Alpha, BA: 11L), 0.452 (Alpha, BA: 47R)). However, neutral does not exist in the situation. EEG research has revealed that increased relative right fronto-cortical activity tends to emerge during the processing of negative information and emotions [6]. Furthermore compared with neutral block, the difference in motor area of emotion block is more apparent(Log of ratio of averages of emotional block: −0.649 (theta); Log of ratio of averages of neutral block: −0.403 (theta)). Beck's cognitive model has indicated that depressed patients have a bias towards the negative, especially depressed mood [25].

## 4   Conclusion

In summary, source location results suggest mild depressed patients' left PFC exists hypoactivation. The phenomenon indicates that mild depressed subjects exists disorder of process positive information. And the higher activity in motor cortex reveals that mild depressed subjects pay more attention to negative face expressions.

In our future work, the analysis of mild depression will be correlated to structural and functional abnormalities of brain regions. It is hoped that we can generalize these findings to help diagnosis and treatment of depression.

**Acknowledgements.** This work was supported by the National Basic Research Program of China (973 Program) (No. 2014CB744600), the Program of International S&T Cooperation of MOST (No. 2013DFA11140), the National Natural Science Foundation of China (grant No. 61210010, No. 61300231).

# References

1. http://www.who.int
2. Davidson, R.J., Pizzagalli, D., Nitschke, J.B., Putnam, K.: Depression: perspectives from affective neuroscience. Ann. Rev. Psychol. **53**, 545–574 (2002)
3. Ochsner, K.N., Ray, R.D., Cooper, J.C., Robertson, E.R., Chopra, S., Gabrieli, J.D., Gross, J.J.: For better or for worse: neural systems supporting the cognitive down-and up-regulation of negative emotion. Neuroimage **23**, 483–499 (2004)
4. Giannakopoulos, P., Missonnier, P., Gold, G., Michon, A.: Electrophysiological markers of rapid cognitive decline in mild cognitive impairment (2009)
5. Parvinnia, E., Sabeti, M., Jahromi, M.Z., Boostani, R.: Classification of EEG Signals using adaptive weighted distance nearest neighbor algorithm. J. King Saud Univ. – Comput. Inf. Sci. **26**, 1–6 (2014)
6. Davidson, R.J., Hugdahl, K.E.: Brain Asymmetry. The MIT Press, Cambridge (1995)
7. Davidson, R.J., Slagter, H.A.: Probing emotion in the developing brain: functional neuroimaging in the assessment of the neural substrates of emotion in normal and disordered children and adolescents. Mental Retard. Dev. Disabil. Res. Rev. **6**, 166–170 (2000)
8. Pössel, P., Lo, H., Fritz, A., Seemann, S.: A longitudinal study of cortical EEG activity in adolescents. Biol. Psychol. **78**, 173–178 (2008)
9. Henriguez, J., Davidson, R.: Regional brain electrical asymmetries discriminate between previously depressed and healthy control subjects. J. Abnorm. Psychol. **99**, 22–31 (1990)
10. Hale, T.S., Smalley, S.L., Dang, J., Hanada, G., Macion, J., McCracken, J.T., McGough, J. J., Loo, S.K.: ADHD familial loading and abnormal EEG alpha asymmetry in children with ADHD. J. Psychiatr. Res. **44**, 605–615 (2010)
11. Stuhrmann, A., Suslow, T., Dannlowski, U.: Facial emotion processing in major depression: a systematic review of neuroimaging findings. Biol. Mood Anxiety Disord. **1**, 1 (2011)
12. Fogel, J., Eaton, W., Ford, D.: Minor depression as a predictor of the first onset of major depressive disorder over a 15-year follow-up. Acta Psychiatr. Scand. **113**, 36–43 (2006)
13. Beck, A.T., Steer, R.A., Ball, R., Ranieri, W.F.: Comparison of beck depression inventories-IA and-II in psychiatric outpatients. J. Pers. Assess. **67**, 588–597 (1996)
14. Lu, B., Hui, M., Yu-Xia, H.: The development of native Chinese affective picture system–a pretest in 46 college students. Chin. Mental Health J. **19**, 719–722 (2005)
15. Ohira, H., Nomura, M., Ichikawa, N., Isowa, T., Iidaka, T., Sato, A., Fukuyama, S., Nakajima, T., Yamada, J.: Association of neural and physiological responses during voluntary emotion suppression. Neuroimage **29**, 721–733 (2006)
16. Lévesque, J., Joanette, Y., Mensour, B., Beaudoin, G., Leroux, J.-M., Bourgouin, P., Beauregard, M.: Neural basis of emotional self-regulation in childhood. Neuroscience **129**, 361–369 (2004)
17. Phan, K.L., Fitzgerald, D.A., Nathan, P.J., Moore, G.J., Uhde, T.W., Tancer, M.E.: Neural substrates for voluntary suppression of negative affect: a functional magnetic resonance imaging study. Biol. Psychiatry **57**, 210–219 (2005)

18. Beer, J.S., Knight, R.T., D'Esposito, M.: Controlling the integration of emotion and cognition the role of frontal cortex in distinguishing helpful from hurtful emotional information. Psychol. Sci. **17**, 448–453 (2006)
19. Carr, L., Iacoboni, M., Dubeau, M.-C., Mazziotta, J.C., Lenzi, G.L.: Neural mechanisms of empathy in humans: a relay from neural systems for imitation to limbic areas. Proc. Natl. Acad. Sci. **100**, 5497–5502 (2003)
20. Carmichael, S., Price, J.: Limbic connections of the orbital and medial prefrontal cortex in macaque monkeys. J. Comp. Neurol. **363**, 615–641 (1995)
21. Öngür, D., Price, J.: The organization of networks within the orbital and medial prefrontal cortex of rats, monkeys and humans. Cereb. Cortex **10**, 206–219 (2000)
22. Jaworska, N., Blier, P., Fusee, W., Knott, V.: Alpha power, alpha asymmetry and anterior cingulate cortex activity in depressed males and females. J. Psychiatr. Res. **46**, 1483–1491 (2012)
23. Saletu, B., Anderer, P., Saletu-Zyhlarz, G.: EEG topography and tomography (LORETA) in diagnosis and pharmacotherapy of depression. Clin. EEG Neurosci. **41**, 203–210 (2010)
24. Stewart, J.L., Coan, J.A., Towers, D.N., Allen, J.J.: Resting and task-elicited prefrontal EEG alpha asymmetry in depression: support for the capability model. Psychophysiology **51**, 446–455 (2014)
25. Beck, A.T.: The evolution of the cognitive model of depression and its neurobiological correlates. Am. J. Psychiatry **165**, 969–977 (2008)

# Evaluation of Depression Severity in Speech

Zhenyu Liu, Bin Hu(✉), Fei Liu, Huanyu Kang, Xiaoyu Li,
Lihua Yan, and Tianyang Wang

Ubiquitous Awareness and Intelligent Solutions Lab,
Lanzhou University, Lanzhou, China
{liuzhy12, bh, fliu14, kanghy15,
yanlh14, tywang14}@lzu.edu.cn, li461547885@163.com

**Abstract.** Depression is a frequent affective disorder, leading to a high impact on patients, their families and society. Depression diagnosis is limited by assessment methods that rely on patient-reported or clinician judgments of symptom severity. Recently, many researches showed that voice is an objective indicator for depressive diagnosis. In this paper, we investigate a sample of 111 subjects (38 healthy controls, 36 mild depressed patients and 37 severe depressed patients) through comparative analysis to explore the correlation between acoustic features and depression severity. We extract features as many as possible according to previous researches to create a large voice feature set. Then we employ some feature selection methods to form compact subsets on different tasks. Finally, we evaluate depressive disorder severity by these acoustic feature subsets. Results show that interview is a better choice than reading and picture description for depression assessment. Meanwhile, speech signal correlate to depression severity in a medium-level with statistically significant ($p < 0.01$).

**Keywords:** Depression severity · Speech · Acoustic feature · Feature selection · PHQ-9

## 1 Introduction

The increase in the prevalence of clinical depression in human beings has been linked to a range of serious outcomes. It is a common mental disorder lasting for a long period and leads to a high impact on patients, their families and society. Depression is associated with half of all suicides and a significant economic burden [1]. The World Health Organization (WHO) estimated that about 350 million people of all ages suffer from this disease [2]. Moreover, depression is estimated to become the second greatest disease burden in the world by the year 2020.

However, current depression diagnosis methods almost rely on patient self-report and professional interview of symptom severity [3]. The patient self-report, like Self-rating Depression Scale (SDS) [4], risks a range of subjective biases. Similarly, professional interview varies depending on their clinical experience and the diagnostic methods used (e.g., Diagnostic and Statistical Manual of Mental Disorders (DSM-IV) [5]). So, an objective and convenient method for depression evaluation is necessary.

© Springer International Publishing AG 2016
G.A. Ascoli et al. (Eds.): BIH 2016, LNAI 9919, pp. 312–321, 2016.
DOI: 10.1007/978-3-319-47103-7_31

Developments in affective sensing technology (e.g., facial expression, body gesture, speech, motion, eye movement, etc.) will potentially enable an objective depression evaluation method. Among these technologies, speech signals can be collected easily by non-invasive and portable instrument. Voice of depressed individuals reflect the perception of qualities such as monotony, slur, low intensity and less fluctuation [6]. Vocal characteristics have been verified to change with a speaker's mental condition and emotional state [7–9]. Such changes are complicated processes involving coordination of several brain areas and peripheral muscle controls [10]. And, researches support the feasibility and validity of vocal acoustic measures of depression severity [11, 12]. Therefore, we focus on depressed patients' speech analysis.

At early age, many researchers aimed at the correlation between depression and some particular speech features [13, 14]. A lot of experiments have been conducted to reveal relevance between depression and various acoustic features, like pitch, jitter, speaking rate, formants, Mel-Frequency Cepstral Coefficient (MFCC) and so on. Low et al. [15] and Mundt et al. [3] illustrated relation between depressive severity and some acoustic features. Lately, automatic detection approaches of depression have been investigated. Alghowinem et al. investigated and compared different features on depression classification. And, She figured out that spontaneous speech gives better results than reading [16]. Many researchers believe that feature combination optimization may lead to progress of recognition accuracy. Moore et al. proposed new feature sets with good performance on depression classification [7].

In this paper, we speculate speech signal correlate with severity of depression in a way. In order to validate our hypothesis, we take two steps: First, choose a feature set through comparing the classification accuracy in different tasks. Second, explore the correlation between the feature set and severity of depression.

The rest of this paper is organized as follows: Sect. 2 is a presentation of the details of our method and experiment, consisting of seven parts: the participants and their basic information, the procedure of experiment, data collection, data preprocessing and feature extraction, feature selection, classifiers, and correlation analysis. In Sect. 3, we showed the results of our experiment. Following this, we presented a discussion in Sect. 4 and in Sect. 5 conclusions were draw.

## 2   Method

### 2.1   Participants

111 participants' (54 males, 57 females) data from an ongoing study in Beijing and Lanzhou, China, were used for the experimental validation. These participants, with the age range of 18-55, were selected by psychiatrists following Diagnostic and Statistical Manual of Mental Disorders (DSM-IV). All participants were asked to sign informed consent, fill in basic information and a series of scales. These basic information of subjects are summarized in Table 1.

All the participants were interviewed by a psychiatrist to finish the Patient Health Questionnaire-9 (PHQ-9) [17]. They were divided into three groups according to the PHQ-9 scores: 38 healthy control subjects (PHQ-9 < 5), 36 mild depressive patients

**Table 1.** Basic information of subjects

| Parameter | Male subjects | Female subjects |
|---|---|---|
| Number of subjects | 54 | 57 |
| Average age (years) | 36.6 ± 10.3 | 40.5 ± 10.8 |
| PHQ-9 score | 10.8 ± 8.1 | 11.7 ± 8.9 |
| Recordings | 29 | |
| Tasks | Interview, reading, picture description | |
| Native language | Chinese | |

($5 \leq$ PHQ-9 $< 17$) and 37 severe depressive patients (PHQ-9 $\geq 17$). This three groups division can describe the change trend of speech features and keep relative larger subjects of each groups. The results are showed in Table 2.

**Table 2.** Basic information of groups

| Parameter | Male subjects | | | Female subjects | | |
|---|---|---|---|---|---|---|
| | Healthy | Mild | Severe | Healthy | Mild | Severe |
| Number of subjects | 19 | 17 | 18 | 19 | 19 | 19 |
| Average age (years) | 36 ± 9.6 | 37.5 ± 10.9 | 36.2 ± 11 | 40.3 ± 11.1 | 40.5 ± 11.1 | 40.3 ± 10.8 |
| PHQ-9 score | 1.9 ± 1.5 | 10.9 ± 3.7 | 20 ± 3.1 | 1.3 ± 1.5 | 11.9 ± 3.9 | 21.7 ± 3.2 |

## 2.2    The Procedure of Experiment

Our experiment comprises three parts: interview, reading and picture description. Each part can be divided into three groups in terms of its induced emotion: positive, neutral and negative. To counteract the sequence effect of evoked emotion, the emotion order of each participant is assigned randomly. Details of the experiment follows below.

**Interview.** The interview part consisted of 18 questions. These questions are divided into three groups according to emotion valence: 6 positive, 6 neutral and 6 negative. These topics came from DSM-IV and some depression scales which are often used in depressive disorder diagnosis. For examples: What is your favorite TV program? What is the best gift you have ever received [18]? Please describe one of your friends. How do you evaluate yourself? What makes you desperate?

**Reading.** This part consisted of a short story named "The North Wind and the Sun", which was often used in acoustic analysis in international, multilingual clinical research, and three groups words with positive (e.g., outstanding, happy), neutral (e.g., center, since) and negative (e.g., depression, wail) emotion valence. Positive and negative words were selected from affective ontology corpus created by Lin [19], and neutral ones were selected from Chinese affective words extremum table [20]. All of them are commonly used words in Chinese and have close stroke number.

**Picture Description.** This part comprises four pictures. Three of them, which express positive (happy), neutral and negative (sad) faces, were selected from Chinese Facial Affective Picture System (CFAPS) and the last one with a "crying woman" came from Thematic Apperception Test (TAT) [18]. Participants were asked to describe these four pictures freely.

## 2.3  Data Collection

We collected recording data in a clean, quiet and soundproof laboratory. The whole experiment lasted about 25 min for one participant. During the course of recording, the subject was asked not to touch any equipment and keep the distance between mouth and microphone about 20 cm. A NEUMANN TLM102 microphone and a RME FIREFACE UCX audio card with 44.1 kHz sampling rate and 24-bit sampling depth were used for collecting voice signals. All recording data were saved as uncompressed WAV format. During the whole experimental process, ambient noise was required under 60 dB to prevent interference with subject's audio signals.

In the experiment, 29 recordings for every single participant were stored and named as 1 to 29 in a determined sequence. The details were as follows: The positive, neutral and negative interview recordings are named as 1–6, 7–12 and 13–18 separately. The record of the short story is name as 19. The readings of six word groups are named as 20–21, 22–23 and 24–25 in accordance with the sequence of positive, neutral and negative emotion. 26–28 were the picture description with the same order to reading part. The record of TAT was numbered as 29.

## 2.4  Data Preprocessing and Feature Extraction

All recordings are segmented and labeled manually. Only subjects' voice signal are reserved for analysis. Preprocessing mainly includes of filtering (a band-pass filter with 60–4500 Hz), framing, windowing and sometimes endpoint detection for some particular feature extraction. Each frame is 25 ms length with 50 % overlap. Voice characteristics can be divided into two categories: acoustic and linguistic features [21, 22]. The latter will not be analyzed since we are aiming at general characteristics for depressed speech regardless of the language used. Several software tools are employed for extracting sound features. We used the open-source software 'openSMILE' [23], VOICEBOX [24] and Praat [25] to extract 1753-dimension features. These features will be used in the following feature selection, classification and correlation analysis.

There are two steps to get the final acoustic feature subset of the speech signal: First, the signals of story (19) and TAT (29) are excluded in this paper. So, only 27 recordings for every subject were analysed. Second, compute the average value of every feature in the same part and induced emotion for one participant. For example, the speech 1–6 are for interview in positive emotion and we stored the mean values of all features as the Data 1 (in Table 3). The details are presented in Table 3.

**Table 3.** Names of nine data sets

| Task | Positive | Neutral | Negative |
|------|----------|---------|----------|
| Interview | Data_1 | Data_2 | Data_3 |
| Reading | Data_4 | Data_5 | Data_6 |
| Picture description | Data_7 | Data_8 | Data_9 |

## 2.5    Feature Selection

Feature selection refers to selecting effective features for classification in universal feature set. It is a critical problem in preprocess of data mining to cope with the curse of dimensionality [26]. In our experiment, we utilize a two-stage feature selection method by combining a filter and a wrapper method to reduce the feature dimension. Filter approach only utilizes data to decide which features should be kept. In general, filter approach has an efficient searching strategy with a result tradeoff. With "wrapping" accuracy of classifier, wrapper method may lead to a better performance compared to filter. Combining both we may have a high efficient method.

Here are the details about our two-stage feature selection method. We combine the minimal-redundancy-maximal-relevance (mRMR) criterion [27] as the filter approach and the Sequential Forward Floating Selection (SFFS) algorithm [28] as the search strategy of the wrapper approach. On the first stage, a candidate subset is selected from the universal feature set by mRMR. On the second stage, final subset is obtained from the candidate subset by SFFS. The final feature subset is used for the following discussion. In this process, the Support Vector Machine (SVM) [29] and Leave-One-Out Cross-Validation (LOOCV) scheme are be employed for evaluating and testing. This feature selection scheme is carried out on the nine data sets separately, which means nine feature subsets will be gained. We named these nine feature subsets as fs_1, fs_2, … fs_9, etc.

## 2.6    Classifier

We intend to evaluate feature subset in a specific situation to measure the severity of depression by pattern classification approach. Three widely used classifiers were employed in this paper: SVM, Naïve Bayes (NB) [29] and Random Forest (RF) [30]. The Radial Basis Function (RBF) kernel function was chosen in LIBSVM package [31]. Compared with the dimensionality of feature set, the sample size is often so small that we use the LOOCV scheme in testing. LOOCV is a special cross-validation. More specifically, one sample is for testing and the others are for training within a process. This repeated for all the samples and the result is the average accuracy of all repeats.

## 2.7    Correlation Analysis

Our main target is to explore the correlation between vocal features and depression severity. The PHQ-9 is a brief depression assessment instrument with severity categories. It is the depression module of the Primary Care Evaluation of Mental Disorder

[32, 33] that was designed to be used in primary care [34] and provides scores on each of the nine DSM-IV criteria using a severity scale from "0" (not all) to "3" (nearly every day). In our research, one or more feature subsets selected from the nine sets based on classification accuracy are used to explore the relation between voice and depression severity. Principal Component Analysis (PCA) will be applied on the normalized data of these feature subsets. We observe the Pearson's Correlation Coefficient (r) and the corresponding significance level (ρ) between the first principal component (FPC) and the PHQ-9 score with significance being tested with a T-test.

## 3  Result

Table 4 shows the average classification accuracy of three groups with three classifiers on nine feature subsets respectively. Although the accuracy of interview on positive and negative is inferior to reading or picture description for male, interview is with the best performance on average accuracy. And, it has a minimal standard deviation. For both male and female interview is the best choice of three for speech signal collection.

**Table 4.** Classification accuracy using data on nine feature subsets separately

| Gender | Task | Positive | Neutral | Negative | AVG | STDEV |
|---|---|---|---|---|---|---|
| Male | Interview | 0.648 | 0.630 | 0.605 | 0.628 | 0.022 |
| | Reading | 0.537 | 0.525 | 0.605 | 0.556 | 0.043 |
| | Picture description | 0.506 | 0.598 | 0.475 | 0.526 | 0.064 |
| Female | Interview | 0.544 | 0.526 | 0.579 | 0.550 | 0.027 |
| | Reading | 0.444 | 0.432 | 0.608 | 0.495 | 0.098 |
| | Picture description | 0.608 | 0.491 | 0.462 | 0.520 | 0.077 |

Table 5 presents the Pearson correlation coefficients between FPCs from fs_1, fs_2 and fs_3 on interview and PHQ-9 scores separately with significance levels. The values of r and ρ show that these FPCs are related to depression severity at a moderate level and statistically significant for both male and female.

**Table 5.** Pearson's correlation coefficient (r) and corresponding significant level (ρ) between FPC from the data of fs_1, fs_2 and fs_3 in interview and PHQ-9 score separately

| Gender | Parameter | Positive | Neutral | Negative |
|---|---|---|---|---|
| Female | r | −0.400 | 0.501 | 0.543 |
| | ρ | 0.002 | 0.000 | 0.000 |
| Male | r | 0.499 | −0.481 | −0.544 |
| | ρ | 0.000 | 0.000 | 0.000 |

Figures 1, 2 and 3 show the scatter diagram of FPCs from Data_1, Data_2 and Data_3 and PHQ-9 scores in order to observe the linear correlation directly with

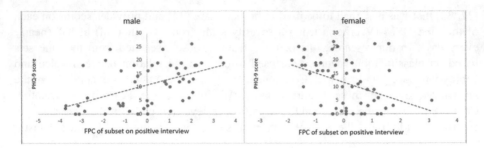

**Fig. 1.** Scatter diagram of FPC and PHQ-9 score on the data of positive interview

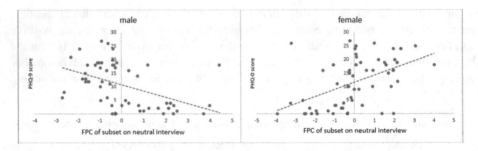

**Fig. 2.** Scatter diagram of FPC and PHQ-9 score on the data of neutral interview

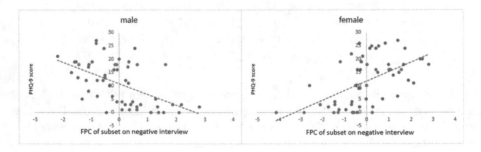

**Fig. 3.** Scatter diagram of FPC and PHQ-9 score on the data of negative interview

different emotion respectively. We can find that the negative questions perform better than positive and neutral on both male and female. All the correlation coefficients have opposite signs between genders.

## 4    Discussion

Our research aims at exploring the correlation between acoustic features and depression to evaluate depression severity. From results above, we get three points: First, the average classification accuracies (male: 0.57, female: 0.52) are probably limited for a real system, nonetheless, they are much higher than chance level. Second, for both male and female, interview is the best pattern among these three ways to pick up the speech signals to evaluate severity of depression. Third, the correlation between the feature subsets from interview and PHQ-9 manifest that depressive severity is related to speech at a moderate level and the correlation is statistically significant.

Recording patterns may influence the classification performance. In our experiment, interview performs better than reading and picture description, which is consistent with the conclusion of Alghowinem et al. [23]. She pointed out that spontaneous speech gives a better results than reading. Both interview and picture description can be considered as spontaneous speech. However, picture description is worse than interview, we speculate that most of interview questions refer to the subject himself so that they are easy to get into emotional state.

In our further study, we intend to seek a more stable feature subset for depression assessment on a larger size of participants. And, we will combine speech features with other physiological feature (e.g. facial expression, gait, head movement etc.) to improve the classification accuracy.

## 5   Conclusion

Our work aims at an objective diagnostic aid supporting clinicians in evaluating severity of depression. The results confirmed our hypothesis by examining subjects' acoustic features on interview, reading and picture description patterns. Speech may be considered as a biomarker on depressive severity. Interview is a proper way to gain effective speech signal for depression assessment. The correlation between the FPC of speech feature subset and PHQ-9 score with statistical significance indicate that there may exist some features sets can be used to evaluate depression severity.

**Acknowledgment.** This work was supported by the National Basic Research Program of China (973 Program) (No. 2014CB744600), the Program of International S&T Cooperation of MOST (No. 2013DFA11140), the National Natural Science Foundation of China (grant No. 61210010, No. 61300231). Grateful acknowledgement is made to my classmates: Xiang Gao, Jinning Zhao, Xin Guo, Fei Heng and Lele He. They gave us considerable help by means of data collection, comments and criticism.

## References

1. Lecrubier, Y.: Depressive illness and disability. Eur. Neuropsychopharmacol **10**, S439–S443 (2000)
2. World Health Organization. http://www.who.int/mediacentre/factsheets/fs396/en/
3. Mundt, J.C., Snyder, P.J., Cannizzaro, M.S., Chappie, K., Geralts, D.S.: Voice acoustic measures of depression severity and treatment response collected via interactive voice response (IVR) technology. J. Neurolinguist. **20**, 50–64 (2007)
4. Zung, W.W., Richards, C.B., Short, M.J.: Self-rating depression scale in an outpatient clinic: further validation of the SDS. Arch. Gen. Psychiatry **13**, 508–515 (1965)

5. American Psychiatric Association: DSM-III-R: Diagnostic and Statistical Manual of Mental Disorders. American Psychiatric Association, Arlington (1980)
6. Horwitz, R., Quatieri, T.F., Helfer, B.S., Yu, B., Williamson, J.R., Mundt, J.: On the relative importance of vocal source, system, and prosody in human depression. In: 2013 IEEE International Conference on Body Sensor Networks (BSN), pp. 1–6. IEEE (2013)
7. Moore, E., Clements, M., Peifer, J., Weisser, L.: Analysis of prosodic variation in speech for clinical depression. In: Proceedings of the 25th Annual International Conference of the IEEE on Engineering in Medicine and Biology Society, pp. 2925–2928. IEEE (2003)
8. France, D.J., Shiavi, R.G., Silverman, S., Silverman, M., Wilkes, D.M.: Acoustical properties of speech as indicators of depression and suicidal risk. IEEE Trans. Biomed. Eng. **47**, 829–837 (2000)
9. Quatieri, T.F., Malyska, N.: Vocal-source biomarkers for depression: a link to psychomotor activity. In: Interspeech, pp. 1059–1062
10. Vicsi, K., Sztaho, D., Kiss, G.: Examination of the sensitivity of acoustic-phonetic parameters of speech to depression. In: 2012 IEEE 3rd International Conference on Cognitive Infocommunications (CogInfoCom), pp. 511–515. IEEE (2012)
11. Harel, B., Cannizzaro, M., Snyder, P.J.: Variability in fundamental frequency during speech in prodromal and incipient Parkinson's disease: a longitudinal case study. Brain Cogn. **56**, 24–29 (2004)
12. Mundt, J.C., Vogel, A.P., Feltner, D.E., Lenderking, W.R.: Vocal acoustic biomarkers of depression severity and treatment response. Biol. Psychiatry **72**, 580–587 (2012)
13. Nilsonne, Å., Sundberg, J., Ternström, S., Askenfelt, A.: Measuring the rate of change of voice fundamental frequency in fluent speech during mental depression. J. Acoust. Soc. Am. **83**, 716–728 (1988)
14. Scripture, E.: A study of emotions by speech transcription. Vox **31**, 179–183 (1921)
15. Ooi, K.E.B., Low, L.-S.A., Lech, M., Allen, N.: Early prediction of major depression in adolescents using glottal wave characteristics and teager energy parameters. In: 2012 IEEE International Conference on Acoustics, Speech and Signal Processing (ICASSP), pp. 4613–4616. IEEE (2012)
16. Alghowinem, S., Goecke, R., Wagner, M., Epps, J., Breakspear, M., Parker, G.: Detecting depression: a comparison between spontaneous and read speech. In: 2013 IEEE International Conference on Acoustics, Speech and Signal Processing, pp. 7547–7551. IEEE (2013)
17. Kroencke, K., Spitzer, R., Williams, J.: The phq-9: validity of a brief depression severity measure [electronic version]. J. Gen. Intern. Med. **16**, 606–613 (2001)
18. Hönig, F., Batliner, A., Nöth, E., Schnieder, S., Krajewski, J.: Automatic modelling of depressed speech: relevant features and relevance of gender. In: INTERSPEECH, pp. 1248–1252
19. DUTIR. http://ir.dlut.edu.cn/Group.aspx?ID=4
20. ShuJuTang. http://www.datatang.com/data/43216
21. Bandura, A., Pastorelli, C., Barbaranelli, C., Caprara, G.V.: Self-efficacy pathways to childhood depression. J. Pers. Soc. Psychol. **76**, 258 (1999)
22. Zhou, G., Hansen, J.H., Kaiser, J.F.: Nonlinear feature based classification of speech under stress. IEEE Trans. Speech Audio Process. **9**, 201–216 (2001)
23. Alghowinem, S., Goecke, R., Wagner, M., Epps, J., Gedeon, T., Breakspear, M., Parker, G.: A comparative study of different classifiers for detecting depression from spontaneous speech. In: 2013 IEEE International Conference on Acoustics, Speech and Signal Processing (ICASSP), pp. 8022–8026. IEEE (2013)
24. Kurniawan, H., Maslov, A.V., Pechenizkiy, M.: Stress detection from speech and galvanic skin response signals. In: 2013 IEEE 26th International Symposium on Computer-Based Medical Systems (CBMS), pp. 209–214. IEEE (2013)

25. De Jong, N.H., Wempe, T.: Praat script speech rate (2008). Accessed 14 Oct 2008
26. Guyon, I., Elisseeff, A.: An introduction to variable and feature selection. J. Mach. Learn. Res. **3**, 1157–1182 (2003)
27. Peng, H., Long, F., Ding, C.: Feature selection based on mutual information criteria of max-dependency, max-relevance, and min-redundancy. IEEE Trans. Pattern Anal. Mach. Intell. **27**, 1226–1238 (2005)
28. Pudil, P., Novovičová, J., Kittler, J.: Floating search methods in feature selection. Pattern Recogn. Lett. **15**, 1119–1125 (1994)
29. Mitchell, T.M.: Machine Learning. WCB/McGraw-Hill, Boston (1997)
30. Quinlan, J.R.: C4. 5: programs for machine learning. Elsevier (2014)
31. Hsu, C.-W., Lin, C.-J.: A comparison of methods for multiclass support vector machines. IEEE Trans. Neural Netw. **13**, 415–425 (2002)
32. Farzanfar, R., Hereen, T., Fava, J., Davis, J., Vachon, L., Friedman, R.: Psychometric properties of an automated telephone-based PHQ-9. Telemed. e-Health **20**, 115–121 (2014)
33. Spitzer, R.L., Kroenke, K., Williams, J.B., Patient Health Questionnaire Primary Care Study Group: Validation and utility of a self-report version of PRIME-MD: the PHQ primary care study. JAMA **282**, 1737–1744 (1999)
34. Löwe, B., Unützer, J., Callahan, C.M., Perkins, A.J., Kroenke, K.: Monitoring depression treatment outcomes with the patient health questionnaire-9. Med. Care **42**, 1194–1201 (2004)

# Brain-Inspired Intelligence
and Computing

# A Noninvasive Real-Time Solution for Driving Fatigue Detection Based on Left Prefrontal EEG and Eye Blink

Jian He[1,2(⊠)], Yan Zhang[2], Cheng Zhang[2], Mingwo Zhou[2],
and Yi Han[3]

[1] Beijing Advanced Innovation Center for Future Internet Technology,
Beijing 100124, China
jianhee@bjut.edu.cn
[2] School of Software Engineering,
Beijing University of Technology, Beijing 100124, China
{875205252,916389805}@qq.com, p_s_i@foxmail.com
[3] China Welfare Lottery Technology Center, Beijing 100010, China
4296288@qq.com

**Abstract.** According to the portable and real-time problems on the driving fatigue prevention based on EEG, a headband integrated with Thinkgear EEG chip, tri-axial accelerometer, gyroscope and Bluetooth is developed to collect the subject's blink, the Attention and Meditation of the left prefrontal EEG. The comparison between Attention and Meditation of the left prefrontal EEG is discussed at first when the subject is in the state of concentration, relaxation, fatigue and sleep. The slide window and k-NN algorithm are introduced to develop a new method for driving fatigue detection based on subject's blink and the correlation coefficient between Attention and Meditation. Lastly, a software running on a smart device is developed based on above technologies, it can issue alarm and play music when it detects driving fatigue. The experiment proves that it has noninvasive and real-time advantages, while its sensitivity and specificity are 73.8 % and 88.6 % respectively.

**Keywords:** Eye blink · Driving fatigue detection · Prefrontal lobe EEG · Ubiquitous computing · k-NN

## 1 Introduction

With the vast amount of vehicles on roads, transportation safety has been of increasing concern. How to avoid or reduce transportation accidents has become a hot research field. Driving fatigue has become a large factor in transportation accidents because of the marked decline in the driver's perception, recognition, and vehicle control while fatigued. The statistical data and survey reports indicate that, if the driver's response time could be half a second faster, 60 % transportation accidents could be avoided [1]. Hence, developing an accurate and noninvasive real-time driving fatigue detection system would be highly desirable [2].

© Springer International Publishing AG 2016
G.A. Ascoli et al. (Eds.): BIH 2016, LNAI 9919, pp. 325–335, 2016.
DOI: 10.1007/978-3-319-47103-7_32

Different research has been reported on driving fatigue detection including methods identifying physiological associations between driver's fatigue and the corresponding patterns of the electroocculogram (EOG) (eye movement), electroencephalogram signals (brain activity), and electrocardiogram (ECG) signals (heart rate) [3]. Schleicher finds that spontaneous eye blink is the most promising biosignal for in-car sleepiness warnings [4]. Besides, many research suggested the EEG was found to be sensitive to changes in alertness and able to predict change in the cognitive state by used significant changes in the EEG frequency bands. However, the existing majority of EEG-based driving fatigue detection needs lots contact sensors, which often makes the subject feel uncomfortable during the driving [5]. So the practical application on EEG-based driving fatigue detection technology faces great challenges, such as portability and real-time requirements. And the accuracy and practicality of the existing majority of EEG-based driving fatigue detection can be further improved.

Eye blink is an important performance of fatigue and decreased attention. Stern found that the frequency of blink and blink duration subject to the direct control of the brain [6]. When the driver awake, blink frequency is normal; when the driver is tired, blink frequency is significantly reduced. Therefore eye blink can be used as parameters in the fatigue detection.

Based on above discussion, an noninvasive real-time method for driving fatigue detection is proposed in this paper, which uses an smart phone, and a headband integrated with ThinkGear EEG chip, tri-axial accelerometer, gyro-scope and Bluetooth to capture the subject's blink, Attention and Meditation so as to detect driving fatigue and issue alarm during the driving.

The rest of this paper is organized as follows. In Sect. 2, it introduces the function of prefrontal lobe and eye blink. The relation between the left prefrontal Attention and Meditation EEG is analyzed, and a new driving fatigue detection method is proposed at last. Section 3 introduces the methodology to deploy a system based on subject's blink and the correlation coefficient of the subject's left prefrontal Attention and Meditation EEG. Section 4, the driving fatigue system based on the above technologies is discussed. Section 5 shows the experiment and its analysis. Section 6 summarizes the study and provides future research ideas.

## 2　Foundation

### 2.1　Function of Prefrontal Lobe and Eye Blink

The cerebral cortex can be divided into four major lobes, among them prefrontal lobe plays a key role for the attentive regulation, thinking and reasoning. It accepts and processes information from sensory, motor and other brain regions, and then sends back the processed message so as to control activities of the related brain regions. Hence, the state of fatigue while driving could be detected as long as the EEG data from the driver's frontal lobe could be real-time monitored.

Normally, eye blink frequency in fatigue is different from that in normal state, when person is in fatigue, the blink frequency is significantly reduced. In driving fatigue detection, blink frequency is rarely used alone as the sole criterion, but it was used in image processing technology to helpfully analyze the parameters such as eye position, blink duration, and blink frequency [7]. In this paper, blink as a parameter is combined with the left prefrontal EEG signals to detect driving fatigue.

MindWave EEG headset integrated ThinkGear EEG chip, can collect the subject's blink and left prefrontal EEG from FP1 [8] with 512 Hz frequency. It can count the number of subject's blink and produce the Attention and Meditation EEG in 1 Hz frequency. The value of attention ranges from 0 to 100, the higher the value indicates that the attention is more concentrated. The value of meditation also ranges from 0 to 100, the higher the value indicates that the brain activity of the user is lower. Therefore, ThinkGear EEG chip is used to collect the subject's blink, the Attention and Meditation EEG from the prefrontal lobe.

## 2.2    The Relation Between the Left Prefrontal Attention and Meditation EEG

According to [9], four kinds of 20 min scenarios (Concentration, Relaxation, Fatigue and Sleep) are designed to analyze the relationship between the subject's left prefrontal Attention and Meditation EEG. And the experimental results shows that there is a symmetrical relationship between Attention and Meditation EEG, hence the correlation coefficient is introduced to analyze the relationship between Attention and Meditation in these four scenarios. The correlation coefficient $r$ can be calculated according to the formula (1).

$$r = \frac{\sum\limits_{i=1}^{n} (Xi - \bar{X})(Yi - \bar{Y})}{\sqrt{\sum\limits_{i=1}^{n} (Xi - \bar{X})^2} \sqrt{\sum\limits_{i=1}^{n} (Yi - \bar{Y})^2}} \tag{1}$$

$Xi$ and $Yi$ present the value of Attention and Meditation EEG from the subject's left prefrontal lobe respectively at $i$ moment, $\bar{X}$ and $\bar{Y}$ present the average value of the Attention and Meditation EEG respectively. The experiment in [9] shows that four correlation coefficients between Attention and Meditation EEG calculated by formula (1) could be identified respectively, as long as an appropriate classifying method is chosen.

Besides the Attention and Meditation of the subject's left prefrontal EEG, the ThinkGear can also detect the subject's blink as well. Hence, both the blink and the correlation coefficient between Attention and Meditation EEG are selected as the features for driving fatigue detection.

## 3   Methodology

Being a lazy learning algorithm, k-NN algorithm has been widely used as an effective classification model. Hence, it is introduced to classify normal and fatigue driving, according to the subject's blink and the correlation coefficient between left prefrontal

Attention and Meditation EEG. In the process of driving fatigue detection, the data of the driver's blink and left prefrontal Attention and Meditation EEG vary in real-time, and then makes up stream data. This causes great challenges in classifying stream data because of its infinite length. Hence, sliding window which just takes the last seen N elements of the stream into account is introduced to maintain similarity queries over stream data.

## 3.1    Feature Extraction

Figure 1 illustrates the conventions that new data elements are coming from the right and the elements at the left are ones already seen. The sliding window covers a time period of $T_S \times n$, which $T_S$ is the sampling period. Each element of sensor data stream has an arrival time, which increments by one at each arrival, with the leftmost element considered to have arrived at time 1. Since the ThinkGear chip produces the Attention and Meditation EEG with 1 Hz frequency. The sample period equals to 1 s. The experiment is carried out respectively when the width of the sliding window is 10, 15, 20...60, and through a lot of experiment proves that the k-NN algorithm has the highest correctness when the length of the sliding window is 53. So n equals to 53.

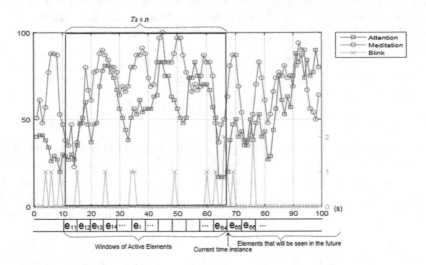

**Fig. 1.** Illustration for the notation and the conventions of sliding window.

For an illustration of this notation, consider the situation presented in Fig. 1. The start time of the sliding window is 11, the current time instant is 11, and the last seen element of the stream data is e64. Each element $ei$ consists of the Blink, Meditation and Attention EEG collected by sensors at time $i$. The input of k-NN algorithm is each sliding window instances in this paper.

## 3.2  K-NN Algorithm for Driving Fatigue Detection

K-NN measures the difference or similarity between instances according to a distance function. Given a test instance x, its k closest neighbors $y1, ..., yk$, are calculated, and a vote is conducted to assign the most common class to x. That is, the class of $x$, denoted by $c(x)$, is determined by the formula (2) [10].

$$c(x) = argmax \sum\nolimits_{n=1}^{k} \delta(c, c(y_i))$$  (2)

Where $c(yi)$ is the class of $yi$, and $\delta$ is a function that $\delta$ (u, v) = 1 if u = v.

Since there are two kinds of features (namely correlation confident $c$, and blink $b$) used for classifying, Euclidean distance defined in formula (3) is selected as the distance function. Among formula (3), $D(x, t)$ is the Euclidean distance, $(cx, bx)$ is a test instance, $(ct, bt)$ is a training instance, and both of them are 2-dimensional real vector.

$$D(x, t) = \sqrt{(c_x - c_t)^2 + (b_x - b_t)^2}$$  (3)

The k-NN algorithm for driving fatigue detection consists of the training and classifying phase. The training phase is as follows:

(A)  Samples the subject's blink, Attention and Meditation EEG in 1 Hz frequency for 53 s when the subject is normally driving, and calculates the correlation coefficient between Attention and Meditation EEG, and labels it as normal drive.
(B)  Samples the subject's blink, Attention and Meditation EEG in 1 Hz frequency for 53 s when the subject is in fatigue drive, calculates the correlation coefficient between Attention and Meditation EEG and the sum of blink, and labels it as fatigue.
(C)  Repeats steps (A) and (B) until enough training samples are produced.

The classifying phase is as follows.

(A)  Constructs sliding window WB [53], WA [53] and WM [53], of which are used to cache the last 53 s of the subject's blink, Attention and Meditation EEG respectively.
(B)  Samples the subject's blink, Attention and Meditation EEG in 1 Hz frequency, and appends them into the tail of WB, WA and WM respectively.
(C)  Judges whether WB, WA and WM are full or not. If they are not full, then goes to (B); otherwise goes to (D).
(D)  Calculates the current correlation coefficient between Attention and Meditation EEG according to formulas (1).
(E)  Judges whether the subject's blink and the current correlation coefficient between Attention and Meditation EEG is fatigue or not according to the formula (2). If the subject in a normal driving state, then it goes to (B); if the subject in a fatigued driving state, then it will issue an alert.

# 4 Implementation

Referencing the Mindwave, a headband integrated with ThinkGear EEG chip, tri-axial accelerometer and gyroscope is developed to collect subject's left pre-frontal EEG, head movement data and blink. Besides, the headband is integrated with Bluetooth module, of which makes it able to wireless send data. Since most smart devices (such as Android smart phone and iPad) are also integrated with the Bluetooth module as well, and they have strong calculation capability. Android smart device integrated with Bluetooth is introduced to receive the left prefrontal EEG, head movement data and blink from the headband, and software running on it is developed based on above technologies to detect driving fatigue and issue alert.

## 4.1 System Architecture

Figure 2 shows the system architecture for driving fatigue detection which mainly includes three parts: headband, Android smart device and Internet. Among them, the headband samples the subject's left prefrontal Attention and Meditation EEG, the resultant acceleration and angular velocity, blink and transfers the data to an Android smart device via Bluetooth. The software running on the Android smart device will calculate the correlation coefficient between the Attention and Meditation EEG and judge whether the subject is fatigue or not by calling the k-NN algorithm, as soon as it receives the subject's blink and left prefrontal Attention and Meditation EEG. The smart device will immediately issue an alert, and call the bus monitor or send a short message to the bus schedule center as long as it detects driving fatigue. Besides, the smart device will automatic play music as soon as it detects the subject's nod with agreement by a threshold algorithm.

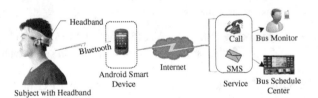

**Fig. 2.** The system architecture for detecting driving fatigue.

## 4.2 Hardware Design

ThinkGear chip is developed by Neurosky, it integrates the functions of the brain wave signal acquisition, filtering, amplification, A/D conversion, data processing and analysis into an ASIC chip. By supporting the dry electrode, it can collect the weak signal of the brain waves, and identify the different states such as the focus, blink, relax and so on.

The sensor board which measures 25 mm × 55 mm × 7 mm (width × length × thick-ness) and is suitable for making a headband. It consists of a high-performance, low-powered microcontroller, and a class 2 Bluetooth module. The Bluetooth module has a range of 10 m, a default transmission rate of 115 k baud. The microcontroller reads the data from the accelerometer, gyroscope and ThinkGear chip. After getting the left prefrontal EEG and the resultant acceleration and angular velocity, it transmits them to the mobile smart device via Bluetooth. The tri-axial accelerometer has a range of ±16 g. The tri-axial gyroscope has a full-scale range of ±2000°/s.

## 4.3   Software Design

Figure 3 shows the flow chart of the program running on the smart device. According to the instance of a Sliding Window of the input stream, the correlation coefficient of the instance is calculated according to the formula (1), and the similarity between the instance and training sample in the training dataset is calculated by calling the k-NN algorithm so as to judge whether it is driving fatigue or not. After detecting driving fatigue, the smart device will immediately issue an alert which will continue five seconds. Meanwhile, the smart device will ask the subject whether he wants to play music or not. The smart device will automatically play music to awake the subject when it detects the subject's nod with agreement, of which means the resultant acceleration $\alpha$ is greater than the threshold $\alpha T$, and the deflection angle $\theta$ is less than the threshold $\theta T$.

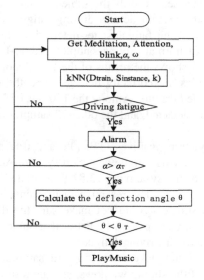

**Fig. 3.** Flow chart of the program running on Android.

## 5   Experimental and Analysis

Although driving fatigues are caused by many reasons such as the geographical context, due to the serious danger of driving fatigue the driving simulation platform (SCANeR Studio) is selected to do the experiment. SCANeR Studio not only provides a real-time driving environment, but also keeps the subject safe. In addition to the SCANeR Studio components, a Samsung Galaxy Note 10.1, which integrates with 3G and Bluetooth and its operating system is Android 4.1, is introduced to run the software to do the experiment.

## 5.1   Experiment and Data Analysis

Seventeen subjects who are aged from 22 to 43, and each of who has at least 1 year driving experience are selected to put on a headband and do one hour experiments to get training samples from SCANeR studio platform after lunch at 12:00. In the same driving environment all subjects will continue to drive for half an hour. During the experiment, an observer sitting at the front passenger seat observes the driving state of the subject and records the state on the driving form while the subject drives. After driving, the subjects should confirm their state of fatigue recorded on the driving form. There are only six subjects who appeared to have fatigue states while driving. Hence, ten sets of normal driving samples and ten sets of fatigued driving samples are selected from those 6 subjects as training samples.

In order to test the driving fatigue detection system, 12 males and 6 females who are aged from 18 to 43, and have at least one year driving experience are selected to drive at Visual SCAN platform after lunch for half an hour. During the test, an observer sitting at the front passenger seat records the subject's state of driving fatigue on the driving form as long as the system detects driving fatigue and issues an alert. The subjects should then confirm their fatigue states detected by the software after driving. In total there are 81 sets of normal driving samples and 170 sets of fatigued driving samples in the test. Table 1 shows the results of the test. Among the 81 sets of normal driving samples, 62 samples are correctly detected, and the other 19 samples were wrongly classified as fatigued driving. Among the 170 sets of fatigued driving samples, 148 samples were correctly detected, and the other 22 samples are wrongly classified as normal driving.

Sensitivity, specificity, true positives (TP) rate and true negatives (TN) rate are introduced to evaluate the driving fatigue detection system. According to Table 1, the sensitivity and specificity of the system are 73.81 % and 88.62 % and the TP rate and TN rate are 76.5 % and 87.1 %. The reason why the sensitivity is only 73.81 % is possibility because some subjects could not make sure the detected state of driving fatigue after their driving. It perhaps will be better that subjects make sure their state soon as the system detects their driving fatigue.

During the test, the system takes only 53 s to sample Attention and Meditation EEG so as to construct the sliding windows, and the response delay time to detect driving fatigue is less than 0.1 ms (millisecond) once the Samsung Galaxy Note

**Table 1.**  Test results

| Detecting results | Total | Correct | Wrong |
|---|---|---|---|
| Normal driving | 81 | 62 | 19 |
| Fatigued driving | 170 | 148 | 22 |

receives the Attention and Meditation EEG data. Meanwhile, the software is also installed on a Moto 525 (a smart phone) whose operating system is Android 2.1, and the response delay time to detect driving fatigue is also less than 0.1 ms. It proves that the system has portable and real-time advantages.

Each of the detected driving fatigue not only triggers an alert in 5 s, but also makes a call to monitor, or sends an emergent message with GPS location to bus schedule center immediately, so as to provide a fast and accurate intervention.

## 5.2  Discussion

Except k-NN algorithm, C4.5, Multilayer Perception (MLP) and Naive Bayes algorithms are selected to process data, so as to compare and analyze their performance on driving fatigue detection. Under the optimal parameters, the accuracy, TN Rate, Sensitivity and Specificity of the four algorithms are summarized which is shown in the Fig. 4. The width of the sliding window is set suitable for each algorithm, and four algorithm models all meet the requirements of accuracy.

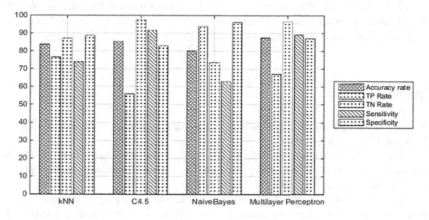

**Fig. 4.** Comparison of four algorithm.

Among the four algorithms, k-NN algorithm not only has a high accuracy, but also it is good at other indicators. Although Sensitivity is relatively low (namely 73.8 %). In the C4.5 decision tree model, TP Rate is low (namely 55.8 %). It shows that the model is biased in favor of one side of the classified data to fatigue driving, and only half of the normal data are correctly classified into the normal category. The reason that the accuracy can reach 85.3 % is that almost all of the fatigue data are correctly classified. Therefore, its Specificity is the lowest in four models. The shortcoming makes it not suitable for application. In the Naive Bayes model, the Sensitivity is 62.8 %, and the TN Rate is 73.5 %. It can be seen that the Naive Bayes model classifies a quarter of fatigue driving to the normal driving. As a result, the Naive Bayes model has the lowest accuracy (namely 80.0 %). MLP model is a little better than the C4.5 decision tree model, because it has higher accuracy. However, its TP Rate is 67.1 %, and the model is also biased in favor of one side of the classified data to fatigue driving.

According to the above comparison, k-NN algorithm is the most one balanced between performance and accuracy, so it is selected to develop the software on Android for driving fatigue detection.

# 6  Conclusion

According to portable and real-time problems for its practical application of EEG based driving fatigue detection, a headband integrated with Thinkgear EEG chip, tri-axial accelerometer, gyroscope and Bluetooth is developed to collect the subject's left prefrontal Attention, Meditation EEG, blink and head movement data. And a new method for detecting driving fatigue is proposed based on k-NN, the correlation coefficient of subject's Attention and Meditation and blink. Meanwhile, a driving fatigue detection system based on the above technologies is implemented on an Android device. The experiment shows that use the correlation coefficient of left prefrontal's Attention and Meditation and blink can pro-vide a relatively accurate method to detect driving fatigue. And it's also proves it has noninvasive and real-time advantages, as well as its sensitivity and specificity are 73.8 % and 88.6 % respectively. In the future, new algorithms will be studied in order to improve the accuracy of system detection.

# References

1. Wu, Y., Li, W., Shi, G., et al.: Survey on fatigue driving detection method research. Chin. J. Ergon. (2003). (in Chinese)
2. Khushaba, R.N., Kodagoda, S., Lal, S., Dissanayake, G., Khushaba, R.N., et al.: Driver drowsiness classification using fuzzy wavelet-packet-based feature-extraction algorithm. IEEE Trans. Biomed. Eng. **58**(1), 121–131 (2011)
3. Lin, C.T., Ko, L.W., Chung, I.F., Huang, T.Y., Chen, Y.C., Jung, T.P., et al.: Adaptive EEG-based alertness estimation system by using ICA-based fuzzy neural networks. IEEE Trans. Circuits Syst. I Regul. Pap. **53**(11), 2469–2476 (2010)
4. Schleicher, R., Galley, N., Briest, S., Galley, L.: Blinks and saccades as indicators of fatigue in sleepiness warnings: looking tired? Ergonomics **51**(7), 982–1010 (2008)
5. Fu, J.W., Li, M., Lu, B.L.: Detecting drowsiness in driving simulation based on EEG. In: Mahr, B., Huanye, S. (eds.) Autonomous Systems – Self-Organization, Management, and Control, pp. 21–28. Springer, Netherlands (2008)
6. Fogarty, C., Stern, J.A.: Eye movements and blinks: their relationship to higher cognitive processes. Int. J. Psychophysiol. Off. J. Int. Organ. Psychophysiol. **8**(1), 35–42 (1989)
7. Holmes, T, Zanker, J.: Eye on the prize: using overt visual attention to drive fitness for interactive evolutionary computation. In: Genetic and Evolutionary Computation Conference, pp. 1531–1538 (2008)
8. American Electroencephalographic Society: Guideline thirteen: guidelines for standard electrode position nomenclature. J. Clin. Neurophysiol. **11**(1), 111–113 (1994). Official Publication of the American Electroencephalographic Society

9. He, J., Hu, C., Li, Y.: An autonomous fall detection and alerting system based on mobile and ubiquitous computing. In: 10th International Conference on Ubiquitous Intelligence & Computing, pp. 539–543 (2013)
10. Erdogan, S.Z., Bilgin, T.T.: A data mining approach for fall detection by using k-nearest neighbour algorithm on wireless sensor network data. IET Commun. 6(18), 3281–3287 (2012)

# Detection of $SNr$ Recordings Basing upon Spike Shape Classes and Signal's Background

Konrad A. Ciecierski[1(✉)] and Tomasz Mandat[2,3]

[1] Institute of Computer Science, Warsaw University of Technology,
00-655 Warsaw, Poland
K.Ciecierski@ii.pw.edu.pl
[2] Department of Neurosurgery, M. Sklodowska-Curie Memorial Oncology Center,
Warsaw, Poland
tomaszmandat@yahoo.com
[3] Department of Neurosurgery, Institute of Psychiatry and Neurology in Warsaw,
Warsaw, Poland

**Abstract.** During deep brain stimulation (DBS) surgery for Parkinson disease, the target is the subthalamic nucleus ($STN$). $STN$ is small, ($9 \times 7 \times 4$ mm) and typically localized by a series of parallel microelectrodes. As those electrodes are in steps advanced towards and through the $STN$, they record the neurobiological activity of the surrounding tissues. The electrodes are advanced until they pass through the $STN$ and/or they reach the Substantia Nigra pars reticulata ($SNr$). There is no necessity of going further as the $SNr$ lies ventral to the $STN$. There are good classification methods for detection weather given recording comes from the $STN$ or not, they still do sometimes falsely identify $SNr$ recordings as $STN$ ones. This paper focuses on method devised for $SNr$ detection, specifically on detection if given recording bears characteristics typical for $SNr$. Presented method relies on spike sorting and assessing characteristics of the obtained spike shape classes together with the enhanced analysis of the signal's background computed by the $STN$ classification methods described in [8–12].

**Keywords:** SNr · DBS · STN · Spike sorting · Spike shape · Signal power

## 1 Introduction

During deep brain stimulation (DBS) surgery for Parkinsons disease, the anatomical target is a small ($9 \times 7 \times 4$ mm) deeply located structure called the Subthalamic Nucleus (STN). It is morphologically similar to the surrounding tissue and as such, not easy to visualize in CT or MRI. The goal of the surgery is precise placement of a permanent stimulating electrode within $STN$. Precision is very important as incorrect by single millimeters placement of the stimulating electrode may lead to various adverse effects such as paraesthesia: muscle contractions, double vision or potentially serious mood disturbances [4,13–15].

© Springer International Publishing AG 2016
G.A. Ascoli et al. (Eds.): BIH 2016, LNAI 9919, pp. 336–345, 2016.
DOI: 10.1007/978-3-319-47103-7_33

To obtain the exact location of the *STN* nucleus, during surgery the stereo-tactic navigation is used. A set of 3 to 5 parallel microelectrodes is inserted into the brain and advanced towards the expected location of the nucleus.

Typically, from a depth of 10 mm above the estimated *STN*, the electrodes are advanced with 1 mm steps. At each step, the activity of the neural tissue surrounding the leads of the electrodes is recorded. The electrodes are advanced in such steps until the ventral *STN* border has been passed and eventually the Substantia Nigra pars reticulata (SNr) is reached. The first five of those steps go through the white matter above the *STN* and typically have low background noise and little spike activity. They are therefore used as negative baseline, referencing point in normalization of background based attributes described in Sect. 3.2.

The *SNr* being ventral to the *STN* is separated from it by structure called Transient Zone (TZ) [3, 4]. While in some patients this structure can be clearly observed in the passage of the electrodes, in other cases the *STN* and *SNr* seems to be virtually adjacent. Distinction between those two structures is important as the *STN* is the target of the stimulation.

The permanent stimulating electrode has four leads on its length. Those leads are separated from each other by 0.5 mm starting from the tip of the electrode. From this, for best coverage of the *STN*, the tip of the stimulating electrode should be at the ventral border of the *STN* – part of the *STN* being the closest to the *SNr*.

The *STN* has some quite distinct physiological properties and so recording coming from it with good certainty can be identified [4,8 12]. Still, the computer based methods in some cases can erroneously classify recordings from *SNr* as those from *STN* [11,12].

It is therefore useful to have an additional classification method targeted at finding recordings registered within *SNr*.

Data presented in this paper, has been obtained from 154 DBS surgeries. As the *SNr* is located ventral to the *STN*, from each pass of the set of micro-electrodes, only recordings from depths ventral to the found dorsal *STN* border were used. That gave a set of 9114 recordings, each typically 10 s long.

## 2     Spike Detection and Shape Classes

What is immediately noticeable when one looks at recording made within the *SNr* (Fig. 1(a)) is the characteristic spiking activity and relatively low – when comparing to *STN* (Fig. 1(b)) – level of background activity. It is therefore natural to look closely at spiking activity when discriminating *SNr* recordings.

### 2.1     Spike Detection

The spike amplitude based detection method described in [11,12] relies on its amplitude crossing the $4\,\sigma_e$ based threshold. In this paper, this threshold has been set to slightly lower value i.e. $3\,\sigma$. This threshold, while being low enough for

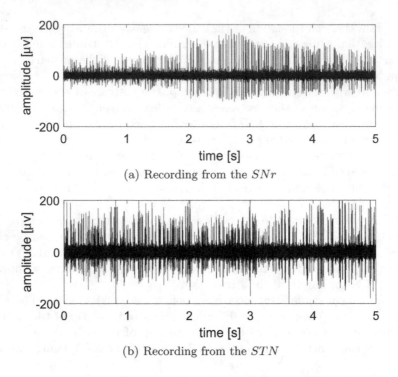

(a) Recording from the $SNr$

(b) Recording from the $STN$

**Fig. 1.** Comparison of recordings from $STN$ and $SNr$

spikes from $STN$ ($n = 2,640,112; \mu = 48.44\,\mu v; \sigma = 28.09\,\mu v$) is of course easily crossed by $SNr$ high amplitude spiking activity ($n = 155,368; \mu = 57.19\,\mu v; \sigma = 30.27\,\mu v$). The $\sigma_e$ is here estimated in the same way as in [5,11,12] as

$$\sigma_e = \frac{1}{0.6745}\, median(|x_1|, \ldots, |x_n|) \tag{1}$$

The spike with positive polarity with its maximal amplitude at $t_0$ above $4\,\sigma_e$ is assumed to last in time interval from $t_0 - 0.5$ ms to $t_0 + 1.1$ ms. The spike with negative polarity with its minimal amplitude at $t_0$ below $-4\,\sigma_e$ is also assumed to last in time interval from $t_0 - 0.5$ ms to $t_0 + 1.1$ ms.

To reflect much higher amplitudes of the $SNr$ spikes, constraints given in [11, 12] regarding spike amplitude in various its phases have had to be modified. In case of spikes with positive polarity the following constraints have also to be met:

$$\forall(t_0 - 0.5\text{ ms} < t < t_0) \cup (t_0 < t < t_0 + 1.1\text{ ms}) \quad f(t) < f(t_0)$$

$$\forall(t_0 - 0.5\text{ ms} < t < t_0 + 1.1\text{ ms}) \quad f(t) >= -20\,\sigma$$

$$\forall(t_0 - 0.5\text{ ms} < t < t_0 - 0.4\text{ ms}) \cup (t_0 + 0.4\text{ ms} < t < t_0 + 1.1\text{ ms}) \quad f(t) <= 8\,\sigma$$

$$\forall(t_0 - 0.5\text{ ms} < t < t_0 - 0.4\text{ ms}) \cup (t_0 + 1.0\text{ ms} < t < t_0 + 1.1\text{ ms}) \quad f(t) >= -8\,\sigma$$

For spikes with negative polarity a appropriately modified set of above restrictions is used.

## 2.2    Sorting Spikes into Shape Classes

After spikes have all been detected they are sorted into shape classes [6]. The most obvious discrimination is into spikes with positive and negative polarity. Spikes with positive polarity have their extremal amplitude positive, those with negative – otherwise.

Later each subset is further divided into subclasses. As our data is sampled with 24 kHz the single spike ranging from $t_0 - 0.5$ ms to $t_0 + 1.1$ ms takes 39 samples with its top amplitude at $13^{th}$ sample.

Assuming that in given recording $k$ spikes were found, they together form an $k \times 39$ array of aligned spike waveforms.

Clustering is then made using K-means technique. Shape classes are not always clearly distinguishable, sometimes decision if a given class should be further split into subclasses can be a very subjective one. Because of that, to obtain the optimal number of clusters that accertain sufficient difference between resulting classes of spike shapes, the decision must be based on objective measure – silhouette value. Selected is this clustering, which has the biggest silhouette value and for which this value is at least 0.4. It is therefore possible, that when all silhouette values were low, no clusters would be detected. This way candidates for shape classes are calculated.

In subsequent steps each shape class candidate is again clustered using waveform samples at which its average has minimum and maximum values. Again the criterion for clustering selection is silhouette based. This time requirement is for more pronounced clusters so the minimum silhouette value is 0.6. This step allows for discrimination between neurons that are similar morphologically but differently distanced from the electrode. Spike from more distant neuron will be detected with lower amplitude. [4,6,7]. Example of such discrimination can be seen between classes A and D. While the width of spikes are similar in both classes, the amplitudes differ between classes and have low variance within each of those classes.

Clusters with less than 25 spikes are discarded.

Finally for each shape class, the $\sigma$ for its maximal absolute value is calculated and all its spikes for whom maximal absolute value does not fit within $<\mu - 3\sigma; \mu + 3\sigma>$ interval are from it removed.

For recording shown on Fig. 1(a) several shape classes have been found, four of them are shown Fig. 2.

## 2.3    Importance of Spike Sorting

For each spike shape class there can be calculated many various characteristic features [6]. They may rely on spike occurrence, its average proportions and amplitude. Those features are described in more detail in the Sect. 3.1. In Table 1 are shown certain features calculated for classes shown on Fig. 2.

It is evident that there are differences between features computed for different shape classes. Some of those classes might be characteristic for the *SNr* while some others might not. It is known that given cell has constant spike

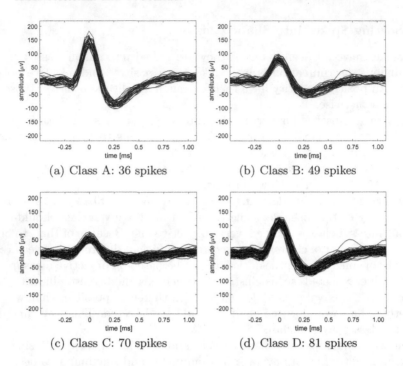

(a) Class A: 36 spikes            (b) Class B: 49 spikes

(c) Class C: 70 spikes            (d) Class D: 81 spikes

**Fig. 2.** Shape classes found in $SNr$ recording shown on Fig. 1(a)

**Table 1.** Example features for spike shape classes

| Class | Figure | Spikes | Maximal amplitude | dy/dx | Burst index | Pause index | Pause ratio |
|-------|--------|--------|-------------------|-------|-------------|-------------|-------------|
| Class A | 2(a) | 36 | 143 | 38 | 0.25 | 0.30 | 1.79 |
| Class B | 2(b) | 49 | 78 | 18 | 0.20 | 0.33 | 5.80 |
| Class C | 2(c) | 70 | 52 | 10 | 0.17 | 0.64 | 4.00 |
| Class D | 2(d) | 81 | 110 | 25 | 0.31 | 0.25 | 2.24 |

shape – it derives from it's morphology [3,4]. Considering all spike shape classes we are looking at separate cells in the vicinity of the electrode, some of those cells might be $SNr$ specific, others might not. If one were to consider all spikes form given recording together those values would become averaged and the information about activities of separate cells/cell types would be lost.

Treating each spike shape class separately allows one to make much finer classifications. Instead of classifying whole recordings, one might classify its sub features.

# 3    Feature Extraction

Hypothesis assumed in this paper is that specific activity of some cell types might be useful in detection whether given recording has been made within the *SNr*. For this purpose spikes are sorted into shape classes and spike based features are calculated for those classes not for whole recordings.

In this way for given recording one might receive five, six or even more shape classes. Some of them might then be labeled as *SNr* characteristic while other as generic ones. Later, proportion of spike shape classes classified for given recording as *SNr* might give medical doctors additional information. In search for *SNr* recordings, beside the spike based attributes, also some background based attributes are used. Those attributes are taken and derived from methods devised for *STN* detection [11,12].

In particular, the information if given recording has been previously classified as recorded in the *STN* is certainly useful. In such case – assuming it is a TP case – this recording is of course not a *SNr* one. Methods for *STN* detection described in those papers have sensitivity 0.94 and specificity 0.97 and have already been successfully applied during many neurosurgical operations.

## 3.1    Spike Based Features

Let's define average shape for a shape class as average of waveforms of its members. The following features [6,8–12] are calculated for each spike shape class:

- Average number of spikes per second of the recording.
- Maximal absolute amplitude of average shape.
- Distance between maximal and minimal amplitude of average shape divided by time distance between those maximal and minimal occurrences.
- Maximal positive amplitude of average shape divided by absolute maximal negative amplitude of average shape.
- Maximal positive amplitude of average shape divided by SD of recording.
- Absolute maximal negative amplitude of average shape divided by SD of the recording.
- Mean number of spikes in 100 ms wide window. For purpose of this and next attribute, the recording is divided into 100 ms adjacent windows. Windows without spikes of given class are discarded.
- Variance of number of spikes in 100 ms wide window.
- Burst index: proportion of number interspike intervals shorter than 10 ms to number of interspike intervals longer than 10 ms.
- Pause index: proportion of number interspike intervals longer than 50 ms to number of interspike intervals shorter than 50 ms.
- Pause ratio: sum of interspike intervals longer than 50 ms to sum of interspike intervals shorter than 50 ms.
- Number of bursts: number of bursts of spikes. Burst is a series of at leats five spikes with all interspike intervals below 50 ms.
- Mean number of spikes in a burst.
- Median number of spikes in a burst.

### 3.2    Background Based Features

The following features are calculated for each recording, as such they are common for all shape classes from given recording

- Q80: $80^{th}$ percentile of the recordings amplitude, this attribute estimates the amplitude of the background noise present in given recordings [2,11,12].
- RMS: Root mean square of the recording, this attribute estimates the amplitude of the background noise present in given recordings and also spiking activity [2,11,12].
- LFB: power of the signal calculated for frequencies below 500 Hz [1,2,11,12].
- HFB: power of the signal calculated for frequencies between 500 Hz and 3 kHz [1,2,11,12].
- temporal meta attributes for four above background attributes.

Temporal attributes holds biggest so far (counting from dorsal to ventral depths) decline of each attribute between two depths separated by 1000 μm and by 2000 μm. Consequently, there are eight temporal attributes.

### 3.3    Classification Based Feature

- STN: attribute being the result of a classification described in [11,12]. Attribute states if given recording has been classified as recorded within $STN$ or not.

## 4    Classification Results

Prior to classification the spike shapes were manually classified into those characteristic for the $SNr$ and not. There were 771 shape classes identified as $SNr$ characteristic and 27815 shape classes deemed not typical for the $SNr$.

Classifications were then made using Random Forest implementation provided by Weka (www.cs.waikato.ac.nz/ml/weka) and additionally also using the TreeBagger class provided by Matlab (www.mathworks.com/). Verification of classification was made using 10 fold cross validation technique.

First the classification was made using spike based features only and 100 trees. The results were very poor:

$$sensitivity = \frac{245}{245 + 526} \approx 0.318 \; specificity = \frac{27731}{27731+84} \approx 0.997$$

After the inclusion of the background attributes together with the STN attribute the results were better but still not acceptable (Tables 2 and 3):

$$sensitivity = \frac{474}{474 + 297} \approx 0.615 \; specificity = \frac{27728}{27728+87} \approx 0.997$$

At this point one must however look at number of shape classes in each category. There are 36 times as many non $SNr$ shape classes than the $SNr$ ones.

**Table 2.** Cross validation results

|  |  | Human classification | | Total |
|---|---|---|---|---|
|  |  | *SNr* | ¬*SNr* |  |
| Classifier | *SNr* | 245 | 84 | 329 |
|  | ¬*SNr* | 526 | 27731 | 28257 |
|  | Total | 771 | 27815 | 28586 |

**Table 3.** Cross validation results

|  |  | Human classification | | Total |
|---|---|---|---|---|
|  |  | *SNr* | ¬*SNr* |  |
| Classifier | *SNr* | 474 | 87 | 561 |
|  | ¬*SNr* | 297 | 27728 | 28025 |
|  | Total | 771 | 27815 | 28586 |

This mean that the data is highly skewed and that it must be taken into account during the construction of the classifier. When the classifier has been constructed with the cost matrix proper for found skewness (36:1), the obtained results were much better (Table 4):

$$sensitivity = \frac{658}{658 + 113} \approx 0.853 \; specificity = \frac{27519}{27519+296} \approx 0.989$$

Increasing the number of random features in trees from default 5 to 15 allowed for even better results:

$$sensitivity = \frac{677}{677 + 94} \approx 0.878 \; specificity = \frac{27476}{27476+339} \approx 0.988$$

The Matlab's TreeBagger class, when taking into account the skewness of data gave sensitivity = 0.82 and specificity 0.99.

The Matlab's RUSBoosted trees algorithm that is tailored for skewed data gave (Tables 5 and 6)

$$sensitivity = \frac{725}{725 + 46} \approx 0.940 \; specificity = \frac{26686}{26686+1129} \approx 0.959$$

**Table 4.** Cross validation results

|  |  | Human classification | | Total |
|---|---|---|---|---|
|  |  | *SNr* | ¬*SNr* |  |
| Classifier | *SNr* | 658 | 296 | 954 |
|  | ¬*SNr* | 113 | 27519 | 27632 |
|  | Total | 771 | 27815 | 28586 |

**Table 5.** Cross validation results

|            |           | Human classification | | Total |
|------------|-----------|------|--------|-------|
|            |           | $SNr$ | $\neg SNr$ |       |
| Classifier | $SNr$     | 677  | 339    | 1016  |
|            | $\neg SNr$ | 94   | 27476  | 27570 |
|            | Total     | 771  | 27815  | 28586 |

**Table 6.** Cross validation results

|            |           | Human classification | | Total |
|------------|-----------|------|--------|-------|
|            |           | $SNr$ | $\neg SNr$ |       |
| Classifier | $SNr$     | 725  | 1129   | 1854  |
|            | $\neg SNr$ | 46   | 26686  | 26732 |
|            | Total     | 771  | 27815  | 28586 |

## 5   Summary

Attributes based on features taken from spike shape classes alone failed to discriminate those of them that were registered within the $SNr$. When taken together with information calculated from signal's background and information about previously detected $STN$ location results were much improved.

Even better results were obtained when the skewness of the input data has been taken into account during construction of the classifier. Here the obtained sensitivity was over 0.85 with specificity over 0.989. The sensitivity can be improved even further but at cost of lowering specificity, is might seem that sensitivity 0.94 with specificity 0.96 might be ok but one must take into account the skewness of the data and fact that even slight lowering of specificity might dramatically increase amount of FP cases as in case of the Matlab's RUSBoosted solution. Described method will have to be further verified in the clinical practice but results achieved so far are optimistic. On Fig. 3 are shown spikes from the shape classes classified as $SNr$ in the recording shown on Fig. 1(a).

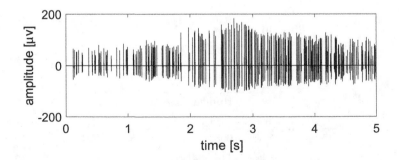

**Fig. 3.** Spikes from $SNr$ shape classes for recording shown on Fig. 1(a)

# References

1. Jensen, A., Cour-Harbo, A.I.: Ripples in Mathematics. Springer, Berlin (2001)
2. Smith, S.W.: Digital Signal Processing. Elsevier, Amsterdam (2003)
3. Nieuwenhuys, R., Huijzen, C., Voogd, J.: The Human Central Nervous System. Springer, Berlin (2008)
4. Israel, Z., Burchiel, K.J.: Microelectrode Recording in Movement Disorder Surgery. Thieme Medical Publishers, Stuttgart (2004)
5. Donoho, D.L.: De-noising by soft-thresholding. IEEE Trans. Inf. Theor. **41**(3), 613–627 (1995)
6. Archer, C., Hochstenbach, M.E., Hoede, C., et al.: Neural spike sorting with spatio-temporal features. In: Proceedings of 63rd European Study Group Mathematics with Industry, Enschede, The Netherlands, pp. 21–45, 28 January–1 February 2008
7. Henze, D.A., Borhegyi, Z., Csicsvari, J., Mamiya, A., Harris, K.D., Buzsk, G.: Intracellular features predicted by extracellular recordings in the hippocampus in vivo. J. Neurophysiol. **84**, 390–400 (2000)
8. Ciecierski, K., Raś, Z.W., Przybyszewski, A.W.: Foundations of recommender system for STN localization during DBS surgery in Parkinson's patients. In: Chen, L., Felfernig, A., Liu, J., Raś, Z.W. (eds.) ISMIS 2012. LNCS, vol. 7661, pp. 234–243. Springer, Heidelberg (2012)
9. Ciecierski, K., Raś, Z.W., Przybyszewski, A.W.: Discrimination of the micro electrode recordings for STN localization during DBS surgery in Parkinson's patients. In: Larsen, H.L., Martin-Bautista, M.J., Vila, M.A., Andreasen, T., Christiansen, H. (eds.) FQAS 2013. LNCS, vol. 8132, pp. 328–339. Springer, Heidelberg (2013)
10. Ciecierski, K.A., Raś, Z.W., Przybyszewski, A.W.: Foundations of automatic system for intrasurgical localization of subthalamic nucleus in Parkinson patients. In: Web Intelligence and Agent Systems, vol. 1, pp. 63–82. IOS Press, Amsterdam (2014)
11. Ciecierski, K.A.: Decision support system for surgical treatment of Parkinsons disease. Ph.D. thesis, Warsaw University of Technology Press (2013)
12. Ciecierski, K.A., Mandat, T., Rola, R., Raś, Z.W., Przybyszewski, A.W.: Computer aided subthalamic nucleus (STN) localization during deep brain stimulation (DBS) surgery in Parkinson's patients. Annales Academiae Medicae Silesiensis **68**(5), 275–283 (2014)
13. Mandat, T., Tykocki, T., Koziara, H., et al.: Subthalamic deep brain stimulation for the treatment of Parkinson disease. Neurologia i neurochirurgia polska **45**(1), 32–36 (2011)
14. Pizzolato, G., Mandat, T.: Deep brain stimulation for movement disorders. In: The Development of Deep Brain Stimulation for Neurological and Psychiatric Disorders: Clinical, Societal and Ethical issues, p. 10 (2012)
15. Novak, P., Przybyszewski, A.W., Barborica, A., Ravin, P., Margolin, L., Pilitsis, J.G.: Localization of the subthalamic nucleus in Parkinson disease using multiunit activity. J. Neurol. Sci. **310**(1), 44–49 (2011)

# Influence of Spatial Learning Perspectives on Navigation Through Virtual Reality Environment

Greeshma Sharma[1], Amritha Abdul Salam[2(✉)], Sushil Chandra[1],
Vijander Singh[3], and Alok Mittal[3]

[1] Bio Medical Engineering Department,
Institute of Nuclear Medicine and Allied Science, New Delhi, Delhi, India
[2] Bio Medical Engineering Department,
Manipal Institute of Technology, Manipal, Karnataka, India
amrithasalam@gmail.com
[3] Netaji Subhas Institute of Technology, New Delhi, Delhi, India

**Abstract.** In navigation with virtual reality, spatial knowledge can be acquired through both route and survey perspective. Our study correlates the influence on spatial knowledge while navigating in a virtual reality environment after gaining information with different spatial perspectives. We measured brain activations while the participants navigated through a complex spatial environment, using the analysis tool of sLORETA. In the experimental condition, the participant watched a simulated video feed of either route perspective (front view) or survey perspective (top view) of the virtual environment. Distance travelled, path efficiency and time efficiency of the participants were measured while they navigated through nine successive landmarks. We obtained significant differences between the brain activation patterns while comparing both conditions. Higher activations in inferior frontal gyrus, parahippocampal gyrus, superior temporal gyrus and insula were observed for the theta band in route perspective when compared to survey perspective. Higher activations in the inferior parietal lobule, angular gyrus and precuneus were observed in survey perspective when compared to route perspective. Results showed higher path efficiency and time efficiency and lower distance travelled to reach the destination in survey perspective when compared to route perspective. The result indicates that survey perspective is better for navigation in a far spaced virtual reality environment.

**Keywords:** Spatial perspective · Navigation · Virtual reality · sLORETA · EEG

## 1 Introduction

Spatial cognition is a critical component for planning, spatial configuration, and orientation while navigating in unfamiliar locations. We rely on a multitude of spatial information such as landmarks, relative location information, route distance estimation, depth information etc. during navigation. Exploring environment through different perspectives either route or survey imparts different types of spatial information. Route

© Springer International Publishing AG 2016
G.A. Ascoli et al. (Eds.): BIH 2016, LNAI 9919, pp. 346–354, 2016.
DOI: 10.1007/978-3-319-47103-7_34

perspective characterizes a within the environment viewpoint whereas the survey perspective reflects a bird's eye viewpoint. These perspectives build a topographic mental representation of the environment that provides the spatial knowledge required to reach the destination. The spatial judgment is influenced by the spatial knowledge acquired through different perspectives. Accuracy and precision of spatial judgment depend on the spatial cognition skills of the individual. Accurate spatial judgment is critical for soldiers and rescue operators who constantly undertake missions in unfamiliar terrains after acquiring the spatial overview of the region by studying a map. Seminal research (Brunyé et al. [11]) examining the effect of spatial learning perspectives while navigating through virtual urban environment demonstrated that route perspective supported a restricted range of local navigation whereas the survey perspective supported far-space navigation. Further, survey perspective also supports navigation through unexpected detours.

Behavioral analysis study of human spatial cognition [1, 2] gave the evidence for two types of spatial information, route based knowledge and survey based knowledge. Differences in spatial perspective may result in different behavioral consequences. Research by [3] demonstrated that map learners are superior for judgments of relative location and location of straight line distances among objects whereas navigation learners are superior for orienting oneself with unseen objects and estimating route distances. A neuroimaging study [4] on spatial mental imagery after route and survey learning showed right hippocampus activation for both route and survey imagery, and bilateral activation of parahippocampal gyrus for route imagery alone. Another study analyzed the neural mechanism of route and survey knowledge encoded in the brain. Their results suggested that the differences in brain activation in different perspectives are associated with differences in memory performance for the two types of spatial information.

Virtual navigation elicits a strong sense of presence while navigating in virtual environments [5]. As [6] remarked: "Presence in a virtual environment necessitates a belief that the participant no longer inhabits the physical space but now occupies the computer generated virtual environment as a 'place'". A recent study measured brain activations due to a sense of presence in a virtual environment [7] using sLORETA. They found higher activation of the Insula for alpha and theta bands while navigating, when comparing a common desktop screen and a high-resolution power wall screen. The sense of presence and spatial perspectives are factors that affect spatial cognition.

Several studies have been made combining virtual reality with EEG to measure the spatial cognition experienced by subjects while navigating through the virtual environment. For example, a study on brain oscillatory activity during spatial navigation demonstrated theta and gamma activity link with medial temporal and parietal regions [8]. Their results suggest that theta activity on the medial temporal parietal source is positively correlated with more efficient navigation. Another study using a VR town navigation task showed increased theta power during periods of navigation was localized to temporal and parietal regions using a single current dipole model [9]. A recent study aimed to localize current sources of event related potential associated with spatial updating specifically using sLORETA [10]. Their result indicated activation of brain regions in the test phase that are associated with place and landmark recognition (entorhinal cortex/hippocampus, parahippocampal and retrosplenial cortices, fusiform, and lingual gyri), detecting self motion (posterior cingulate and posterior insular cortices), motor planning (superior frontal gyrus, including the medial frontal cortex) and regions that process spatial attention (inferior parietal lobule).

In our study, we explored the differences in brain activity after being exposed to survey and route perspective. Since learning from different perspectives exhibits different behavioral features, we compared the pattern activation in both the groups. We also investigated the path efficiency, time efficiency and distance traveled by both groups while navigating through the virtual environment based on either route or survey perspective. We expect differences in brain activations in areas related to perspective learning and a sense of presence during navigation in virtual reality. Our hypothesis is that survey and route perspective would cause differences in brain activations. We are specifically interested in the efficiency of navigation in an urban virtual environment while navigating with different perspective information.

## 2    Materials and Methods

### 2.1    Subjects

For the study, 20 undergraduate students (12 males and 8 females, age range 20–25 years) were recruited. The participants were divided into two groups of 10 subjects each. The first group learned the virtual reality environment in route perspective while the second group learned the virtual reality environment in survey perspectives. All the participants had no history of neurological diseases. Participants were informed about the recording procedure and virtual navigation environment. A signed informed consent was obtained from each participant before the onset of the navigation task. Gender was equally represented in both groups. All the participants were familiar with video game experiences.

### 2.2    Materials

#### 2.2.1    Virtual Environment

A large-scale virtual reality environment similar to a previous research work [11] was created using the Unity game engine (Unity 5.3.1 by Unity Technologies), displayed on a 20″ widescreen LCD display. The overall environment measured approximately 628,000 square feet with several landmarks. Two videos were designed to present the route perspective and survey perspective respectively. The route perspective shows a forward view of traveling through the environment (See Fig. 1A). The view starts with entrance through the bank and continuing straight passing through the graveyard and turning right immediately after the record store reaching the Hotel. A left turn from the hotel leads to the market place followed by a left circular turn heading towards Hospital and Police Station. Following landmarks are encountered during the subsequent section of the stimulated journey: University, Library, Radio station, Construction Site, Theatre, Compound, City Hall, Courtyard Mosque, Mountain Pass. The journey ends at the Mountain Pass. Survey perspective (See Fig. 1B) depicts a top view of the landmarks from a bird's eye viewpoint following the same route as described above.

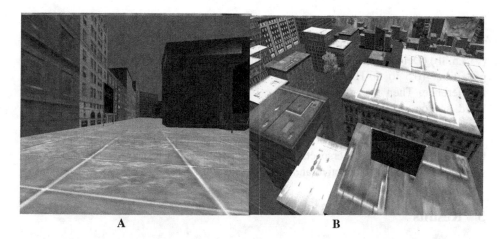

**Fig. 1.** The route perspective video 1 (A) and the survey perspective video 1 (B)

### 2.2.2 Tasks and Measures

Each subject participated in 9 successive trials with at least two possible pathways to consider in each trial. The first trial begins at the bank and ends at the city hall. The second trial starts from city hall and ends at the hotel and then proceeds to construction site, hospital, mosque, radio station, police station, record store, and theatre. Proximal and distal landmarks were included in the trials to evaluate the participant's spatial cognition. Prior to the perspective based learning from videos the participants study a map view showing all the labeled landmarks with approximate locations. For maximum efficiency, the participant should choose the optimal path to increase both path and time efficiency. The unity software measures position in xy coordinates and automatically output these xy coordinates into a text file. The software calculates path efficiency, time efficiency and distance travelled to reach each landmark automatically. Path efficiency is the ratio of the optimal path length to the actual path length travelled by the participants between starting point and destination. If the path efficiency is high then the spatial knowledge gathered from a particular perspective is also high. Time efficiency is the ratio of the optimal time period required to reach the destination to the actual time taken by the participants. Distance travelled by the participants during each trial is also measured.

### 2.2.3 Method

When participants arrived in the lab they were given a learning session in which they learn the locations and pathways to reach each landmark. This is followed by a video viewing session in which the participant view either a route perspective video or survey perspective video depicted at 1920 * 1080 resolution. All videos are of 1 min 20 s duration. After viewing the video the participants are introduced into the virtual reality environment. During the successive trials, the participant views their objective, which appears on the screen for 2 s. The Participants then navigates through the environment until the destined landmark is reached.

## 2.3  Data Analysis

The EEG signals were preprocessed and artifacts were removed using EEGLAB (v13.5.4b) (Delorme and Makeig, 2004). Initially, EEG signals were filtered using band pass filter (0.5 to 60 Hz) followed by notch filtering to remove 50 Hz power line interference. Then the artifacts such eye blinks, muscle artifacts are removed using blind source separation technique. For analysis of activations in brain areas, the standardized low-resolution electromagnetic tomography (sLORETA) tool is used [12–14]. The pair wise t-test is used to analyze the brain areas activated while navigating through different spatial perspectives. Moreover, the same test was used to compare survey versus route perspective and route versus survey perspective for two groups.

## 3  Results

The built in programs in the software compute the indices of navigation measures such as path efficiency, time efficiency and distance travelled. For analysis we compared the indices with SPSS using paired sample t-test for each trial. We tested path efficiency, time efficiency and distance travelled for both video conditions. T-test comparison of path efficiency depicted significant differences in Trial 1 $t(9) = 7.616$, $p < 0.05$ and Trial 5 $t(9) = 3.456$, $p < 0.01$. Time efficiency show significant difference in Trial 8 t $(9) = 3.8$, $p < 0.05$. Survey perspective showed numerically higher performance when compared to route perspective. For distance travelled there is a significant difference in Trial 5 $t(9) = 4.05$, $p < 0.05$. Path efficiency and time efficiency of survey perspective subjects were high. Distance travelled by survey perspective group was lower when compared to route perspective group. Comparison between survey and route perspective using voxel-wise t-test revealed significant differences in theta band (4–7 Hz), for $p < 0.05$. There were significant differences in Para hippocampal gyrus of limbic lobe and insula of sub lobar in Theta band, $p < 0.01$ (Fig. 2).

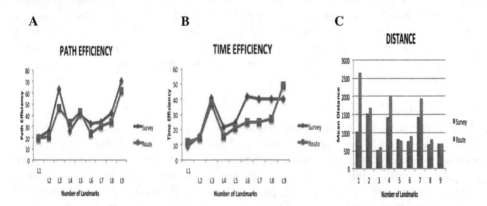

**Fig. 2.** Mean Path Efficiency (A), Mean Time Efficiency (B), and Distance (C) for all navigation trials in survey and route perspective.

# 4  Discussion

The comparison between the route versus survey navigation condition showed significant differences in frontal and temporal areas and in parahippocampal gyrus. We have found significant differences in the parahippocampal gyrus of limbic lobe and insula of sub lobar in the Theta band (See Table 1). When London taxi drivers recalled familiar routes, there was greater activation of the right hippocampus, bilateral parahippocampal cortex, and bilateral precuneus [15]. The activation of the parahippocampal gyrus is related to memory encoding and retrieval [16]. The activation of parahipocampal gyrus is crucial for navigation and spatial mapping [17]. The parahippocampal gyrus is active in the encoding of an environment when salient landmarks were present but not when landmarks were lacking [18]. The activations in the frontal areas, the subcallosal gyrus is related to the parahippocampal activation, and both areas work together in the periarcheocortex; while the BA47 of the inferior frontal gyrus has been implicated in the processing of syntax in oral, sign and musical languages [19]. The Insula is related to emotion and regulation of the body's homeostasis, which includes among other functions self-awareness or the sense of agency and body ownership [20]. A previous study has reported a parametric increase in the right insula activations while comparing the three experimental conditions: photographs, video, and free navigation through a virtual environment [7]. Activation in the superior temporal gyrus is related to the perception of emotions [21]. According to the literature the topographic representation built from route learning and survey learning exhibit different or similar behavioral consequences [3, 22, 23] (Fig. 3).

**Table 1.** Comparison of route versus survey perspective

| Group | Brain area | Band | Hemisphere | p |
|---|---|---|---|---|
| RS | Frontal lobe, Inferior frontal gyrus (BA 47) | Theta | Right | <0.05 |
| RS | Sub lobar, Extra Nuclear, Insula (BA 13) | Theta | Right | <0.05 |
| RS | Frontal lobe, subcallosal gyrus (BA 34) | Theta | Right | <0.05 |
| RS | Limbic Lobe, Parahippocampal gyrus, (BA 34) | Theta | Right | <0.05 |
| RS | Temporal lobe, Superior temporal gyrus, (BA 38) | Theta | Right | >0.1 |
| RS | Limbic lobe, Uncus (BA 20) | Theta | Right | >0.1 |
| RS | Limbic lobe, Parahippocampal gyrus (BA 36) | Theta | Right | >0.1 |

A                           B

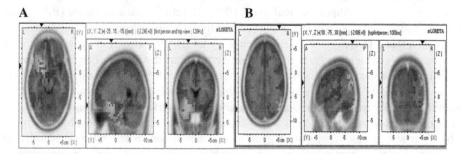

**Fig. 3.** (A) Result of route perspective versus survey perspective and (B) survey perspective versus route perspective condition for the navigation condition for theta band.

**Table 2.** Comparison of survey versus route perspective

| Group | Brain area | Band | Hemisphere | p |
|-------|------------|------|------------|---|
| TF | Temporal lobe, Angular gyrus (BA 39) | Theta | Right | <0.05 |
| TF | Parietal lobe, Angular gyrus, (BA 39) | Theta | Right | <0.05 |
| TF | Temporal lobe, superior temporal gyrus (BA 39) | Theta | Right | <0.05 |
| TF | Parietal lobe, Supramarginal gyrus, (BA 40) | Theta | Right | <0.05 |
| TF | Parietal lobe, Inferior parietal lobule, (BA 40) | Theta | Right | <0.1 |
| TF | Parietal lobe, Precuneus, (BA 19) | Theta | Right | <0.1 |
| TF | Frontal lobe, Inferior Frontal gyrus, (BA 47) | Theta | Right | >0.1 |
| TF | Sub-lobar, Extra Nuclear, (BA 13) | Theta | Right | >0.1 |
| TF | Frontal lobe, Middle frontal gyrus, (BA 9) | Alpha | Right | <0.1 |
| TF | Frontal lobe, Middle frontal gyrus, (BA 46) | Alpha | Right | <0.1 |
| TF | Frontal lobe, Superior frontal gyrus, (BA 9) | Alpha | Right | <0.1 |
| TF | Parietal lobe, Inferior parietal lobule, (BA 39) | Alpha | Right | >0.1 |

The comparison between the survey versus route perspective showed a tendency of significance for theta band in the right temporal and parietal lobe (See Table 2). We have found activations in the inferior parietal lobules, precuneus, and the angular gyrus. The inferior parietal lobule has been involved in the interpretation of sensory information [21], which is processed by the subject during navigation. The precuneus has been widely related to presence and navigation, being involved in directing attention in space [24]. The angular gyrus is related to the sense of self-awareness and the developing of out-of-body experiences [25]. A previous study reveals that the activation of a parietofrontal network composed of the intraparietal sulcus, the superior frontal sulcus, the middle frontal gyrus, and the pre-supplementary motor area (among other areas) were observed in common for both mental navigation and mental map topographic representations and is likely to reflect the spatial mental imagery components of the tasks [4].

There was a higher activation for route encoding in parahippocampal gyrus (BA 34 and BA 36), superior temporal gyrus (BA 38), subcallosal gyrus (BA 34), inferior frontal gyrus (BA 47) and Insula (BA 13). There was greater activation in survey encoding in Angular gyrus (BA 39), in the temporal and parietal area, Superior temporal gyrus (BA 39), Supramarginal gyrus (BA 40), inferior parietal lobule (BA 40 and BA 39) and Precuneus (BA 19). Significant activity is also observed at middle frontal gyrus (BA 9 and BA 46) and superior frontal gyrus (BA 9). This is in agreement with a previous study which suggests that, the properties that distinguish between the route and survey perspectives are sense of immersion and the form of updating involved i.e. route perspectives facilitate a sense of immersion relative to survey perspectives; to learn the spatial layout from a route perspective, the observer must continuously update changes in the local environment based on movements through and within the space [26]. A previous study [4] also suggested that activation in the bilateral entorhinal/parahippocampal cortex is observed when subjects mentally explore an environment built from a route perspective, while these regions were not involved when the environment had been learned in a survey mode. Activation of Insula is related to a greater sense of presence while navigating in a virtual environment [7].

Survey learning perspective group showed higher path efficiency and time efficiency in most of the trials. Previous research indicates that learning solely from route perspective requires more time relative to learning from survey perspective [27]. This is in agreement with previous research where the survey perspective appeared to promote higher efficiency navigation and support far-spaced navigation while route perspective support a restricted range of local navigation [11]. This work has much applicability for soldiers and emergency rescuers who navigate in unfamiliar terrains after learning maps in different topographical representations.

## 5 Conclusion

Our study aimed to demonstrate the influence of different spatial perspectives for effective navigation. Furthermore, we analyzed the neural correlates underlying different spatial perspectives. The results obtained demonstrate the effectiveness of using distinct spatial perspective for spatial navigation through a virtual reality environment. The differential suitability of each perspective can be used to support navigation through far spaced and restricted space navigation. These differences can be tapped to guide the navigators in different terrains effectively. These techniques should be applied in real time environment to study the effectiveness of spatial acquisition of knowledge through visualization for navigators in unfamiliar terrains. Future work should elaborately explore the effectiveness of spatial knowledge acquired with different perspectives in real time applications.

## References

1. Siegel, A.W., White, S.H.: The development of spatial representations of large-scale environments. Adv. Child Dev. Behav. **10**, 9 (1975)
2. Tversky, B.: Spatial mental models. Psychol. Learn. Motiv.: Adv. Res. Theory **27**, 109–145 (1991)
3. Thorndyke, P.W., Hayes-Roth, B.: Differences in spatial knowledge acquired from maps and navigation. Cogn. Psychol. **14**(4), 560–589 (1982)
4. Mellet, E., et al.: Neural correlates of topographic mental exploration: the impact of route versus survey perspective learning. Neuroimage **12**(5), 588–600 (2000)
5. Slater, M., Usoh, M., Steed, A.: Depth of presence in virtual environments. Presence: Teleoper. Virtual Environ. **3**(2), 130–144 (1994)
6. Barfield, W., Weghorst, S.: The sense of presence within virtual environments: a conceptual framework. Adv. Hum. Factors Ergon. **19**, 699 (1993)
7. Clemente, M., et al.: Assessment of the influence of navigation control and screen size on the sense of presence in virtual reality using EEG. Expert Syst. Appl. **41**(4), 1584–1592 (2014)
8. White, D.J., et al.: Brain oscillatory activity during spatial navigation: theta and gamma activity link medial temporal and parietal regions. J. Cogn. Neurosci. **24**(3), 686–697 (2012)
9. De Araújo, D.B., Baffa, O., Wakai, R.T.: Theta oscillations and human navigation: a magnetoencephalography study. J. Cogn. Neurosci. **14**(1), 70–78 (2002)

10. Nguyen, H.M., et al.: sLORETA current source density analysis of evoked potentials for spatial updating in a virtual navigation task. Front. Behav. Neurosci. **8**, 66 (2014)
11. Brunyé, T.T., et al.: Going to town: visualized perspectives and navigation through virtual environments. Comput. Hum. Behav. **28**(1), 257–266 (2012)
12. Pascual-Marqui, R.D.: Standardized low-resolution brain electromagnetic tomography (sLORETA): technical details. Methods Find. Exp. Clin. Pharmacol. **24**(Suppl. D), 5–12 (2002)
13. Fuchs, M., et al.: A standardized boundary element method volume conductor model. Clin. Neurophysiol. **113**(5), 702–712 (2002)
14. Jurcak, V., Tsuzuki, D., Dan, I.: 10/20, 10/10, and 10/5 systems revisited: their validity as relative head-surface-based positioning systems. Neuroimage **34**(4), 1600–1611 (2007)
15. Maguire, E.A., Frackowiak, R.S., Frith, C.D.: Recalling routes around London: activation of the right hippocampus in taxi drivers. J. Neurosci. **17**(18), 7103–7110 (1997)
16. Epstein, R., Kanwisher, N.: A cortical representation of the local visual environment. Nature **392**(6676), 598–601 (1998)
17. Aguirre, G.K., Zarahn, E., D'Esposito, M.: Neural components of topographical representation. Proc. Nat. Acad. Sci. **95**(3), 839–846 (1998)
18. Maguire, E.A., et al.: Knowing where things are: parahippocampal involvement in encoding object locations in virtual large-scale space. Cogn. Neurosci. **10**(1), 61–76 (1998)
19. Levitin, D.J., Menon, V.: Musical structure is processed in "language" areas of the brain: a possible role for Brodmann Area 47 in temporal coherence. Neuroimage **20**(4), 2142–2152 (2003)
20. Karnath, H.O., Baier, B., Nägele, T.: Awareness of the functioning of one's own limbs mediated by the insular cortex. J. Neurosci. **25**(31), 7134–7138 (2005)
21. Radua, J., et al.: Neural response to specific components of fearful faces in healthy and schizophrenic adults. Neuroimage **49**(1), 939–946 (2010)
22. Taylor, H.A., Tversky, B.: Spatial mental models derived from survey and route descriptions. J. Mem. Lang. **31**(2), 261–292 (1992)
23. Ferguson, E.L., Hegarty, M.: Properties of cognitive maps constructed from texts. Mem. Cogn. **22**(4), 455–473 (1994)
24. Cavanna, A.E., Trimble, M.R.: The precuneus: a review of its functional anatomy and behavioural correlates. Brain **129**(3), 564–583 (2006)
25. Arzy, S., et al.: Induction of an illusory shadow person. Nature **443**(7109), 287 (2006)
26. Shelton, A.L., Gabrieli, J.D.: Neural correlates of encoding space from route and survey perspectives. J. Neurosci. **22**(7), 2711–2717 (2002)
27. Brunyé, T.T., Taylor, H.A.: Extended experience benefits spatial mental model development with route but not survey descriptions. Acta Psychol. **127**(2), 340–354 (2008)

# Brain-Inspired Obstacle Detection Based on the Biological Visual Pathway

Yi Zeng[1,2(✉)], Feifei Zhao[1,2], Guixiang Wang[1,2], Lingyu Zhang[1,2], and Bo Xu[1,2]

[1] Institute of Automation, Chinese Academy of Sciences, Beijing, China
{yi.zeng,zhaofeifei2014}@ia.ac.cn
[2] Center for Excellence in Brain Science and Intelligence Technology, Chinese Academy of Sciences, Shanghai, China

**Abstract.** Obstacle detection is crucial for intelligent systems (e.g. robots, unmanned ariel vehicle) that interact with the real world. This paper proposes a brain-inspired rasterization algorithm for obstacle detection. Rasterization algorithm is inspired by the information processing mechanism of the biological brain (including arthropod brain and human brain). Obstacle detection relies on feed forward and feed backward information processing mechanism. Receptive fields in every level of abstraction transmit different sizes of image regions to higher levels. Feedback is related to modulating attention about the position and size of target receptive field. Inspired by the circuit in human vision system, this paper provides a computational model for obstacle detection. Good performance on the experiments supports the proposed theoretical model. The major contribution of the proposed brain-inspired rasterization algorithm is that it can detect obstacle in any size from any direction without any preprocessing.

**Keywords:** Obstacle detection · Biological visual pathway · Rasterization algorithm · Brain-inspired intelligence

## 1 Introduction

Obstacle detection is a fundamental and basic cognitive ability, and is of vital importance for moving intelligent systems, such as various robots, unmanned ariel vehicle, etc. It is critical for intelligent agents to keep safety while they are performing any other tasks. As a result, the ability to accurately detect obstacle is essential in order to avoid obstacle. Two main problems are mostly studied in the obstacle detection field: one is to find obstacle in real time; and the other is to detect obstacle accurately.

In practice, obstacle detection algorithms can be divided into two parts: sensor-based methods and vision-based methods. Sensor-based methods need sensors information for obstacle detection. Sometimes they are unstable because of the environment influence. Vision-based methods are usually used for detecting featured obstacle. It still has large space to improve for obstacle detection.

© Springer International Publishing AG 2016
G.A. Ascoli et al. (Eds.): BIH 2016, LNAI 9919, pp. 355–364, 2016.
DOI: 10.1007/978-3-319-47103-7_35

In this paper, our motivation is to get inspirations from human visual information processing mechanism to propose a brain-inspired algorithm for automatic obstacle detection. We purely use visual information from single camera to address the problem of automatic obstacle detection. In fact, human visual mechanism is based on a circuit from retina to visual cortex [1]. The obstacle detection process is an integration of bottom-up transmission with top-down feedback. The top-down feedback hopes to find the smallest receptive field which contains the obstacle. The bottom-up transmission follows the feedback signal to modulate the position and the size of receptive fields.

Major contributions of this paper are as the following:

**Feedback Signal Analysis.** For the problem of obstacle detection, top-down feedback controls the attention to the position and size of obstacle. Because the characterization of obstacle must be enlarged over time, we propose an effective edge motion rule and calculate a scalar collision for evaluating every receptive field. The feedback signal is used to modulate the position and size of target receptive field.

**The Brain-Inspired Rasterization Algorithm for Obstacle Detection.** Considering that the arthropod can quickly detect the obstacle from any direction. This powerful function depends on the compound eye, which is composed of many ommatidia. Every ommatidium concentrates on a small part of the visual field [2]. It is to some extent similar to the receptive fields in human retina. We rasterize the images to many squares to simulate receptive fields in lowest level. In low level, there are many small receptive fields. The receptive fields in high level consist of the adjacent receptive fields in low level. From low level to high level, we calculate collision coefficient for every receptive field until it goes beyond the threshold.

**Experimental Validations on Effectiveness.** We implement our algorithm to verify our theoretical results. Experiment shows that our method can detect obstacle accurately in both immobile and mobile camera. We also test the algorithm on Unmanned Ariel Vehicle (UAV) obstacle avoidance experiment. It can detect obstacle in real time.

This paper is organized as follows. Section 2 introduces the related researches about obstacle detection and biological vision mechanism. Section 3 describes the proposed algorithm inspired by the human visual circuit and the arthropod visual circuit. Section 4 presents the details of real-time obstacle detection experiment. Section 5 presents result analysis, and Sect. 6 concludes the paper.

## 2    Related Work

### 2.1    Computational Models for Obstacle Detection

Obstacle detection has been studied for decades. Most of algorithms focus on sensor-based methods and vision-based methods. Various sensors such as ultrasonic and sonar have been used for obstacle detection [3–5]. They can measure direction and determine position of obstacle. Although it is simple and inexpensive, many factors such as air density can distort a sensor's result.

This paper focuses on the vision-based methods. Most researches of vision-based obstacle detection can be classified into two categories:

**Stereo Vision.** Stereo vision is widely used for obstacle detection [6–8]. It can construct disparity image, and estimate depth distance for the objects in image. However, it is so time-consuming that it may not suitable for the real-time detection. It is not robust because the accuracy depends on the environment.

**Background and Foreground Separation.** Most of the obstacle detection methods are based on background and foreground separation. Some methods focus on colour classification and clustering algorithm [9]. They are limited to some images that are easy to distinguish between obstacle and background. Some methods combine background subtraction with optical flow to detect obstacle [10–12]. Others focus on the Gaussian Mixture Model (GMM) background modelling methods [13]. These methods consider that obstacle is the foreground of an image. They are not always sufficient because sometimes foreground is not an obstacle. As a result, it is sometimes inaccurate for obstacle detection by separating background and foreground methods.

Other obstacle detection methods focus on the bio-inspired methods. A lobula giant movement detector (LGMD) neuron which is sensitive to the enlarging objects in locusts has been discovered [14]. Yue et al. proposed a feed forward network to simulate the enlarging object detection of LGMD [15].

## 2.2 Human Visual Circuit

When light projects to the retina, ganglion cells process it. The ganglion cells mainly project to the lateral geniculate nucleus. The lateral geniculate nucleus directly projects to primary visual cortex (V1). Other visual cortical regions are also involved in the bottom-up transmission [16].

What people notice is not simply a transmission from retina to visual cortex. The visual cortex combines the information in human brain to decide which one is a person really interested in [17]. The visual cortex feedback controls the attention of bottom-up information transmission. Attention plays a key role in obstacle detection.

In the circuit, receptive fields exist in every level to represent information. The receptive fields in higher level consist of integrated adjacent receptive fields in lower level. Nearby receptive fields correspond to nearby locations in the visual inputs [18]. This hierarchical structure is useful for representing visual inputs in different level of abstractions.

# 3   The Brain-Inspired Obstacle Detection Algorithm

The human visual system is with bottom-up transmission and top-down feedback. Under selective attention, receptive fields of low level converge to high level ones based on the selective attention of high level. The top-down feedback modulates the attention of the receptive field which contains the obstacle. The bottom-up transmission follows the feedback signal to modulate the attention about the position and size of receptive fields.

## 3.1   Top-Down Feedback

In this subsection, we will discuss the influences of top-down processing and propose the calculation of feedback signal.

Hierarchical theory allows cells at one level to be influenced by feedbacks from higher levels [19]. The feedback modulates the information carried by neurons [20]. After receiving such feedback inputs, neurons execute the instruction based on the feedback signal from higher level [21].

In the obstacle detection task, feedback from high level back to low level could mediate selective attention on the visual inputs [22]. We divide the feedback analytical process into three steps:

**Enlargement-Based Motion Detection.** No matter an obstacle is static or dynamic, it must be enlarged over time in the vision system of an moving agent. The motion of the object is the key of the feedback. The evidence shows that the medial superior temporal (MST) area is responsible for detecting motion [23]. MST belongs to high level in the circuit. The feedback from MST carries obstacle motion information controls the low-level attention.

**Edge Motion Detection.** In the visual cortex, cells are more sensitive to the contours of an object [24]. We assume that obstacle's edge motion can be used for describing the obstacle's enlargement. This will be verified in Sect. 4.1. The correct rules are described as the following: The left part of receptive field moves towards left direction. The right part of receptive field moves towards the right direction. The upper part of receptive field moves towards upper direction. The bottom part of receptive field moves towards bottom direction. The agents pay attention to the receptive fields which conform to these rules.

**Collision Coefficient Calculation.** Based on the edge motion rules, we evaluate every receptive field by a scalar collision coefficient. We use $l$, $r$, $u$, $d$ to present the left, right, upper, nether part of the receptive field, and the function $D_l$, $D_r$, $D_u$, $D_d$ measure the degree of the left, right, up, and down motion. For example, $D_l(l)$ represents the degree of left part moves towards left, and $D_l(r)$ represents the degree of left part moves towards right. The Eq. 1 represents the collision coefficient of the receptive field. It is a warning signal about the criticality of obstacle. Generally, the nearer the obstacle, the greater the $Col$ value.

Every time, we take two adjacent frames to calculate the collision coefficient. In the same receptive field, the rule is that if the left part moves towards left, we give a positive number to $D_l(l)$, and $D_l(r)$ is equal to zero. The bigger the size of receptive field, the greater the value of $D_l(l)$. The others will be assigned in the same way. They are calculated by subtracting two adjacent frames. If the four parts of the field are all conform to the rule and the obstacle is big enough, then the collision coefficient exceed the threshold. At this time, the whole receptive field contains the obstacle.

$$Col = D_l(l) + D_r(r) + D_u(u) + D_d(d) - D_l(r) - D_r(l) - D_u(d) - D_d(u) \quad (1)$$

## 3.2   Bottom-Up Transmission

Receptive fields exist in neurons of all levels of the visual system. Small, adjacent receptive fields in low level can be combined to larger receptive fields in higher levels. Features in the low level are combined in some way to form the features recognized in higher level regions.

For the obstacle detection task, we propose a brain-inspired rasterization algorithm. It is shown in Algorithm 1.

---

**Algorithm 1.** The brain-inspired rasterization algorithm.

---

**Input:** A current image $I_c$; The previous image $I_p$; The threshold of the collision coefficient $Th_c$; Variable initialization $i = 2$;

**Output:** The obstacle region $O_c$;

1: Rasterize the images $I_c$ and $I_p$ to $N_x \times N_y$ squares;
2: Choose all the regions with the size of $i \times i$ pixels in the image $I_c$ and $I_p$;
3: Calculate the collision coefficient of $Col$ for all regions. Compare $Col$ with $Th_c$;
4: $i = i + 1$.
5: Repeat Step 2 to Step 4 until $Col > Th_c$;
6: Output the region $O_c$ that contains an obstacle;
7: **return** $O_c$;

---

The arthropod compound eye has thousands of ommatidia. Every ommatidium represents different region of visual field [2]. We use center points to represent the different locations of ommatidia. Based on the large amount of center points, arthropod can detect the obstacle from any direction. We map the compound eye to the receptive fields in lowest level. Every receptive field corresponds to the ommatidium of compound eye. The images can be rasterized to many receptive fields, then the information is transmitted to the receptive fields in higher level. In the high level, the receptive fields are composed of several adjacent receptive fields from low level. They are many bigger image regions. The algorithm rasterizes the image to $N_x \times N_y$ squares. The size of receptive fields in the bottom level are squares with the size of $2 \times 2$ pixels, the number of the center points is $(N_x - 1) \times (N_y - 1)$. The size of receptive fields in $k$th level are $(k + 1) \times (k + 1)$ pixels, the number of the center points is $(N_x - k) \times (N_y - k)$. In the top level,

$k = \min(N_x, N_y) - 1$. From bottom to up, the judgement processes are executed in every receptive field of every level until the collision coefficient goes beyond threshold. Because the size and position of the receptive field is changeable in our method, we can judge flexible size to detect obstacle on the image.

## 4    Experiments and Validations

### 4.1    Edge Motion Judgment and Collision Coefficient Calculation

When obstacle moves towards the agent from arbitrary direction, a sequence of images are generated. Figure 1 is an example of image sequences. It is obvious that the obstacle is enlarged over time. If the position of the object is fixed or farther compared to the agent, it is not an obstacle.

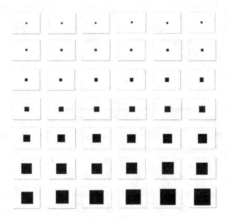

**Fig. 1.** The image sequences of the obstacle. We use the black block to simulate the obstacle. It is flying towards the camera.

Based on the idea in Sect. 3.1, we conduct experiments to test the edge motion change in the image sequences. We take out the left field of frame 17 to test the response of movement towards different directions for one small step. Frame 18 and frame 16 can describe the images after movement. We minus the RGB values of former frame with the latter frame. Just like Fig. 2 shows. Figure 2(a) is the left field of frame 18 which represents moving towards left for one small step, and the strongest response is the edge. Figure 2(b) is the left field of frame 16 which represents moving towards right for one small step, and there is no response at all. We also test this phenomenon for the right field, up field and bottom field. The reaction of edges are strongest only when one field moving towards the enlargement direction. Then, the results are assigned to the functions in Eq. 1. As the collision coefficient introduced in Sect. 3.1, we calculate the collision coefficient of fist attack image sequences. This is a simulation of the true environment. The result is shown in Fig. 3. The x-axis represents frames, and the y-axis represents the value of collision coefficient. It is obvious that the

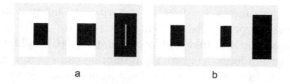

**Fig. 2.** (a) The left field of frame 17 and frame 18. We get the strong response in edge. (b) The left field of frame 17 and frame 16. There is no response at all.

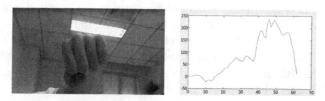

**Fig. 3.** The fist towards cameras and the change of collision coefficient. In the right picture, x-axis is the frame and y-axis is the collision coefficient. The collision coefficient is increasing as the fist gets closer to the camera.

collision coefficient is almost increasing along with the fist as it gets close to the camera. Collision coefficient can be used to measure whether the receptive field precisely contains an obstacle. We set a threshold for the collision coefficient. When collision coefficient exceed the threshold, the corresponding receptive field precisely contains an obstacle.

## 4.2   Experimental Validation

Based on the bottom-up mechanism in Sect. 3.2, we divide the image into $11 \times 16$ squares that represent the receptive fields in lowest level, as shown in Fig. 4(a). We pay attention to the enlarged edge motion by subtracting two adjacent frames. In this area, we calculate the collision coefficient for every receptive field based on Algorithm 1. This process will be circulate until the collision coefficient of the receptive field goes beyond the threshold. Figure 4(b) shows the ultimate receptive field which is the smallest one that contains the obstacle. For threshold parameters, we use 100 for the collision coefficient.

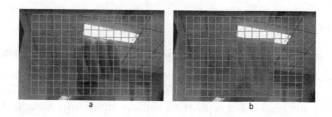

**Fig. 4.** (a) The beginning of the rasterization algorithm. We divide the image into many squares to simulate the compound eye. (b) The end of the rasterization algorithm. The receptive field of obstacle displayed by a rectangle.

The images from camera are directly rasterized to many squares. We don't need any preprocessing procedure and feature extraction. The rasterization algorithm is implemented on a ThinkPad laptop computer (CPU 2.60 GHz). We test our approach in two different conditions: immobile camera and mobile camera. We test the obstacle from various directions and positions. Some immobile camera results are shown in Fig. 5(a). Camera STEBOO t16 catches the images in Hd 12 million pixels and concurrently detects obstacle. Figure 5(b) shows the results in mobile camera. We use the 2.4 GHz wireless digital video camera (1/4 CCD) to test the mobile experiment. Under these setups, our method can detect the enlarged obstacle in 0.008 s at the resolution of 640 * 480 pixels. To test the real-time detection, we use the 2.4 GHz wireless digital video camera (1/4 CCD) on unmanned ariel vehicle (UAV) to test the obstacle detection and avoidance. The UAV is DJI MATRICE 100 with guidance in 0.5 m stable precision. Figure 5(c) shows the UAV obstacle detection experiment.

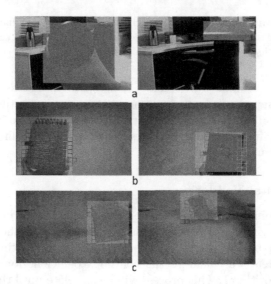

**Fig. 5.** The red rectangle areas are the obstacles. (a) The obstacle detection results in immobile camera. (b) The obstacle detection results in mobile camera. (c) The obstacle detection results on UAV. (Color figure online)

## 5    Discussion

The advantages of the proposed model is summarized as the following:

- Simple visual information acquisition setup. Just one camera is enough to support the visual information acquisition for obstacle detection. The proposed algorithm do not need other sensors to achieve more information. Preprocessing or feature extraction are also not needed. This can be to some extend compared to human brain from the obstacle detection perspective, since human also rely on visual information processing to detect obstacles.

- Low computational complexity. Our method uses the feedback signal to catch the candidate obstacle area. In the candidate area, we calculate collision coefficient for every receptive field to get the exact obstacle position. The computational complexity of collision coefficient is low since it only rely on plus and minus operations.
- Robustness. Based on the feedback mechanism, the method can find the correct receptive field adaptively from any direction and any size. Compared with other methods which are not Brain-inspired, the rasterization algorithm catches the obstacle based on the feedback signal. It pays attention to the enlarged object which is the real obstacle.
- Multi-level of Abstraction. The receptive field in different scales represent different level of abstractions. So, it can detect the obstacle precisely.

## 6    Conclusion

This paper investigate on the obstacle detection problem based on inspirations from human visual circuit and arthropod visual circuit. In the human brain, the obstacle detection converge the top-down feedback with bottom-up transmission. Under the context of obstacle detection, the feedback is about the attention of obstacle edge motion. We consider the feedback signal as a scalar collision coefficient to focus on the interesting receptive field. A rasterization algorithm is used to transmit the receptive fields in different directions and different scales. Based on the experimental evaluations, our model can detect the obstacle in arbitrary direction and arbitrary scales correctly.

Currently, the proposed method is efficient for both static and moving cameras when the background is simple. If the background is complex (e.g. with many objects), the current algorithm is efficient for static cameras. In the future, we would like to improve the algorithm to deal with more complex background for moving cameras.

**Acknowledgments.** This study was funded by the Strategic Priority Research Program of the Chinese Academy of Sciences (XDB02060007), and Beijing Municipal Commission of Science and Technology (Z151100000915070, Z161100000216124).

## References

1. DiCarlo, J.J., Zoccolan, D., Rust, N.C.: How does the brain solve visual object recognition? Neuron **73**(3), 415–434 (2012)
2. Mayer, G.: Structure and development of onychophoran eyes: what is the ancestral visual organ in arthropods? Arthropod Struct. Dev. **35**(4), 231–245 (2006)
3. Menezes, P., Dias, J., Araújo, H., de Almeida, A.: Low cost sensor based obstacle detection and description. In: Khatib, O., Kenneth Salisbury, J. (eds.) Experimental Robotics IV. Lecture Notes in Control and Information Sciences, vol. 223, pp. 231–237. Springer, Heidelberg (2005)
4. Mejias, L., McNamara, S., Lai, J., Ford, J.: Vision-based detection and tracking of aerial targets for UAV collision avoidance. In: Proceedings of the 2010 IEEE/RSJ International Conference on Intelligent Robots and Systems, pp. 87–92 (2010)

5. Heidarsson, H.K., Sukhatme, G.S.: Obstacle detection and avoidance for an autonomous surface vehicle using a profiling sonar. In: Proceedings of 2011 IEEE International Conference on Robotics and Automation, pp. 731–736 (2011)
6. Wedel, A., Franke, U., Klappstein, J., Brox, T., Cremers, D.: Realtime depth estimation and obstacle detection from monocular video. In: Franke, K., Müller, K.-R., Nickolay, B., Schäfer, R. (eds.) DAGM 2006. LNCS, vol. 4174, pp. 475–484. Springer, Heidelberg (2006)
7. Labayrade, R., Aubert, D., Tarel, J.P.: Real time obstacle detection in stereovision on non flat road geometry through "v-disparity" representation. In: Proceedings of the 2002 IEEE Intelligent Vehicles Symposium, vol. 2, pp. 646–651 (2002)
8. Badal, S., Ravela, S., Draper, B., Hanson, A.: A practical obstacle detection and avoidance system. In: Proceedings of 2nd IEEE Workshop on Applications of Computer Vision, pp. 97–104 (1994)
9. Omkar, S.N., Tripathi, S., Kumar, G., Gupta, I.: Vision based obstacle detection mechanism of a fixed wing UAV. Int. J. Adv. Comput. Res. 4(1), 2249–7277 (2014)
10. Low, T., Wyeth, G.: Obstacle detection using optical flow. In: Proceedings of the 2005 Australasian Conference on Robotics & Automation, pp. 1–10 (2005)
11. Ess, A., Leibe, B., Schindler, K., Van Gool, L.: Moving obstacle detection in highly dynamic scenes. In: Proceedings of 2009 IEEE International Conference on Robotics and Automation, pp. 56–63 (2009)
12. Sagar, J., Visser, A.: Obstacle avoidance by combining background subtraction, optical flow and proximity estimation. In: Proceedings of the 2014 International Micro Air Vehicle Conference and Competition, pp. 142–149 (2014)
13. Qian, S., Tan, J.K., Kim, H.: Videotaped obstacle extraction from a moving camera. Int. J. Innov. Comput. Inf. Control 10, 717–728 (2014)
14. Rind, F.C., Simmons, J.P.: Orthopteran DCMD neuron: a reevaluation of responses to moving objects. I. Selective responses to approaching objects. Neurophysiology 68(5), 1654–1666 (1992)
15. Yue, S., Rind, F.C.: Collision detection in complex dynamic scenes using an LGMD-based visual neural network with feature enhancement. IEEE Trans. Neural Netw. 17(3), 705–716 (2006)
16. Brewer, A.A., Barton, B.: Visual cortex in aging and Alzheimer's disease: changes in visual field maps and population receptive fields. Front. Psychol. 5, 74 (2014)
17. Carlson, N.R.: Physiology of Behavior. Allyn & Bacon, Boston (1986)
18. Wandell, B.A., Dumoulin, S.O., Brewer, A.A.: Visual field maps in human cortex. Neuron 56(2), 366–383 (2007)
19. Hubel, D.H., Wiesel, T.N.: Receptive fields, binocular interaction and functional architecture in the cat's visual cortex. J. Physiol. 160(1), 106–154 (1962)
20. McAlonan, K., Cavanaugh, J., Wurtz, R.H.: Guarding the gateway to cortex with attention in visual thalamus. Nature 456(7220), 391–394 (2008)
21. Gilbert, C.D., Li, W.: Top-down influences on visual processing. Nat. Rev. Neurosci. 14(5), 350–363 (2013)
22. Ungerleider, L.G., Haxby, J.V.: 'What' and 'where' in the human brain. Curr. Opin. Neurobiol. 4(2), 157–165 (1994)
23. Ichikawa, M., Masakura, Y., Munechika, K.: Dependence of illusory motion on directional consistency in oblique components. Perception 35(7), 933–946 (2006)
24. Wurtz, R.H., Kandel, E.R.: Central visual pathways. In: Principles of Neural Science, 4 edn, pp. 523–545. McGraw-Hill (2000)

# Workshop on Brain and Artificial Intelligence (BAI 2016)

# A Probabilistic Method for Linking BI Provenances to Open Knowledge Base

Jing Wang[1,2(✉)], Yongchuan Yu[1,2], Jianzhuo Yan[1,2], Jianhui Chen[1,2,3,4,5], Zhongcheng Zhao[1], and Dongsheng Wang[3,6]

[1] Beijing Advanced Innovation Center for Future Internet Technology,
Beijing University of Technology, Beijing 100024, China
{yuyongchuan,yanjianzhuo,chenjianhui}@bjut.edu.cn, zhaozhongch@163.com,
dkwangjing@emails.bjut.edu.cn
[2] College of Electronic Information and Control Engineering,
Beijing University of Technology, Beijing 100024, China
[3] International WIC Institute, Beijing University of Technology, Beijing, China
dswang@bjut.edu.cn
[4] Beijing International Collaboration Base on Brain Informatics
and Wisdom Services, Beijing, China
[5] Beijing Key Laboratory of MRI and Brain Informatics, Beijing, China
[6] Institute of Intelligent Transport System,
School of Computer Science and Engineering,
Jiangsu University of Science of Technology, Zhenjiang 212003, China

**Abstract.** Owing the explosive growth of unstructured cognitive big data, provenances become a core issue in Brain informatics. In order to construct a open and sharing knowledge graph about cognitive big data, Brain informatics provenances cannot be isolated. All entities, which were extracted from biomedical literatures, web documents, information systems, etc., should be linked to open knowledge bases, such as DBpedia. However, the entity ambiguity is a key obstacle with the linking task. This paper proposes a probabilistic method for linking BI provenances to open knowledge base. Both the popularity knowledge and context knowledge are considered to solve the entity ambiguity. The experimental results shows the proposed method is effective.

## 1 Introduction

The development of brain science has led to a vast increase of brain data. At present, Brain informatics (BI) focuses on two kinds of important brain data, ERP (event-related potential) data and fMRI (functional magnetic resonance imaging) data. [14] Because both of them are unstructured data, provenances become a core issue in Brain informatics. The biomedical literature is the main knowledge source for BI provenances. Since the BI provenances can be isolated and heterogeneous on the Web, for the purpose of constructing a open and sharing knowledge graph in the brain informatics domain, and for the sake of systematic research of brain informatics, linking BI provenances to open knowledge bases can be very important and pivotal.

© Springer International Publishing AG 2016
G.A. Ascoli et al. (Eds.): BIH 2016, LNAI 9919, pp. 367–376, 2016.
DOI: 10.1007/978-3-319-47103-7_36

DBpedia data set is an open database extracted from the Wikipedia structured data, it is an interdisciplinary, multi-language supported and widely accepted knowledge base. In DBpedia dataset each entity has a globally unique identifier, all identifiers are in strict accordance with the Linked Data dissemination standard definition. In recent years, more and more publishers linked their data with entities in DBpedia, which makes DBpedia the hub of the Linked Open Data (LOD). Since DBpedia data set is such a big and wide-covering data set, in brain informatics domain, linking BI provenances to DBpedia has great significance for constructing a open and sharing knowledge graph. However, the name ambiguity is a key obstacle with the linking task. For example, the term "Schizophrenia" in DBpedia is involved with three entities, including a name of a mental disease, an album of music and a method of programming. For solving this problem, this paper proposes a probabilistic method for linking BI provenances to DBpedia.

The rest of this paper is organized as follows. Section 2 discusses background and related work, mainly about BI provenance and entity linking. Section 3 illustrates the details of the proposed method. Section 4 shows the experimental results and discussion. Finally, Sect. 5 gives conclusion and future work.

## 2   Background and Related Work

### 2.1   BI Provenance

Data provenance, also called data lineage or data pedigree, records sources as well as a set of processing steps applied to sources [16]. Data provenance provides important information for users to determine the reliability of data products, and helps users to reproduce and validate the data products [17]. Current data provenance of brain cognitive data have made great achievement.

Systematic Brain Informatics (BI) study produces various original data, deriving data and data features, which include a large number of unstructured data. Aiming at different purposes of data sharing and data utilization, the metadata need to include different contents. The metadata describing the origin and subsequent processing of biological images is often referred to as provenance. Similarly, we call BI Provenances, which include data provenances and analysis provenances. A BI data provenance is a metadata set that describes the BI data origin by multi-aspect experiment information, including subjects information, how experimental data of subjects were collected, what instrument was used, etc. [15]. Furthermore, a BI analysis provenance is a metadata set that describes what processing in a brain dataset has been carried out, including what analytic tasks were performed, what experimental data were used, what data features were extracted, and so on [15]. BI provenance contains brain function data content itself, data generation and data processing.

As the explosive growth of biomedical literature, biomedical literature mining is not only the way for the collection and integration of domain knowledge, but also the effect means for identifying potential knowledge and promoting biomedical research breakthroughs. For the above reasons, the biomedical literatures are the main knowledge source for constructing BI provenances. Constructing BI provenance with the biomedical literatures involves a lot of work such as terminology recognition, relationship found as well as the integration of terminology and relationship, so we adopt term recognition technology based on heuristic rules and machine learning to achieve automatic extraction of brain information content. In the Web of Data environment, linking data provenance to open knowledge base can make it easier for knowledge sharing and integration.

## 2.2  Entity Disambiguation

Entity disambiguation plays an important role in natural language processing applications. With the development of the information age, the deepening of research on text mining, information retrieval system and other fields has made the application of entity disambiguation popular. The existing methods on entity disambiguation can be divided into the following two types:

- The first type is single entity disambiguation method, which deal with one name mention in textual data one time without considering the influence from other entities in the same document. The first part of this kind of methods is local compatibility based approach which is also the initial method by extracting the discriminative features of an entity from its textual description, then linking a name mention to the entity which has the highest contextual similarity with it. Mihalcea and Csomai [21] proposed a bag of words (BoW)-based methods, where the compatibility between a name mention and an entity was measured as the cosine similarity between them. One of its largest problems is that the dimension of vectors of the words sometimes becomes too big to calculate. The second part is simple relation approaches. Considering the entity linking decisions in one document have no influence with each other, we can utilize the semantic relations between different entities in one document for linking decision. The core assumption is that the referent entity of a name mention should have a strong semantic relationship with its unambiguous contextual entities [18]. The main problem of this method is that they can only exploit pairwise interdependence between a name mention and its unambiguous contextual entities.
- The second type is global entity disambiguation method. Owing to the entities appears in the same document are related to the same topic or provided with some relatedness, the core assumption is that disambiguation of different name mentions in the same document should have dependencies with each other. Alhelbawy [24] modeling dependencies between name mentions by Hidden Markov model. Yang et al. [20] proposed a method using Graph model which is constructed by candidate entities of name mentions. This model needs to model the global semantic relations by iterate methods in one document which is not as efficient as the first method.

Based on the above background, in this issue, we use a probability-based entity linking model by considering an entity alleged visibility and situational judgment context of the alleged corresponding entities, eliminate ambiguity of named entity.

## 3    A Probabilistic Method for Entity Linking

As stated in [1], an entity linking process often needs to consider the three factors, including the popularity of entities, the name knowledge and the context knowledge. BI provenances often have standard entity names because they are mainly extracted from biomedical literatures. Thus, it only needs to consider the popularity of entities and the context knowledge for linking BI provenances with the open knowledge base. By means of the study of literatures related to entities linking, and combining with the characteristics of this research, pros Links task in this paper can be summarized as shown in Fig. 1.

Our method consists of three parts: entity popularity knowledge for entity linking task, entity context knowledge for entity linking task, and then combine the two knowledge mentioned above for the entity linking task, finally evaluate the results of our method by the accuracy of entity disambiguation. The details will be discussed as follows.

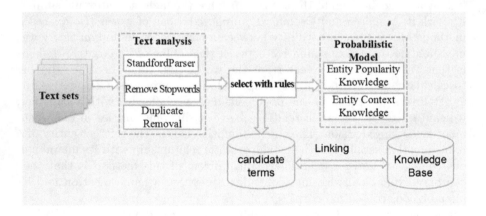

**Fig. 1.** Framework of entity disambiguation

### 3.1    Modeling Popularity Knowledge of Entities

The popularity knowledge of entities reflects the likelihood of an entity appearing in the BI provenance. In entity linking, the popularity knowledge can be used as an empirical judgment [1]. The higher popularity the entity has, the greater chance it appears in the BI provenance. We use the distribution $p(e)$ as a description of popularity knowledge of entities. If entity $e_1$ is more popular than the entity $e_2$, then the value of $p(e_1)$ will be larger than the value of $p(e_2)$.

Given a term $m_0$, if there are N entities in the knowledge base are referent to the $m_0$, in its simplest form, we can assume that these entities have equal popularity, we can estimate $p(e)$ as:

$$p(e) = \frac{1}{N} \tag{1}$$

It is obviously that it can't reflect the objective facts, because different entities of the same name may represent different things in the world, there must be some difference of their popularity and their application rate.

To get a more precise estimation, we observed that a more popular entity often appears more times than a less popular entity in the open knowledge base. For example, in DBpedia the entity <http://dbpedia.org/resource/Anxiety> appears 4 times while the entity *<http://dbpedia.org/resource/Anxiety_(Smile Empty Soul album)* appears only 2 times, under the circumstance that we don't have any other information, the popularity knowledge can tell us that the entity <http://dbpedia.org/resource/Anxiety> will be more likely to refer to the term "Anxiety" than the entity *<http://dbpedia.org/resource/Anxiety_(Smile Empty Soul album)*. Based on the above observation, our entity popularity knowledge uses the frequencies the entity appears in knowledge base to calculate. So the distribution $p(e)$ can be estimated as follows:

$$p(e) = \frac{Count_{ei}(m_0)}{Count_e(m_0)} \tag{2}$$

where $Count_e(m_0)$ is the count of entities with the name mention $m_0$, and $Count_{ei}(m_0)$ represents the count of one of its entities. Here is the popularity of entities with the name "Anxiety" in Table 1.

**Table 1.** Examples of name mentions with ambiguity problem

| Name | Entity | Count of entity in DBpedia | Popularity |
|------|--------|---------------------------|------------|
| Anxiety | *<Anxiety>* | 4 | 57.1 % |
| | *<Anxiety_(Smile_Empty_Soul_album)>* | 2 | 28.6 % |
| | *<Anxiety_(film)>* | 0 | 0 % |
| | *<Anxiety_(Ladyhawke_album)>* | 1 | 14.3 % |
| | *<Anxiety_(Munch)>* | 0 | 0 % |

### 3.2 Modeling Context Knowledge of Entities

It occurs to us that we can't understand the meaning of a word when we read an article. The meaning of the term can be judged based on the context information. Such as when we read the word "Schizophrenia", we may not be able to determine the meaning, but to see its context with words like "disorder", "disease", "mental health", we can determine that it may represent a mental illness. The context of different entities usually appear very different, hence, the context knowledge is crucial in solving the name ambiguities.

Let $M = \{m_1, m_2, ..., m_k\}$ donate a collection of name mentions extracted from BI provenances. Each name mention in the M is characteristic by its name $m$, its local surrounding context $c$. There are a set of entities $E = \{e_1, e_2, ..., e_m\}$ in DBpedia. Each entity e in E is characteristic by its description found in DBpedia, the terms in the description are treated as the context of entity $e$. The distribution $p(e|c)$ encodes the context knowledge of entities, i.e., it will assign a high $p(e|c)$ value if the name mention is more likely referent to the entity $e$, and will assign a low $p(e|c)$ value if the name mention rarely referent to the entity $e$. To estimate the distribution of $p(e|c)$, we propose a method based on probability with context knowledge. Generally speaking, the context knowledge of an entity $e$ can be described in an unigram language model as stated in [1]:

$$M_e(t) = \{p_e(t)\} \tag{3}$$

where $p_e(t)$ is the frequently of an term in the context of $m$ appearing in the context of entity $e$, in our research, the term may indicate a word. Now, given a name mention $m$, its surrounding context is described as a corpus in unigram language model, we donate it as $c$, and the context of its referent entity contains k words $t_1, t_2, ..., t_k$, so the $p(e|c)$ can be estimated as:

$$p(e|c) = p(t_1 t_2 ... t_k|c) \tag{4}$$

Due to the context of term and the context of entity are independent from each other, so $p(e|c)$ can also be estimated as follows:

$$p(c|e) = p(t_1|c)p(t_2|c)...p(t_k|c) \tag{5}$$

So the main problem is to estimate $p(t_i|c)$, based on a method for the calculation of the similarity of context, the estimation of $p(t_i|c)$ as follows:

$$p(t_i|c) = \frac{Count_e(t_i)}{\sum_t Count_e(t)} \tag{6}$$

where $Count_e(t_i)$ is the frequency of occurrences of a word $t_i$ in the context of the entity which is referent to the term $m$.

### 3.3    Entity Linking Based Two Knowledge

Binding the popularity knowledge and context knowledge, the probability of the term $m_0$ referring to the entity e can be calculated as follows:

$$P = \alpha * p(e) + \beta * p(e|c) \tag{7}$$

Based on experiences, the optimal value of $\alpha$ and $\beta$ is set to be 0.5 and 0.5. So the entity with the highest value of $P$ will be the objective entity.

# 4    Experiments

## 4.1    Knowledge Base

This article adopts the DBpedia version of 2015 as the entity disambiguation knowledge base. This is a multilingual knowledge base extracted from Wikipedia by DBpedia community. We used the English version of DBpedia, since it has the richest entity information including about 500 million facts and 4.5 million things. DBpedia is constructed by a series of disparate data set forms, different sets of data drawn from different parts of the Wikipedia page.

In order to solve the entity ambiguity problem, we chose the *long − abstractsen.nt* file from DBpedia. This data set is stored in the form of triplets, for example, a row of data in data set is shown as below (here show it in three lines):

---

$< http : //dbpedia.org/resource/26th\_century\_BC >$
$< http : //dbpedia.org/ontology/abstract >$
The 26th century BC is a century which lasted from the year 2600 BC to 2501 BC.

---

The subject of this triplet represents an entity. The object of the triplet represents the description of the entity, we treat it as the contexts of entity. The predicate of a data set is identical, so we can ignore the predicate part.

## 4.2    Candidate Data Selection

As mentioned above, we use the biomedical data sets to build BI provenance. According to the characteristics of the data set, we define a rule to find ambiguous terms in BI provenances, as well as their corresponding entities in the DBpedia. The rules of candidate selection is shown in Table 2:

**Table 2.** The algorithm of research recommendation

| Candidate Data Set Selection |
| --- |
| Input: literature from pubmed |
| Output: words with ambiguity problem and their entities find from DBpedia |
| 1. Perform part-of-speech tagging and syntactic parsing by using the Stanford parser to extract all noun phrases as terms |
| 2. Remove adjectives, articles and other stop words from obtained terms |
| 3. IF there is a word $A$ in the word set and we can find more than two entities like $A$ or $A\_() >$ in the DBpedia data set |
| 4. Then we choose the word $A$ as the word with name ambiguity problem in our candidate word set |
| 5. And, the entities associated with the word $A$ will be added to our candidate entity set |

## 4.3    Evaluation Criteria

We adopted the accuracy of entity disambiguation as the evaluation, and the correctness of disambiguation result is judged by domain expert. Here is the calculation of accuracy:

$$p = \frac{the\ number\ of\ correct\ disambiguation}{the\ number\ of\ name\ mentions\ used\ in\ experiment} \tag{8}$$

## 4.4    Experiment Results and Evaluation

We compared our method with existing disambiguation algorithm. we choose traditional Bag of Words based method. [18] we denoted this method as BOW. And there is a method described in [19], which find the unambiguous entity of a name mention by calculating the commonness of entities and the semantic relatedness of name mention and entity. We denoted this method as C&R. Also, we adopt the Graph-based method for entity disambiguation [20], We denoted this method as Graph. We conduct experiments on our data set with several methods: the BOW, the C&R, the Graph, and the method we proposed using entity popularity knowledge(*popu*) $p(e)$, the method we proposed using entity context knowledge(*context*) $p(e|c)$. And also the combination of entity popularity knowledge and entity context knowledge (PM)

Experimental results shows in Table 3 tells the accuracy of linking performance. As we can see, when only using the entity popularity knowledge, our method can achieve 52 % accuracy. And when only using the entity context knowledge, the accuracy turned to be 78 %. In order to improve the link accuracy and get a better consequence, as both the entity popularity knowledge and the entity context knowledge contribute to the accuracy of link consequence, we can combine the two method. With the accuracy of 80 %, which is better than other methods we choose for comparation, we can know that our method can be useful for solving the problem we met when linking BI provenance with open knowledge base.

**Table 3.** Consequence of entity linking with entity popularity knowledge

| Method | Accuracy |
|--------|----------|
| BOW | 0.35 |
| C&R | 0.60 |
| Graph | 0.74 |
| *popu* | 0.52 |
| *context* | 0.78 |
| PM | 0.80 |

# 5 Conclusion and Future Work

This paper adopt two knowledge based on probability to solve the name ambiguity problem. The main advantage of our research is that it can link the term with the only right entity in the knowledge base, it is significance for constructing sharing and open knowledge graph in brain informatics domain, which is helpful for the research of brain informatics based on the large scale of data, and is good for the systematic research in brain science. Experimental results show that our method can reach our target in advance. Also, there is also a lack in our research. In the course of our study, we discovered that there are many acronyms in the literatures, such as EEG, ERP. These acronyms also have ambiguity problem. For example, the ERP can not only be the acronym of "event-related potential" but also the acronym of "enterprise resourse planning", this ambiguity problem also has effect on the entity linking. So for the future work, we can take the ambiguity of acronym into our account and make our research more comprehensive.

**Acknowledgments.** The work is supported by National Key Basic Research Program of China (2014CB744605), National Natural Science Foundation of China (61272345), Research Supported by the CAS/SAFEA International Partnership Program for Creative Research Teams, the Japan Society for the Promotion of Science Grants-in-Aid for Scientific Research (25330270).

# References

1. Han, X.P., Sun, L.: A generative entity-mention model for linking entities with knowledge base. In: Meeting of the Association for Computational Linguistics: Human Language Technologies, pp. 945–954 (2011)
2. Huai, B.X., Bao, T.F., Zhu, H.S., Liu, Q.: Topic modeling approach to named entity linking. Ruan Jian Xue Bao/J. Softw. **25**(9), 2076–2087 (2014). (in chinese). http://www.jos.org.cn/1000-9825/4642.htm
3. Wu, C., Lu, W.: Context feature based entity linking for short text. Inf. Sci. **2**, 144–147 (2016)
4. Wu, Y.G.: Named Entity Linking Based on Multisource Knowledge
5. Zhu, M., Jia, Z., Zuo, L., Wu, A.J., Chen, F.Z., Bai, Y.: Research on entity linking of Chinese micro blog. Acta Sci. Naturalium Universitatis Pekinensis **1**, 73–78 (2014)
6. Wang, H., Fang, Z., Zhang, L., Pan, J.Z., Ruan, T.: Effective online knowledge graph fusion. In: Arenas, M., et al. (eds.) ISWC 2015. LNCS, vol. 9366, pp. 286–302. Springer, Heidelberg (2015). doi:10.1007/978-3-319-25007-6_17
7. Zhou, Y., Nie, L., Rouhani-Kalleh, O., Vasile, F., Gaffney, S.: Resolving surface forms to Wikipedia topics. In: Proceedings of the 23rd International Conference on Computational Linguistics, pp. 1335–1343 (2010)
8. Pedersen, T., Purandare, A., Kulkarni, A.: Name discrimination by clustering similar contexts. In: Gelbukh, A. (ed.) CICLing 2005. LNCS, vol. 3406, pp. 226–237. Springer, Heidelberg (2005)
9. Bagga, A., Baldwin, B.: Entity-based cross-document coreferencing using the vector space model. In: Proceedings of EMNLP 2008, pp. 79–85. HLT/ACL, Stroudsburg (2008)

10. Witten, I., Milne, D.: An effective, low-cost measure of semantic relatedness obtained from Wikipedia links. In: Proceedings of the AAAI Workshop on Wikipedia and Artificial Intelligence: An Evolving Synergy, pp. 25–30. AAAI Press (2008)

11. Hachey, B., Radford, W., Nothman, J., Honnibal, M., Curran, J.R.: Evaluating entity linking with Wikipedia. Artif. Intell. **194**, 130–150 (2013)

12. Zheng, J., Mao, Y.H.: Word sense tagging method based on word relationships. J. Tsinghua Univ. **41**, 117–120 (2001)

13. Yuan, J., Yue, P., Gong, J.Y., Zhang, M.D.: A linked data approach for geospatial data provenance. IEEE Trans. Geosci. Remote Sens. **51**(11), 5105–5112 (2013)

14. Zhong, N., Chen, J.H.: Constructing a new-style conceptual model of brain data for systematic brain informatics. IEEE Trans. Knowl. Data Eng. **24**(12), 2127–2142 (2012)

15. Chen, J., et al.: Data-Brain driven systematic human brain data analysis: a case study in numerical inductive reasoning centric investigation. Cogn. Syst. Res. (2011). doi:10.1016/j.cogsys.2010.12.014

16. Woodruff, A., Stonebraker, M.: Supporting fine-grained data lineage in a database visualization environment. In: Proceedings of 13th International Conference on Data Engineering, pp. 7–11 (1997)

17. Yue, P., Wei, Y., Di, L., He, L., Gong, J., Zhang, L.: Sharing geospatial provenance in a service-oriented environment. Comput. Environ. Urban Syst. **35**(2), 333–343 (2011)

18. Medelyan, O, Witten, I.H., Milne, D.: Topic indexing with Wikipedia. In: Proceedings of the AAAI WikiAI Workshop (2008)

19. Wang, H.F., Fang, Z.J., Zhang, L., Pan, J.Z., Ruan, T.: Effective online knowledge graph fusion. In: Arenas, M., et al. (eds.) ISWC 2015. LNCS, vol. 9366, pp. 286–302. Springer International Publishing, Switzerland (2015)

20. Yang, G., Liu, B.Q., Liu, M.: Graph based method for named entity disambiguation. Intell. Comput. Appl. 5(5) (2015)

21. Mihalcea, R., Csomai, A.: Wikify! Linking documents to encyclopedic knowledge. In: Proceedings of the Sixteenth ACM CIKM

22. Cucerzan, S.: Large-scale named entity disambiguation based on Wikipedia data. In: Proceedings of EMNLPCoNLL (2007)

23. Bunescu, R., Pasca, M.: Using encyclopedic knowledge for named entity disambiguation. In: Proceedings of EACL, vol. 6 (2006)

24. AGaizauskas, A.: Named entity disambiguation using HMMs. In: 2013 IEEE/WIC/ACM International Joint Conferences on Web Intelligence (WI) and Intelligent Agent Technologies(IAT), pp. 159–162. IEEE Computer Society, Atlanta (2013)

# Using Decision Trees to Analyse Brain Signals in Spacial Activities

Narúsci S. Bastos(✉), Diana F. Adamatti, and Cleo Z. Billa

Programa de Pós-Graduação em Computação, Universidade Federal do Rio Grande,
Rio Grande, Rio Grande do Sul, Brazil
naruscibastos@gmail.com, dianaada@gmail.com, cleo.billa@gmail.com

**Abstract.** The goal of this work is to use decision trees for knowledge discovery in brain data signals. We use a dataset of blind and sight people during an activity of spatial patterns recognition. The dataset was acquired through a BCI System, when individuals have to identify 3D geometric objects. The collected brain signals were preprocessed and used as input in Weka data mining software, more specifically the J48 algorithm. In our tests, we find decisions trees which indicate that blind people do not have significant activities in the occipital lobe (visual memory) to identify the objects. Sight people, instead, have significant activities in the occipital lobe, even when they are blindfolded.

**Keywords:** Decision trees · Neuroscience · Brain Computer Interface · Brain signals

## 1 Introduction

Blindness is a severe or total change of one or more elementary functions of vision that affects irremediably the ability to perceive color, size, distance, shape, position or movement in a given space [1]. The expression "visual impairment" refers to the spectrum ranging from blindness to low vision. There are two types of blind: congenitally blind and acquired blind. The congenitally blind has the cognitive system from birth, made on the basis of other senses and without reference to visual elements. Unlike the blind acquired, which has cognitive changes related to the reduced abilities of efficiency and previous habits [3].

The nervous system is primarily used for the reception, storage and release information. It is a complex system that consist of various structures and specialized organs with different functions [2], and it can be divided in: sensory system, which presents information about the organism and the environment; motor system, that organizes and executes actions; and the associative system. In this work we stand out the sensory system, since it is known that individuals with visual impairment have their orientation and mobility capabilities compromised [4]. Stimulate the capacity of other senses as touch, hearing, smell and taste, it is very important for individual adaptation in the world that people live.

© Springer International Publishing AG 2016
G.A. Ascoli et al. (Eds.): BIH 2016, LNAI 9919, pp. 377–385, 2016.
DOI: 10.1007/978-3-319-47103-7_37

BCI (Brain Computer Interface) systems are tools (hardware and software) that allow a way of communication between the brain and the computer. They are based on neural activities of the brain, and they do not require other stimuli, such as muscle movements [5]. The electroencephalogram (EEG) is based on brain electrical activity records that are measured on the surface of the scalp, usually presented in the form of waves. It is widely used because it has a high temporal resolution, that is capable of measure the activity every millisecond.

Data mining (DM) is the process of extracting or mining knowledge from a large volume of data. DM involves the study of tasks and techniques. Tasks are a specific class of problems defined by studies in the area. Techniques are groups of solutions to solve these tasks [6]. This work uses decision trees for knowledge discovery in a dataset of brain signals of blind (visual impairment) and sight people during an activity with spatial abilities.

This work is divided into five sections. Section 2 presents some concepts that addresses issues for this study as brain areas and their actions, visual impairment, BCI systems and data mining. Section 3 provides the materials and methods used. Section 4 presents the obtained results, and finally Sect. 5 presents conclusions and future works.

## 2 Theoretical Background

### 2.1 Brain Areas and Their Functions

The brain is the main component of the nervous system. It is responsible for all mental operations as concentration, thinking, learning and motor control. These capabilities are implemented through neurons, which can currently be explained by neuroscience.

Human brain is divided into two hemispheres, right and left. Initially, there was a belief that there was one dominant hemisphere and the other was dominated. However, this concept has become outdated, and now there is a belief that there are actually two specialized hemispheres. Thus, each hemisphere is responsible for a set of functions that end up working together.

Anatomists usually divide the brain into major regions, called lobes, whose boundaries are not always accurate, but transmit an initial idea of regional location. There are five lobes: four visible externally and one positioned inside the large grooves of the brain, the lateral sulcus [9]. The four visible lobes are: frontal, which is located in the forehead; parietal, which is located under the cranial bone with the same name; temporal, which is associated with the temple; and occipital, which is located in the occipital cranial bone. The fifth lobe, the insular lobe can only be seen when the lateral sulcus is opened [7,9]. There are many other structures situated in the central nervous system (CNS), but in this work we investigate only the four visible lobes.

Each one of these regions have specialized functions: the occipital lobe is primarily concerned with the sense of sight, it is divided into multiple distinct visual areas, in which the biggest one is the primary visual cortex. The parietal lobe is partially dedicated to the sense of touch, it is responsible for body sensitivity functions and spatial recognition. The temporal lobe contains the primary auditory cortex, it processes audio data, specific aspects of vision, language understanding and some aspects of memory. Finally, the frontal lobe which is responsible for cognitive actions, memory and movement [7,8].

## 2.2    Visually Impaired

Visual impairment, in any degree, impairs a person's ability to orient and move in space with security and independence [12]. So, people with visual impairment or blindness compensate these visions lack of information using other senses hearing, smell, touch and taste [10].

## 2.3    Brain Computer Interface (BCI Systems)

BCI systems are a set of tools that enable a communication method between the brain and the computer based on neural activity. They acquire electrical signals detected on the scalp of the cortical or subcortical surface areas. The main objective of BCI systems is to provide interaction between the user and the external device, as computers, switches or prostheses, using only brain signals [5].

One way to capture neural activity is the electroencephalography (EEG). The EEG is based on detecting the brain electrical activity through electrodes applied to the scalp.

The signals that are captured by an EEG equipment are the potential differences between regions of the cortex. These electrical signs are generated due to the flow of ions between the different neurons of the brain. When a neuron is activated, it is polarized, generating a potential action that can be propagated to other neurons, provoking a flow of information [14].

The records acquired through the electrodes represent the intensity of brain waves. They can vary between 0 μV and 200 μV, and they have frequency ranging from 0.3 Hz to 100 Hz. The resulting signal of an EEG shows peaks related to existence of electric activity, indicating a general spatial location of brain activity, because this signal is the sum of the activity of a large number of neurons communicating with each other [13].

## 2.4    Data Mining

Data mining (DM) is the process of extracting or mining knowledge from a large volume of data. DM involves the study of tasks and techniques, where tasks are a specific class of problems and techniques are the groups of solutions to solve them [6].

Alencar [16] points out that one of the most accepted definition of data mining by researchers in the field is the one given by Fayyad et al. [17], which states: "database knowledge extraction is the process of identifying valid, new, potentially useful and understandable patterns embedded in the data."

Data mining is a step in a broad process known as KDD (Knowledge Discovery in Database). KDD is the process of finding knowledge in data, in this context, DM is the step to obtain the information [6].

The methods and techniques of data mining are divided in two ways: supervised (predictive) and unsupervised (descriptive) learning. Descriptive tasks are focused on discovering patterns that describe data in a way that human being can understand. The main descriptive tasks are: association rules and clustering. Predictive tasks search for patterns to infer new information about the existing data, or to predict the behavior of new data. The main predictive tasks are classification and regression [6,15].

The difference between predictive and descriptive methods consists in the fact that descriptive methods do not require a pre-categorization of records, i.e., it is not necessary target an attribute; in predictive methods, the dataset has a predefined target variable and records are categorized basing in this target.

## 3    Proposed Methodology

In our approach, we are working with the following hypothesis: sight people primarily use the **occipital lobe** because it is associated with vision, and blind people primarily use the **parietal lobe**, that is associated with the sense of touch.

According to Kastrup [3], the sense of touch is considered the most appropriate way to provide references of the space when there is a lack of the sense of vision. Viveiros [11] points out that the blindness drives the individual to create internal compensation mechanisms to overcome the obstacle of vision lack.

Figure 1 presents the steps of our methodology during the development of this work.

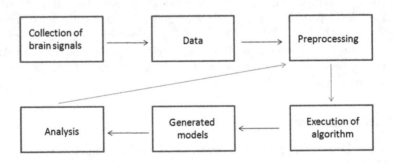

**Fig. 1.** Proposed methodology.

### 3.1    Collection of Brain Signals

We have collected the brain signals during the execution of a protocol on 4 female individuals: 2 sight people (with blindfolded), and 2 blind people. They should identify different solid geometric shapes, in order to stimulate the spacial abilities in each individual. In our protocol, we used three objects: sphere, cube and parallelogram. All tests were performed with the approval of the Research Ethics Committee at the Health Area in Brazil - CCAAE: 344172114.3.0000.5324.

The data are collected in the following way:

1. In a specific room, only the person and the researcher are;
2. With the Actichamp tool properly works, the Easycap is inserted on the head of the person;
3. Therefore, the electrodes are stimulated until they show enough impedance to make possible to start the data collection;
4. Since the impedance is good, these electrodes are connected an audio recorder and Openvibe software is used for the acquisition and monitoring of brain signals;
5. The eyes of sight are blindfolded and we drop the first object in the person hands;
6. The person touch the object and verbalize the name of the form;
7. When the verbalization is done, we return to step 5, and other object is given (until the third object).

**Tool to Collect Brain Signals.** The Actichamp tool developed by Brain Vision LLC, it is modular amplification system that incorporates large components for electrophysiological analysis as EEG, ERP (Event-related brain potentials), and BCI systems. It is used in conjunction with Easycap electrodes, which is a cap that engages the electrode 32 and it is inserted into the scalp of the person. It has the channels exposed on the international standard "10–20". The Easycap is connected to the Actichamp amplifier, so that there is the transmission of data captured by the electrodes.

Table 1 shows the brain areas, the channels that constitute each area and the proprietary functions (abilities) of each region.

**Table 1.** Brain region, electrodes and proprietary functions.

| Brain region | Electrode | Proprietary functions |
|---|---|---|
| Frontal lobe | Fp1, Fp2, Fz, F7, F3, Fz, F4, F8, FC5, FC1, FC2, FC6, FT9, FT10. | Executive functions (management of cognitive/emotional resources on a given task) |
| Temporal lobe | T7, TP9, T8, TP10. | Perception of biological motion |
| Parietal lobe | P7, P3, Pz, P4, P8. | Somatosensory perception, spatial representations and tactile perceptions. |
| Occipital lobe | O1, Oz, O2. | View images (including during a dialogue). |

**OpenVibe Software.** Openvibe is a software platform dedicated to designing, testing and using brain-computer interfaces. The configuration for use with Actichamp is pre-defined, the research just selects the amplifier's name and automatically the software communicates with the signal capture tool. The Openvibe presents a very simple interface, where the user can set through an algorithm (Automata) features that meet the needs of the job.

### 3.2 Preprocessing

The main steps of data preprocessing are:

1. Balance: to avoid an unbalanced tree, all class have the same amount of instances.
2. Data group: we group a set of 10 instances into one to represent brain activity in a larger portion of time. Each attribute receives the highest value of the 10 instances.
3. Normalization: The normalization step is done in Weka software, applying the filter "normalized", which transforms the values of the instances on a scale of 0 to 1.

### 3.3 Decision Trees

The Weka (Waikato Environment for Knowledge Analysis) is a collection of machine learning algorithms for data mining tasks. It was developed by the Department of Computer Science of the University of Waikato, New Zealand [18]. Weka can be used directly as tool, or it can be used by Java programs. It provides functionality for preprocessing, classification, regression, clustering and association rules [15].

In this work, we used the J48 algorithm of decision trees to analyse our dataset. The J48 (Known as C4.5)) is an algorithm that uses the method of division and conquer to increase the predictive ability of decision trees. In this way, it always uses the best step evaluated locally, without worrying if this step will produce the best solution in the end. It takes a problem and divides into several sub-problems, creating sub-trees between the root and the leaves.

We are choose the J48 algorithm because it is a decision tree technique developed for use in WEKA. The decision tree technique has the time and processing efficiency. Additionally, it presents intuitive features to analyze the results, because it shows as results a simple form of symbolic representation and generally easy to interpret, which facilitates the understanding of problwm in analysis [19].

## 4    Results

During our research, we performed several experiments using the J48 algorithm with different settings. Firstly, we use all electrodes (32 channels), later we use only the electrodes that are directly associated with our areas of interested (12 channels). We also change the "minNumObj" parameter, which is the minimum number of instances per leaf. We tested with the values 1 %, 5 % and 10 % of the total number of instances for each test. In all tests the number of instances of each class was balanced and the other parameters were set weka's default.

In the initial tests, we could not infer any conclusion because the generated trees were very large. In this way, they were very specific and difficult interpretation. Probably, we were getting an overfitting since each leaf of the tree classifies the minimum amount of possible instances.

To avoid this overfitting, we group a subset of 10 consecutive instances. Each attribute received the highest value of its set (as mentioned in Sect. 3.2). In these tests, each instance contains the peak of each electrode in larger period of time, representing in one instance a set with the highest values for each electrode during 1 second (approximately). We executed them with the minimum number of objects set to 1 %, because we have a small amount of instances to each class, and 32 channels. The generated decisions trees are showed in Figs. 3 and 2, and they classify 100 % correctly all the instances.

```
FT10 <= 0.615                                    (1)
|   C4 <= 0.97
|   |    PZ <= 0.165: parallelogram (3.0)
|   |    PZ > 0.165
|   |    |    PZ <= 0.726: cube (4.0)
|   |    |    PZ > 0.726: parallelogram (1.0)
|   C4 > 0.97: inactive (1.0)
FT10 > 0.615
|   OZ <= 0.875: ball (4.0)
|   OZ > 0.875: inactive (3.0)
```

```
F3 <= 0.708                                      (2)
|   O1 <= 0.451
|   |    F7 <= 0.768: inactive (4.0)
|   |    F7 > 0.768
|   |    |    FP1 <= 0.389: cube (1.0)
|   |    |    FP1 > 0.389: ball (1.0)
|   O1 > 0.451
|   |    C3 <= 0.529: ball (3.0)
|   |    C3 > 0.529: parallelogram (4.0)
F3 > 0.708: cube (3.0)
```

**Fig. 2.** Decision trees generated by the J48 algorithm. (1) A1 Person (2) A2 Person, both sighted people.

```
FZ <= 0.889                                      (1)
|   FP1 <= 0.563
|   |    CP2 <= 0.241: parallelogram (3.0)
|   |    CP2 > 0.241
|   |    |    FT9 <= 0.724: cube (4.0)
|   |    |    FT9 > 0.724: ball (1.0)
|   FP1 > 0.563
|   |    F7 <= 0.773: inactive (4.0)
|   |    F7 > 0.773: parallelogram (1.0)
FZ > 0.889: ball (3.0)
```

```
P4 <= 0.35: parallelogram (4.0)                  (2)
P4 > 0.35
|   P7 <= 0.786
|   |    F7 <= 0.18
|   |    |    FP1 <= 0.187: cube (1.0)
|   |    |    FP1 > 0.187: ball (3.0)
|   |    F7 > 0.18: cube (3.0)
|   P7 > 0.786
|   |    FP1 <= 0.074: ball (1.0)
|   |    FP1 > 0.074: inactive (4.0)
```

**Fig. 3.** Decision trees generated by the J48 algorithm. (1) B1 person (2) B2 person, both congenital visual impairment.

The Fig. 2 shows the tree generated by the J48 algorithm for sighted people. Figure 2(1) represents one sighted individual (A1) and Fig. 2(2) represents the other sighted individual (A2). Figure 3 is similar, 3(1) represents one blind individual (B1), and 3(2) represents other blind individual (B2).

In Fig. 2, we can see that the channels with a significant brain activity correspond to the frontal lobe (A1: FT10; A2: F3, F7, Fp1), the parietal lobe (A1: Pz), the occipital lobe (A1: Oz; A2: O1) and the core lobe (A1: C4; A2: C3). The high activity in the frontal and the parietal lobe were expected since they are responsible, respectively, for planning and the sense of touch. The occipital lobe is responsible for vision skills and visual memory. In this way, we can infer that these individuals (A1 and A2) use the sense of touch and visual memory to identify the objects during the experiment.

The Fig. 3 shows that individuals B1 and B2 present significant activity in the parietal lobe (B1: P4, P7; B2: CP2) and in the front lobe (B1: F7, Fp1; B2: Fz, Fp1, FT9, F7). As we mentioned before, the parietal lobe is responsible for the sense of touch, and the frontal lobe that coordinates motor activities. In this case, the occipital lobe does not present significant activity. In this way, we can infer that these individuals used basically the sense of touch to identify the objects during the experiment.

## 5    Conclusion

This work analyzed the brain signs of four individuals, including two sighted people and two people with congenital visual impairment, during a 3D geometric recognition activity. For this analysis, we collected the brain signals with Actichamp tool and processed these data with the Weka software to data mining. We choose the J48 data mining technique classification that generates decision trees to analyse the created models.

In our results, we can observe that the sighted people showed significant activity in the occipital lobe, which is responsible for the sense of vision, even when they are blindfolded. Therefore, blind people showed no significant activity in the occipital lobe in the model created by J48 algorithm. In this way, our hypothesis was confirmed: sighted people primarily use the **occipital lobe** because it is associated with vision, and blind people primarily use the **parietal lobe**, that is associated with the sense of touch.

As future works, we intend to expand the study with a larger number of people, and apply other data mining techniques in all dataset.

## References

1. de Sá, E.D., de Campos, I.M., Silva, M.B.C.: Atendimento educacional especializado: deficiência visual. MEC, SEESP (2007) (in Portuguese)
2. Eyzaguirre, C.: Fisiologia do sistema nervoso. Rio de Janeiro (1977) (in Portuguese)
3. Kastrup, V.: A invenção na ponta dos dedos: a reversão da atenção em pessoas com deficiência visual. Psicologia em Revista **13**(1), 69–90 (2007) (in Portuguese)

4. Gil, M.: Cadernos da TV Escola-Deficiência Visual. Ministério da Educação - Secretária de Educação a Distância. [S.l.] (2000) (in Portuguese). http://www. smec.salvador.ba.gov.br/site/documentos/espaco-virtual/espacoeducar/educacao-especial/publicacoes/caderno%20da%20tv%20escola
5. Machado, S., Cunha, M., Velasques, B., Minc, D., Hugo, V., Bastos, H.B., Ribeiro, P.: Interface cérebro-computador: novas perspectivas para a reabilitação. Revista Neurociências, **17**(4), 329–335 (2009) (in Portuguese)
6. Deveza, C.H.: Minerando Padrões Sequenciais para Base de Dados de Lojas Virtuais. Monografia (Curso de Bacharelado em Ciência da Computação), UFOP (Universidade Federal de Ouro Preto) (2011) (in Portuguese)
7. Gazzaniga, M.S., Heatherton, T.F., Veronese, M.A.V.: Psychological Science: Mind, Brain and Behavior. W.W. Norton, New York (2006)
8. Lent, R.: Cem bilhões de neurônios: conceitos fundamentais de neurociência. [S.l.]: Atheneu (2004) (in Portuguese)
9. Lent, R.: Neurociência da mente e do comportamento. RJ: Guanabara Koogan, [S.I.] (2008) (in Portuguese)
10. Silveira, N.S., da, Lomonaco, J.F.B.: Desenvolvimento de conceitos em cegos congênitos: caminhos de aquisição do conhecimento, [S.I.], **12**(1), 119138 (2008) (in Portuguese)
11. Viveiros, E.R.D.: Mindware semiótico-comunicativo: campos conceituais no ensino de física para deficientes visuais utilizando uma interface cérebro-computador, [S.l.] (2013) (in Portuguese)
12. Brasil: Subsídios para a Organização e Funcionamento de serviços de educação especial. [S.l.] Ministério da Educação e do Desporto, Secretária de Educação Especial (1995) (in Portuguses)
13. Oliveira, I., Carric, O., L., Guimaraes, N., Chambel, T., Teixeira, C.: Interfaces Computador-Cérebro: Extracção e Processamento de Características de Electroencefalogramas. Department of Informatics, University of Lisbon, [S.l.] (2008) (in Portuguese)
14. Kugler, M.: Uma Contribuição ao Desenvolvimento de Interfaces Cérebro-computador Utilizando Potenciais Visualmente Evocados. (Doctoral dissertation, Masters thesis, Graduate School in Electrical Engineering and Industrial Computer Science, Federal Technological University of Parana, Curitiba) (2003) (in Portuguese)
15. Camilo, C.O., Silva, J.C., d.: Mineração de dados: Conceitos, tarefas, métodos e ferramentas. Goiania: Universidade Federal de Goias, [S.l.] (2009) (in Portuguese)
16. Alencar, A.B.: Mineração e visualização de coleções de séries temporais.Instituto de Ciências Matemáticas e de Computação (2007) (in Portuguese)
17. Fayyad, U., Piatetsky-Shapiro, G., Smyth, P.: From data mining to knowledge discovery in databases. AI Mag. **17**(3), 37 (1996)
18. Ferreira, J.: DATA MINING em banco de dados de eletrocardiograma. Universidade de São Paulo, Tese de Douturado Instituto Dante Pazzanese de Cardiologia (2014) (in Portuguese)
19. Garcia, S.C.: O uso de rvore de deciso na descoberta de conhecimento na rea da sade. Tese de Doutorado em Cincia da Computação - Universidade Federal do Rio Grande (2003) (in Portuguese)

# Author Index

Printed in the United States
By Bookmasters